Transalveolar Extraction of the Mandibular Third Molars

This practical manual provides details on the clinical and radiographic evaluation, classification, principles of suturing and flaps, intricacies of the transalveolar surgery, newer advances in mandibular third molar surgery and complications that may be encountered during mandibular third molar exodontia. It presents vital surgical skills for the mandibular third molar exodontia in a concise and to-the-point manner. This book is a user-friendly resource for students of dentistry and maxillofacial surgery, as it brings together information from various reputable resources to one single platform for easier understanding and application.

Key features:

- Addresses the necessary gap in the literature with a concise yet comprehensive approach.
- Overhauls and updates the content to provide an exam-oriented text with practical tips for students of oral and maxillofacial surgery, and professionals.

Transalveolar Extraction of the Mandibular Third Molars

Edited by

Dr. Darpan Bhargava
MDS, MOMS RCPS(Glasg.), PGDHM, PhD,
Consultant Maxillofacial Surgery

Professor, Oral and Maxillofacial Surgery, People's University,
Bhopal, Madhya Pradesh, India
Clinical Director, TMJ Consultancy Services,
Bhopal, Madhya Pradesh, India

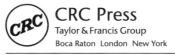

CRC Press
Taylor & Francis Group
Boca Raton London New York

CRC Press is an imprint of the
Taylor & Francis Group, an **informa** business

First edition published 2023
by CRC Press
6000 Broken Sound Parkway NW, Suite 300, Boca Raton, FL 33487-2742

and by CRC Press
4 Park Square, Milton Park, Abingdon, Oxon, OX14 4RN

CRC Press is an imprint of Taylor & Francis Group, LLC

Library of Congress Cataloging-in-Publication Data
Names: Bhargava, Darpan, editor.
Title: Transalveolar extraction of the mandibular third molars / edited by Dr. Darpan Bhargava.
Description: First edition. | Boca Raton, FL : CRC Press, 2023. |
Includes bibliographical references and index. |
Summary: "This practical manual provides details on the clinical and radiographic evaluation, classification, principles of suturing and flaps, intricacies of the transalveolar surgery, newer advances in mandibular third molar surgery and complications that may be encountered during mandibular third molar exodontia"— Provided by publisher.
Identifiers: LCCN 2022042627 (print) | LCCN 2022042628 (ebook) |
ISBN 9781032348315 (pbk) | ISBN 9781032348322 (hbk) | ISBN 9781003324034 (ebk)
Subjects: MESH: Molar, Third—surgery | Tooth Extraction—methods | Alveolar Process—surgery | Tooth, Impacted—surgery
Classification: LCC RK531 (print) | LCC RK531 (ebook) | NLM WU 605 |
DDC 617.6/6—dc23/eng/20221026
LC record available at https://lccn.loc.gov/2022042627
LC ebook record available at https://lccn.loc.gov/2022042628

ISBN: 9781032348322 (hbk)
ISBN: 9781032348315 (pbk)
ISBN: 9781003324034 (ebk)

DOI: 10.1201/9781003324034

Typeset in Minion
by codeMantra

Dedicated to

William Harry Archer
Geoffrey L. Howe
A. J. MacGregor
For their exemplary contribution towards the art and science of mandibular third molar surgery

Contents

Foreword   xi
Preface   xii
Acknowledgements   xiii
About the Book   xiv
Editor   xvi
Contributors   xvii

1   Prologue to "Transalveolar extraction of the mandibular third molars"   1
    M. Anthony Pogrel
    References   2
2   Antiquity and introduction to the third molar or the "wisdom" tooth   3
    Beena Sivakumar and Darpan Bhargava
    Role of genetics in relevance to third molar tooth   3
    Current trends   5
    References   5
3   Applied surgical anatomy for transalveolar extraction of the mandibular third molar   7
    V. Vidya Devi and Darpan Bhargava
    Mucosa and mucoperiosteum   7
    Skeletal anatomy   8
    Adjacent muscles and ligaments   10
    Regional blood vessels   12
    Adjacent nerves and innervation   12
    Adjacent teeth and periodontium   15
    Buccal fat pad   15
    Spaces involved with the mandibular third molars   16
    References   16
4   Indications and contraindications for surgical extraction of the mandibular third molars   17
    Preeti G. Bhargava, Vivianne Ibrahim Shehata Sobh, and Darpan Bhargava
    Definition   17
    Causes for third molar impaction   17
    Theories of tooth impaction   18
    Indications for extraction of mandibular third molars   18
    Contraindications for extraction for mandibular third molars   21
    References   21
5   Classification for impacted mandibular third molars   23
    Puneet Wadhwani, Sapna Tandon, Darpan Bhargava, and Pramod Kumar Gandra
    Introduction   23
    Classification systems for impacted mandibular third molar   23
    Difficulty index   30
    References   31
6   Basics of radiology for impacted mandibular third molars   33
    Sonam Khurana, Prashant Jaju, and Darpan Bhargava
    Introduction   33

Conventional intraoral periapical radiograph 3

Tube shift intraoral radiographic technique 3

Panoramic radiographs 3

Cone-beam computed tomography 3

Magnetic resonance imaging 3

Conclusion 3

References 3

7   Clinical and radiographic assessment for impacted mandibular third molars 3

Darpan Bhargava

Clinical assessment 39

Radiographic assessment 3

Summary of difficulty assessment indices 4

References 49

8   Armamentarium for transalveolar extraction of third molars 51

Elavenil Panneerselvam, Sasikala Balasubramaniam, and Arun Vignesh

Introduction 51

Classification of instruments 51

Instruments for diagnosis 52

Instruments for preparation of the surgical site 53

Instruments used to maintain mouth opening 55

Instruments for administration of local anaesthesia 58

Instruments for clear surgical site 59

Instruments for placing incision 60

Instruments for reflection 63

Instruments for retraction 64

Instruments for bone removal and odontotomy 66

Instruments for tooth delivery 72

Instruments for socket management 75

Instruments and materials for haemostasis and wound closure 78

Instruments and materials for post-operative dressing 84

Instruments for sterilization and storage 84

Advances 85

Acknowledgement 85

References 85

9   Principles and flaps for mandibular third molar surgery 87

Darpan Bhargava

Introduction 87

Principles of tooth extraction 87

Use of dental elevators for third molar surgery 89

Flaps for the mandibular third molar extraction 92

Principles of suturing 95

Ergonomics 97

References 98

10   Surgical techniques for transalveolar extraction of the mandibular third molars 99

Darpan Bhargava

Asepsis and patient preparation 99

Local anaesthesia 99

Incision and mucoperiosteal flap 104

Bone removal 105

Alternative techniques for special scenarios 106

Tooth division and removal of the tooth (odontectomy) 111

Socket toilet 117
Suturing 117
Post-operative care and follow-up 118
Conclusion 119
Transplantation of mandibular third molars 119
References 121

11 Periodontal considerations for impacted mandibular third molars 123
Sumedha Srivastava, Jaideep Mahendra, and Khushboo Desai
Introduction 123
Impaction as a risk factor for periodontal tissues distal to second molar 123
Effects on periodontium with various impaction type 124
Treatment 124
Periodontal risk predictors 125
Preoperative and intraoperative considerations 125
Post-operative management of the periodontal defects 126
Conclusion 129
References 129

12 Complications with impacted mandibular third molar surgery 133
Kishore Moturi, Anil Budumuru, and R. S. G. Satyasai
Preoperative complications 133
Intraoperative complications 137
Post-operative complications 144
References 149

13 Healing after mandibular third molar extraction 153
Einstein A, Shubhangi Durgakumar Mishra, and Darpan Bhargava
Introduction 153
Healing of an extraction socket 153
Healing following mandibular third molar extraction 154
Assessment of wound healing after mandibular third molar extraction 154
Complications in healing of extraction socket 156
Advanced biologic approaches to enhance wound healing after
mandibular third molar extraction 157
References 162

14 Advances in surgical extraction of the mandibular third molars 163
Sundar Ramalingam and Darpan Bhargava
Surgical flaps for mandibular third molar removal 163
Lingual nerve protection during third molar removal surgery 165
Inferior alveolar nerve preservation during third molar removal surgery 165
Lasers in mandibular third molar surgery 169
Piezosurgery for mandibular third molar removal 172
Current perspectives in decision making for the asymptomatic mandibular third molar 173
References 174

15 Medico-legal considerations and informed consent for mandibular third molar extractions 177
George Paul
Introduction 177
Does surgical removal of third molars need informed consent? 177
What are material risks that need to be disclosed? 178
The informed consent document should include 178
Some common benefits and risks of mandibular third molars 178
Validity of informed consent 179
Negligence related to non-disclosure 179

	Conclusion	17
	References	17
	Prototype consent format	18
	Declaration	18
16	Pharmacology relevant to mandibular third molar surgery	18
	Georgakopoulou Eleni and Darpan Bhargava	
	Introduction	18
	Local anaesthesia	18
	Inhalational sedation	18
	Anxiolytics and sedatives	18
	Antibiotics	18
	Analgesics	18
	Corticosteroids (to supress post-surgical oedema, pain and for neuropraxic nerve injury)	18
	Enzyme preparations	18
	Topical oral agents	187
	Topical wound dressings	187
	Styptics	188
	Obtundents	188
	Surgical irrigant	189
	Gaba analogues	189
	References	189
17	Case history: Transalveolar extraction of the mandibular third molars	193
	Darpan Bhargava	
	Prototype case history format	193
18	Appendix of clinical cases: Transalveolar extraction of the mandibular third molars	199
	Vankudoth Dal Singh and Darpan Bhargava	
Index		**203**

Foreword

Surgery for mandibular third molars has long awaited a thorough update. This textbook titled *Transalveolar Extraction of the Mandibular Third Molars* published by the Taylor & Francis Group and CRC Press, with renowned contributors is intended for international readership. This manual is useful for education in the field of maxillofacial surgery and will find its academic place as an authoritative teaching resource. The book is edited and mentored by Professor Darpan Bhargava, Consultant in Oral and Maxillofacial Surgery, who is a renowned academician in the field. This book has received its prologue from M. Anthony Pogrel, Professor, Department of Oral and Maxillofacial Surgery, University of California, San Francisco.

Kandasamy Ganesan
BDS, MDS (OMFS), MFDSRCS (Eng),
FFD RCSI (Oral Surg Oral Med)
Consultant Oral Surgeon, Department of Oral and Maxillofacial Surgery, Southend University Hospitals NHS trust, United Kingdom
Honorary Senior Lecturer, University of Leeds, West Yorkshire, England

Preface

Let us start this journey to the *Transalveolar Extraction of the Mandibular Third Molars* by thanking the Almighty, the supreme power, that keeps us driving to the limits we ourselves don't realize.

त्वं ज्ञानमयो विज्ञानमयोऽसि

You are wisdom and knowledge personified

It was the need of the hour to compile the updated basics on the topic. As I was a student of Oral and Maxillofacial Surgery, it was necessary to refer to extensive literature from various sources to master the art and science of the *Transalveolar Extraction of the Mandibular Third Molars*. Pioneers such as Charles Edmund Kells, George Winter, Kurt Thoma, William Kelsey Fry, Wilfred Fish, Warwick James, Ward, Gustav Kruger, William Harry Archer, Geoffrey L. Howe, A. J. MacGregor and many others have laid a very strong foundation for the exodontia practice. The responsibility lies on our shoulders to take this science forward.

In a race to learn fascinating advanced surgical skills that involve craniofacial surgery, head and neck surgery, temporomandibular joint-related surgeries and microvascular surgery, the importance of the basics in oral surgery is usually underestimated. "Good" exodontia is the "backbone" of dentistry and it is the life and soul of oral and maxillofacial surgical practice. To knock off someone's tooth and still receiving a compliment of doing a "great job" is the best and satisfying experience. Understanding the importance of learning and executing a refined minor oral surgery practice is a matter of prolonged experience and is usually understood very late by the current generation of oral and maxillofacial surgeons. The art and science of *Transalveolar Extraction of the Mandibular Third Molars* not only involves executing the surgical procedure in the limitations of the oral cavity in a less accessible area of the posterior mandible but also, the understanding of right indications and managing the complications, when they arise.

I hope this compilation is a reader's delight to understand and master the art and science of the *Transalveolar Extraction of the Mandibular Third Molars* and also, provides a single point reference.

My piece of advice to a learner or student of maxillofacial surgery is that:

In the practice of maxillofacial surgery, only reading a book hardly helps. Reading a book, applying it to your surgical practice under the guidance and supervision of an experienced wise teacher is the key to refine the skills, until you are skilled enough to pass on the science to your future generation. Fundamentals and basics to any science including surgical exodontia are static, only the advances remain dynamic. If one develops a strong static base, which no one can shake, the pace of the fast-growing advanced dynamics can be easily matched.

Professor Darpan Bhargava BDS, MDS, MOMS
RCPS (Glasg.), PGDHM, PDCR, PhD

Oral & Maxillofacial Surgery,
India

Acknowledgements

I would take this opportunity to express my heartfelt gratitude to my parents, Ragini Bhargava and Dr. Madan Mohan Bhargava, for all their efforts and dedication towards my making. I would not have completed this endeavour without the tireless support of my wife Dr. Preeti G. Bhargava and patience of my son Dear Darsh.

I am thankful to Ms. Shivangi Pramanik, Senior Editor for Medicine, CRC Press and Ms. Himani Dwivedi, Editorial Assistant for Medical, CRC Press and Taylor & Francis Group for their constant support for this project. In spite of their existing commitments and busy schedule, they pursued the project to make it a reality today. I am also grateful to Ms. Miranda Bromage, Publisher, Surgery and Medicine, Taylor & Francis, Oxfordshire, United Kingdom, for having confidence and belief in this work.

I would not miss the opportunity to acknowledge the efforts from Mr. Vijay Shanker P, Sr. Project Manager from codeMantra, for swiftly coordinating and organising the contents of this book.

About the Book

TRANSALVEOLAR EXTRACTION OF THE MANDIBULAR THIRD MOLARS

Impacted tooth is completely or partially unerupted and is positioned against another tooth, bone or soft tissue so that its further eruption is unlikely, described according to its anatomic position. There are several different radiological evaluation protocols that can be used prior to transalveolar extraction of the mandibular third molars. Conventional intraoral radiography provides surgeons with an overview of the basic information at the surgical site without detailed three-dimensional spatial relationship of the anatomic structures. The incorporation of the cone-beam computer tomography remains new to the field considering acquisition is simple with clinically acceptable exposure to radiation for complicated cases. The manual describes practically oriented details regarding the clinical and radiographic evaluation, classification, principles of suturing and flaps, intricacies of the transalveolar surgery, newer advances for mandibular third molar surgery and complications that may be encountered while mandibular third molar surgical exodontia. The manual presents the vital surgical techniques for the mandibular third molar exodontia in a concise and to-the-point manner. This compilation will be a delight to the student of dentistry and maxillofacial surgery considering that it will have an amalgamation of information from various resources of repute at a single terminus. The text will serve as a ready reckoner and clinical notes for undergraduate and postgraduate maxillofacial surgery education.

UNIQUE ABOUT THIS MANUAL

1. Based on available historic oral and maxillofacial surgical literature
2. Short and concise
3. Compilation for undergraduate and postgraduate education as a manual with practical notes
4. Amalgamation of information from various resources of repute in a single compilation
5. Based on exam-oriented approach co-centred on clinical principles and practice

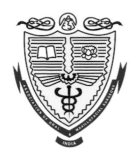

Association of Oral and Maxillofacial Surgeons of India (AOMSI)

PRESIDENTIAL MESSAGE

It is a pleasure to recommend the manual titled *Transalveolar Extraction of the Mandibular Third Molars* dedicated to the international community of oral and maxillofacial surgeons published by the Taylor & Francis Group and CRC Press. This compilation edited by Professor Darpan Bhargava would provide a comprehensive academic teaching and learning material. The text has received contributions in the form of 18 sections from 26 renowned international clinical and surgical specialists in the field adding to the excellence in the academic content. I wish and hope this compilation serves as an important and vital surgical learning tool in the field of maxillofacial surgery.

Jai Hind
Yours Faithfully,

Professor Manjunath Rai BDS, MDS,
MOSRCS(Edinburgh), LLB, PGDMLE
President, Association of Oral and
Maxillofacial Surgeons of India
India

Editor

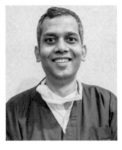

Dr. Darpan Bhargava MDS, MOMSRCPS (Glasg.), PGDHM, PhD, Consultant Maxillofacial Surgery; Professor, Oral and Maxillofacial Surgery, People's University, Bhopal, Madhya Pradesh, India; Clinical Director, TMJ Consultancy Services, Bhopal, Madhya Pradesh, India.

Professor Bhargava completed his bachelor's in dental surgery and master's in oral and maxillofacial surgery from Meenakshi Ammal Dental College and Hospital, Chennai, India. He is a distinction holder and gold medallist from The Tamil Nadu Dr. MGR Medical University (Undergraduation) and Meenakshi Academy of Higher Education, Chennai (Postgraduation). He has also successfully completed Diploma of Membership in Oral and Maxillofacial Surgery from Royal College of Physicians and Surgeons, Glasgow. He holds postgraduate diploma in Hospital Management and Clinical Research. He is credited with introduction of twin-mix nerve block for mandibular anaesthesia. Currently, he is serving as a professor and clinical consultant in the Department of Oral and Maxillofacial Surgery at People's University, Bhopal, Madhya Pradesh, India. He is the founding director of TMJ Consultancy Services, Bhopal, Madhya Pradesh, India. He has more than 100 national and international scientific publications to his credit. He holds first-ever Indian patent for temporomandibular joint prosthesis. He is awarded PhD from Meenakshi University, Chennai for his acclaimed research on "Predictability and Feasibility of Total Alloplastic Temporomandibular Joint Reconstruction Using DARSN TM Joint Prosthesis for Patients in Indian subcontinent". He is the author of the authoritative book *Temporomandibular Joint Disorders: Principles and Current Practice*, published by Springer Nature, Singapore.

Contributors

Sasikala Balasubramaniam, MDS
Department of Oral and Maxillofacial Surgery
SRM Dental College
Chennai, Tamil Nadu, India

Darpan Bhargava, MDS, MOMSRCPS (Glasg.), PGDHM, PhD
Department of Oral and Maxillofacial Surgery
People's University
Bhopal, Madhya Pradesh, India and
TMJ Consultancy Services
Bhopal, Madhya Pradesh, India

Preeti G. Bhargava, MDS
Oral and Maxillofacial Surgery
TMJ Consultancy Services
Bhopal, Madhya Pradesh, India

Anil Budumuru, MDS
Department of Oral and Maxillofacial Surgery
Vishnu Dental College
Bhimavaram, India

Khushboo Desai, MDS
Department of Periodontology
Ahmedabad Dental College and Hospital
Ahmedabad, Gujarat, India

Einstein A, MDS
Department of Oral and Maxillofacial Pathology
Thai Moogambigai Dental College and Hospital
Dr. MGR Educational and Research Institute
Chennai, Tamil Nadu, India

Georgakopoulou Eleni, PhD, MD, DDS, MSc
Consultant Oral Medicine
Néa Ionía, Attiki, Greece

Pramod Kumar Gandra, MDS, MPhil
Department of Oral and Maxillofacial Surgery
Sri Balaji Dental College
Hyderabad, India

Prashant Jaju, MDS
Department of Oral Medicine and Radiology
Rishiraj College of Dental Sciences and Research Centre
Bhopal, Madhya Pradesh, India

Sonam Khurana, MDS, MSc & Cert.
Oral and Maxillofacial Radiology
University of Texas Health Science Center
San Antonio, TX, USA and
Department of Oral and Maxillofacial Pathology
Radiology and Medicine
New York University College of Dentistry
New York, NY, USA

Jaideep Mahendra, MDS, PhD, Post Doc (USA), FIABMS, PGDHM, FABMS
Department of Periodontics
Meenakshi Ammal Dental College and Hospital,
Meenakshi Academy of Higher Education and Research
Chennai, Tamil Nadu, India

Shubhangi Durgakumar Mishra, MDS
Department of Oral and Maxillofacial Pathology
Bhabha College of Dental Sciences
Bhopal, Madhya Pradesh, India

Kishore Moturi, MDS, FTMJF
Department of Oral and Maxillofacial Surgery
Vishnu Dental College
Bhimavaram, India

Elavenil Panneerselvam, MDS
Department of Oral and Maxillofacial Surgery
SRM Dental College
Chennai, Tamil Nadu, India

George Paul, MDS, DNB, LLB, PG Dip.
Consultant Oral and Maxillofacial Surgery
Salem, Tamil Nadu, India

M. Anthony Pogrel, DDS, MD, FRCS
Department of Oral and Maxillofacial Surgery
UCSF School of Dentistry
UCSF Dental Center
San Francisco, CA, USA

Sundar Ramalingam, MDS, FFDRCS (Ire.), FDSRCPS (Glasg.)
Department of Oral and Maxillofacial Surgery
College of Dentistry, King Saud University
Riyadh, Kingdom of Saudi Arabia

R. S. G. Satyasai, MDS
Department of Oral and Maxillofacial Surgery
Vishnu Dental College
Bhimavaram, India

Vankudoth Dal Singh, MDS
Department of Oral and Maxillofacial Surgery
Lenora Institute of Dental Sciences
Rajahmundry, India

Beena Sivakumar, MDS, FTMJF
Oral and Maxillofacial Surgery
TMJ Consultancy Services
Bhopal, Madhya Pradesh, India

Vivianne Ibrahim Shehata Sobh, BDS, FEOMFS
Department of Oral and Maxillofacial Surgery
Cairo University, Ministry of Health
Nasr City Hospital, Egypt

Sumedha Srivastava, MDS
Department of Periodontics
People's College of Dental Sciences and
Research Centre, People's University
Bhopal, Madhya Pradesh, India

Sapna Tandon, MDS
Department of Oral and Maxillofacial Surgery
Career Post Graduate Institute of Dental
Sciences and Hospital
Lucknow, Uttar Pradesh, India

V. Vidya Devi, MDS
Department of Oral and Maxillofacial Surgery
Kamineni Institute of Dental Sciences
Telangana, India

Arun Vignesh, MDS
Department of Oral and Maxillofacial Surgery
SRM Dental College
Chennai, Tamil Nadu, India

Puneet Wadhwani, MDS
Department of Oral and Maxillofacial Surgery
Career Post Graduate Institute of Dental
Sciences and Hospital
Lucknow, Uttar Pradesh, India

Prologue to "Transalveolar extraction of the mandibular third molars"

M. ANTHONY POGREL

It gives me the greatest pleasure to write this prologue for this volume entitled *Transalveolar Extraction of the Mandibular Third Molars*.

Problems associated with third molars are one of the most common issues that confront oral and maxillofacial surgeons. In much of the world, it appears that issues related to third molars account for approximately 60% of the business of many oral and maxillofacial surgeons and sometimes over 65% of income. It is therefore a subject of great importance. It does appear that the occurrences of wisdom tooth problems, particularly impactions, have increased considerably over the last 50 years, and there would appear to be a number of reasons for this.

1. There is some evidence that the human jaws have become smaller over the last 200–300 years while the teeth have stayed the same size. Since the third molars are the last teeth to erupt, they are the ones that are pushed out of the arch and become impacted. The reason for the decrease in size of the jaws is not genetic but is more to do with the equivalent of disuse atrophy as we move to a softer diet that requires less chewing, and therefore there is less muscle development and less bone development.
2. As we move to a more processed diet, requiring less chewing, and causing less abrasion, interproximal wear on the teeth is decreased, and there is less mesial drift, allowing less space for the third molars to erupt.
3. Until relatively recently, it was not uncommon for first molars to be extracted between the ages of 8 and 10 due to gross caries, and therefore, the second and third molars would drift forward. Similarly, second molars were sometimes extracted around the age of 13 or 14 and the third molars would again often drift forward and not become impacted.
4. Orthodontic treatment has moved from being carried out in combination with dental extractions to becoming non-extraction cases where the arches are expanded, widened, and proclined. This reluctance to remove any teeth again means that the last teeth to erupt, which are the third molars, are the ones that are most likely to become impacted.

When third molars need to be removed, I have watched a transition of techniques. In times when drills were expensive and unreliable, reliance was placed on the mallet and chisel and the lingual split technique was often employed, taking away a portion of the lingual plate and delivering the third molar on the lingual side.[1] This technique required less bone removal than the buccal technique and healing was generally straightforward. However, removal of bone with a mallet and chisel is less predictable than with a drill, and there is higher lingual nerve involvement, although this is often attributed to the use of a narrow lingual retractor, such as a Howarth's nasal raspatory, rather than a broader lingual retractor, such as Walter's

DOI: 10.1201/9781003324034-1

retractor,[2] specifically designed for third molar removal. From the 1980s, as surgical drills became more reliable, it was suggested that third molar removal should be carried out from the buccal approach, carrying out all incisions and surgery on the buccal side of the mandible and avoiding the lingual side altogether in order to attempt to decrease the incidence of lingual nerve involvement. This is the technique largely taught today, though proponents of the lingual technique would state that providing a wide enough retractor is utilized, the incidence of permanent lingual nerve involvement is the same as with the buccal approach, though temporary involvement may be greater.

More recently, alternative techniques to conventional removal of the third molar have been suggested. These include coronectomy or intentional root retention,[3] orthodontic extrusion of the third molar,[4] and sequential removal of the impacted portion of the crown of the tooth to allow it to partially erupt.[5] All three of these techniques are proposed to decrease the problem of inferior alveolar nerve involvement when there is evidence of a close relationship between the roots of the third molar and the inferior alveolar nerve. The advent of the cone-beam computed tomography (CBCT) technique allows accurate three-dimensional imaging of the third molar and all associated structures at a relatively low price with low radiation dosage and is now widely employed.

The technique of lateral trepanation also has its advocates where third molar follicles are "scooped out" of the crypt from a lateral approach at the age of 13 or 14. One must accurately assess radiographically the exact state of teeth development in this case, and the correct choice of anaesthesia can be an issue at that age.

I hope this gives the reader some flavour of the subjects to be covered in this volume and the scope of issues related to third molars and their removal.

REFERENCES

1. Ward TG. The split bone technique for removal of lower third molars. *Br Dent J*. 101: 297–304, 1956.
2. Walters H. Reducing lingual nerve damage in third molar surgery: A clinical audit of 1350 cases. *Br Dent J*. 178: 140–144, 1995.
3. Pogrel MA. Coronectomy: Partial odontectomy or intentional root retention. *Oral Maxillofac Clin North Am*. 27: 373–382, 2015.
4. Bonetti GA, Bendandi M, Checci V, Checci L. Orthodontic extraction: Riskless extraction of impacted lower third molars close to the mandibular canal. *J Oral Maxillofac Surg*. 65: 2580–2586, 2007.
5. Tolstunov L, Javid B, Keyes L, Nattestad A. Pericoronal ostectomy: An alternative surgical technique for management of mandibular third molars in close proximity to the inferior alveolar nerve. *J Oral Maxillofac Surg*. 69: 1858–1866, 2011.

Antiquity and introduction to the third molar or the "wisdom" tooth

BEENA SIVAKUMAR AND DARPAN BHARGAVA

Treatment of a decayed tooth dates back to prehistoric evidence in the Neolithic era (10,000–4,500 BC). The first documented tooth extraction was performed by Hippocrates with an instrument named "Plumbeum odontogagon". Aristotle was the first person to use a forceps for teeth extraction and described the forceps in detail in his book titled "Mechanics". Aulus Cornelius Celsus was the first physician who proposed the technique of gingival detachment from the bone to extract a tooth. He also explained that incomplete tooth/root removal from the socket can lead to a possible swelling in the maxilla or mandible [1].

The procedure of third molar extraction gained popularity towards the end of the 18th century. The initial techniques to remove the third molar can be traced to being developed in Germany in the 1800s. In early 1903, National Dental Association published the first official manuscript on third molar extraction. But it is Charles Edmund Kells (1856–1928) who fostered a comprehensive technique for a wisdom tooth removal. Kells in 1918 opined that clinicians should think of them as an engineer to design their extraction technique in such a way that it should be tailor-made for every individual requiring the extraction. Although there are numerous contributors to this science, a few vital ones towards various techniques and procedures to remove the third molar and various soft tissue access incisions to facilitate the tooth removal have been summarized in Table 2.1 [1,2,3,4].

ROLE OF GENETICS IN RELEVANCE TO THIRD MOLAR TOOTH

The natural history of the eruption of third molars is such that it is not possible to foresee the fate predictably among individuals. Various factors, such as adequate space between the anterior mandibular border and the distal of the mandibular second molar, are necessary to allow successful eruption of the wisdom tooth to reach the occlusal plane [1,3,4].

Third molar teeth are unique as they erupt last in the oral cavity with their eruption time ranging from 17 to 24 years, depending on the ethnographic region and race. Understanding various regulatory mechanisms of its variable development patterns is of great clinical importance in terms of decision-making regarding the timing of third molar surgical removal, autologous transplantation, orthodontic treatment planning, and chronological age estimation for medico-legal purposes. Several studies have demonstrated the role of genetics in the agenesis of lateral incisors, central incisors, or second bicuspids, but this aspect is not clearly understood in regard to the hereditary influence on third molars, which could possibly be highly different from the other teeth because of their course of unique development. This area still needs further research to obtain conclusive evidence [5].

DOI: 10.1201/9781003324034-2

Table 2.1 Contributions to the art and science of exodontia

S. No.	Technique	Year	Described by
1	First documented extraction	Between 500 and 300 BC	Hippocrates – Using an instrument named plumbeu odontogagon
2	Forceps extraction	(384–322 BC)	Aristotle
3	Detaching the gingiva from bone	–	Aulus Cornelius Celsus
4	Incisions for difficult extractions	late 1700s	Walter Harris
5	Published first official manual for extraction of third molars	1903	National Dental Association
6	First to foster a comprehensive approach to third molar removal	1856–1928	Charles Edmund Kells
7	Described a more "humane" approach to removal of third molars	1918	Kells
8	Published *Principles of Exodontia as Applied to the Impacted Mandibular Third Molar* Described three flap designs for the extraction of lower third molars depending on the axial orientation of the teeth	1926	George B. Winter
9	Proposed the term odontectomy to describe the surgical removal of teeth	1932	Kurt H. Thoma
10	Split bone technique	1933	William Kelsey Fry
11	Officially published split bone technique	1956	Terrence George Ward
12	Concept of sectioning the tooth with a chisel and mallet	1957	Wilfred Fish
13	Wide flaps were to be sutured only once and with little tension	1937	Warwick James
14	Described three incisions that are widely used today for both upper and lower third molar surgery	1956	Ward
15	First to compare the use of chisel and mallet, low-speed burr, and high-speed burr	-	Harold C. Kilpatrick
16	Described an envelope flap where a distal-buccal incision is made and continued into a crevicular incision Described an approach for distally angled maxillary third molars	1959	Gustav Otto Kruger
17	Provided an in-depth description of all of the surgical approaches to the impacted lower third molar	1960	Guillermo Ries-Centeno
18	Described a flap that provided a good blood supply, vision for instrumentation and minimum trauma	1966	Alistair Berwick
19	Described numerous techniques to section impacted lower molars to facilitate extractions	1971	Lucian Szmyd
20	Published an approach for third molar that was a novelty at the time	1972	Walt W. Magnus
21	Published a minimally invasive incision	1999	Donlon and Triuta
22	Proposed comma-shaped incision	2002	Iyer Nageshwar
23	Introduction of twin-mix anaesthesia for transalveolar mandibular extractions	2013	Darpan Bhargava

CURRENT TRENDS

Some additional therapies being investigated which can be beneficial to the patient for uneventful post-operative outcomes are ozone gel, cryotherapy, platelet-rich plasma (PRP), platelet-rich fibrin (PRF), piezoelectric surgery, and lasers. Ozone gel has shown beneficial outcomes after third molar surgery, but it is not a popular choice owing to the cost factor involved and lack of evidence-based literature currently. There has been renaissance on studies related to cryotherapy or ice application causing vasoconstriction, thereby decreasing post-operative swelling. It diminishes the nerve conduction velocity producing an analgesic effect. However, its use is controversial in relation to third molar surgery. Benefits of cold fomentation or cold compress following a third molar surgical extraction are well documented and clinically demonstrated. PRP and PRF are proven to be effective in third molar surgery in terms of enhanced post-operative outcomes. Low-level laser therapy (LLLT) is a therapeutic laser evoking cellular bio-stimulation, thereby accelerating wound healing and tissue regeneration. LLLT is being studied for its effects to reduce discomfort post-operatively and promote healing following wisdom tooth extraction. Piezoelectric surgical interventions are being studied and incorporated for the transalveolar mandibular extraction surgeries with the benefit of minimal damage to the soft tissues including abating the chances of nerve damage [6,7] Recently, "Twin-Mix Anaesthesia" has been studied for surgical removal of impacted mandibular third molars [8–10].

The newer interventions and surgical modifications in terms of technique, equipment, and utilizing pharmacological or physical agents would require a more robust investigation utilizing well-designed multicentric randomized controlled trials for their endorsement for incorporation for these surgical procedures.

The future of third molar surgery is still undergoing transformation to this present day. Advancements with transoral robotic surgery (TORS) may produce a significant paradigm shift and impact on third molar surgery in the future, similar to its use in procedures such as tonsillectomies, retromolar trigone tumours, and base of tongue neoplasms.

The intention towards any surgery remains directed to reduce complications using a single or multimodal approach which includes the administration of antibiotics, analgesics, steroid-based pharmacological agents along with the execution of an appropriately planned surgical procedure. This holds true for transalveolar extractions too. Conventionally, operator considerations in pre-operative planning include flap design, judicious handling of soft and hard tissues followed by appropriate suture placement and drainage are vital aspects for a successful mandibular third molar surgery.

REFERENCES

1. Guerini V. *A History of Dentistry: From the most Ancient Times to the End of Eighteenth Century.* Philadelphia and New York: Lea & Febiger, 1909.

2. Kumar A. Dentistry in historical perspective. *IJOCR.* 2013;1(2):51–54.

3. Koutroumpas, D, Lioumi, E, Vougiouklakis, G. Tooth extraction in antiquity. *J Hist Dent.* 2020;68:127–144.

4. Hussain A, Khan FA. History of dentistry. *Arch Med Health Sci* [Serial online]. 2014;2:106–110. Available from: https://www.amhsjournal.org/text.asp?2014/2/1/106/133850.

5. Haga, S, Nakaoka, H, Yamaguchi, T, et al. A genome-wide association study of third molar agenesis in Japanese and Korean populations. *J Hum Genet.* 2013;58:799–803. doi: 10.1038/jhg.2013.106.

6. Alzahrani AA, Murriky A, Shafik S. Influence of platelet rich fibrin on post-extraction socket healing: A clinical and radiographic study. *Saudi Dent J.* 2017;29(4):149–155. doi: 10.1016/j.sdentj.2017.07.003.

7. Ahrari F, Eshghpour M, Zare R, Ebrahimi S, Fallahrastegar A, Khaki H. Effectiveness of low-level laser irradiation in reducing pain and accelerating socket healing after undisturbed tooth extraction. *J Lasers Med Sci.* 2020;11(3):274–279. doi: 10.34172/jlms.2020.46.

8. Bhargava D, Sreekumar K, Rastogi S, Deshpande A, Chakravorty N. A prospective randomized double-blind study to assess the latency and efficacy of twin-mix and 2% lignocaine with 1:200,000 epinephrine in surgical removal of impacted mandibular third molars: A pilot study. *Oral Maxillofac Surg.* 2013 Dec;17(4):275–280. doi: 10.1007/s10006-012-0372-3.

9. Bhargava D, Sreekumar K, Deshpande A. Effects of intra-space injection of Twin mix versus intraoral-submucosal, intramuscular, intravenous and per-oral administration of dexamethasone

on post-operative sequelae after mandibular impacted third molar surgery: A preliminary clinical comparative study. *Oral Maxillofac Surg*. 2014 Sep;18(3):293–296. doi: 10.1007/ s10006-013-0412-7.

10. Bhargava D, Deshpande A, Khare P, Pandey SP, Thakur N. Validation of data on the use of twin mix in minor oral surgery: Comparative evaluation of efficacy of twin mix versus 2% lignocaine with 1:200000 epinephrine based on power analysis and an UV spectrometry study for chemical stability of the mixture. *Oral Maxillofac Surg*. 2015 Mar;19(1):37–41. doi: 10.1007/ s10006-014-0446-5.

Applied surgical anatomy for transalveolar extraction of the mandibular third molar

V. VIDYA DEVI AND DARPAN BHARGAVA

The "*mandibular third molar region*" associated with the impacted third molar is a clinico-surgically defined area incorporating the impacted tooth itself and its immediate surrounding structures that are of significance while performing a transalveolar extraction of the concerned impacted molar. In-depth understanding of the anatomy of this region is essential to implement an expedient approach for the removal of the third molar while keeping the patient morbidity low and avoiding potential complications.

The impacted third molar may be completely or partially embedded as the tooth may have coverage with only the mucosa or with the bone of the posterior mandible. Depending on its spatial position and depth of impaction, it can extend into the body of the mandible or cross the anterior border of the ramus. Also, the angulation of the third molar determines the course of its eruption which may be completely or partially covered with the overlying mucosa [1–3].

MUCOSA AND MUCOPERIOSTEUM

The mucosa over the impacted third molar region forms the superior surface overlying the tooth. The medial, lateral, and posterior surfaces can be further divided into three areas for better understanding:

a. **Posterosuperior mucosal surface**: A roughly quadrilateral shaped region forming a concave inclined plane from the occlusal level of the maxillary molars to the lower alveolar region and may be further divided into two triangular areas by the elevated pterygomandibular ligament as superolateral and inferomedial triangles (Figure 3.1).

i. *Superolateral or anaesthetic triangle*, which is covered by a thin mucosal lining, characteristically bright red in colour and is the continuation of the buccal mucosa. The shape of this triangle can be altered with the action of the underlying buccinator muscle. This region is remarkable as it is the puncture site for the inferior alveolar nerve block utilized to anaesthetize the inferior alveolar and lingual nerves (Figure 3.1).

ii. *Inferomedial or retromolar triangle*, which is covered by a relatively thicker pale mucosa, and towards its anterior end forms the retromolar pad (piriformis papilla). The retromolar pad is a triangular soft elevation of mucosa that lies distal to the third molar (or the last erupted tooth) [4]. It comprises non-keratinized loose alveolar mucosa covering the glandular tissues, fibres of buccinator muscle, fibres

DOI: 10.1201/9781003324034-3

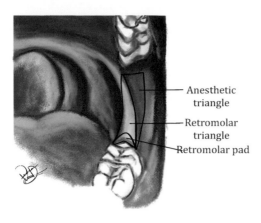

Mucosa of the posteriosuperior surface of third molar region

Figure 3.1 Note the surface anatomy of the retromolar area and mucosa of the posterio-superior surface of the mandibular third molar region.

of superior constrictor muscle, fibres of pterygomandibular raphe, and the terminal part of the tendon of temporalis muscle [5] (Figure 3.1).

In relevance to third molar surgery, the incision starts at the vertex of the retromolar triangle and moves in contact with the bone till the second molar.

b. **Lateral surface**: In the buccal aspect that forms the lateral surface, the mucosa is strongly adherent to the underlying bone forming the mucoperiosteum before it continues further laterally along the posterior floor of the buccal vestibule.

Elevation of the mucoperiosteum at the subperiosteal plane without disturbing the supra-periosteal areas can ensure minimal bleeding while exposing the underlying bone for the exposure and access to the surgical site for the transalveolar extraction of the impacted third molar.

c. **Medial surface**: The mucosa in this area is at its thinnest and adheres firmly to the underlying bone before continuing as the floor of the mouth medially and towards the faucial pillars posteriorly.

The mucosa may be further thinned in cases of lingually rotated impacted tooth that may result in tear of the mucosa during mucoperiosteal elevation.

SKELETAL ANATOMY

Mandibular third molar region is anatomically located at the distal end of the body of the mandible more in a transition zone between the body and the ramus. Relevant anatomical landmarks should be given consideration in understanding the skeletal anatomy of this region with an emphasis on the thickness of the cortical plates and the soft tissue arrangement for better surgical execution and outcome. The skeletal formations include the cortical plates, internal and external oblique ridge, retromolar fossa, retromolar triangle, latero-alveolar canal, and the mylohyoid ridge (Figure 3.2a–d).

Cortical plates, internal and external oblique ridges: The third molar is embedded between a thick cortical plate which is buttressed by the thicker external oblique ridge and the thinner lingual internal oblique ridge. On palpation, the thick buccal cortex may be felt in the buccal vestibular region reinforced by the external oblique ridge lateral to the third molar region. The mylohyoid ridge runs obliquely at the medial surface and extends superiorly over the medial margin of the retromolar triangle. The mylohyoid ridge provides enforcement to the thin lingual cortical plate (Figure 3.2b and d).

The thickness of the lingual plate is also dependent on the position and angulation of the impacted third molar and is more vulnerable to fracture during the elevation of the tooth while applying force in an inappropriate manner and direction. Note the view from the inferior aspect, the third molar remains in proximity to the lingual shelf of the bone (Figure 3.2e). Lingual plate deficiency is a developmental anomaly which may be seen as a dehiscence or fenestration below the lingual crest causing the apices of the third molar to penetrate into the lingual cortex and lie in and adherent to the overlying mucosa.

The external oblique ridge on the buccal side is a bulky prominence that may impede the buccal traction of the mandibular third molar.

Bone trajectories or "grain" of the cortical bone, related to the mechanical stress, run longitudinally in the mandible. This has significance in the removal of the impacted tooth using a chisel where stop cuts are required to prevent transmission of cutting forces beyond what is desired.

Retromolar triangle: Mostly but not always triangular-shaped area is present between the two bony ridges and the distal surface of the posterior

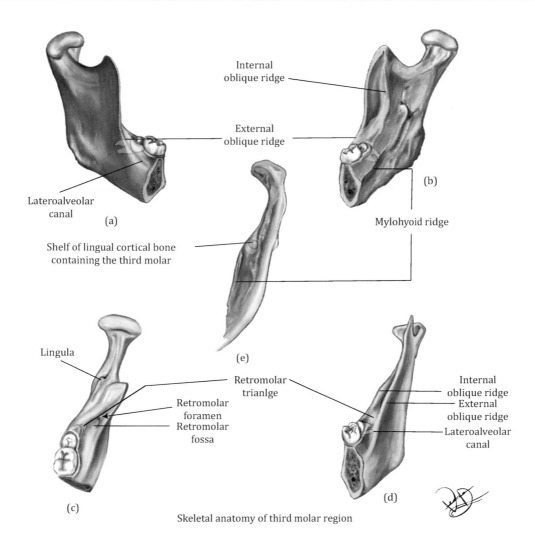

Figure 3.2 Osteology relevant to the mandibular third molar region: (a) Lateral. (b) Medial. (c) Superior. (d) Supero-lateral. (e) Inferior.

most molar. This area is perforated by a number of openings to canals conducting branches of the buccinator artery that anastomose with the inferior alveolar artery (Figure 3.2c and d).

Retromolar fossa: It is a depression bounded medially by the lateral lip of the retromolar triangle and laterally the anterior portion of the mandibular ramus. It owns the insertion of the buccinator muscle. The retromolar foramen is sometimes present in this region conducting blood vessels in the region and facilitating their anastomosis with the inferior alveolar blood vessels. Injury of these anastomosing vessels may lead to abundant bleeding and at times post extraction haematoma (Figure 3.2c).

Lateroalveolar canal: A misnomer describing an elongated depression on the buccal side of the alveolar process extending up to the mental foramen that lacks any muscle attachment (Figure 3.2a and d). Buccal guttering during removal of the third molar stays medial to the lateroalveolar canal. The retromolar fossa and the lateral alveolar canal also form a passage for the spread of infections from the third molar region. This is sometimes referred to as Chompret-L'Hirondel migratory abscess.

Mylohyoid ridge: Rough bony elevation running in an oblique line on the medial surface of the mandible, with its posterior end extending into the third molar region providing insertion to

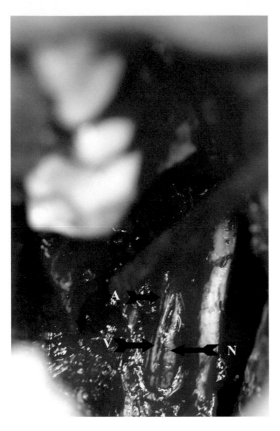

Figure 3.3 The inferior alveolar canal deroofed as part of a marginal mandibular resection showing neurovascular vessels in third molar region. The vein (V) lies superiorly, and the artery (A) lies lingually and superiorly. The inferior alveolar nerve (N) lies below. (Adapted with permission from Pogrel, Dorfman, and Fallah. Inferior alveolar neurovascular bundle. *J Oral Maxillofac Surg.* 2009.)

the mylohyoid muscle and anchorage to mylopharyngeal portion of the upper constrictor muscle (Figure 3.2b).

Mandibular canal (inferior alveolar canal/inferior dental canal): It runs from the mandibular foramen to the mental foramen carrying the inferior alveolar neurovascular bundle. The canal runs from lingual to buccal further anteriorly before ending at the mental foramen. In the third molar region, it has an ovoid shape and lies relatively closer to the lingual cortical plate or rarely between the lingual and buccal plates [1–6]. The variations to the normal anatomy of the mandibular canal are documented with sporadic cases having bifid or trifid canals or accessory canals. Pogrel et al. studied the anatomic structure of the inferior alveolar

neurovascular bundle in the third molar region and demonstrated that the inferior alveolar vein lies superior to the nerve and that there are often multiple veins. The artery appears to be solitary and lies on the lingual side of the nerve, slightly above the horizontal position [7] (Figures 3.3 and 3.4).

Bone is relatively elastic in young individuals and becomes brittle as age advances. This may influence the factors like the choice of method for removal of the impacted tooth and the amount of bone removal that may be required.

ADJACENT MUSCLES AND LIGAMENTS

Three principal muscles are present in the mandibular third molar region (Figure 3.5).

a. **Buccinator:** This muscle contributes to the formation of the muscular wall of the anaesthetic triangle. Part of the muscle originates from the periosteum under the retromolar pad in the retromolar fossa.
b. **Superior pharyngeal constrictor:** The origin of the muscle lay on the lingual side of the mandible below the lingual crest, above the mylohyoid ridge and medial to the third molar forming a part of the third molar region with its buccopharyngeal and mylopharyngeal components. The pterygomandibular ligament (raphe) lies between the superior constrictor and buccinator muscle, which is an important landmark for the anaesthesia in this region.
c. **Temporalis:** The distal fascicle of the temporalis muscle advances downward as the temporalis tendon around the medial and anterior surfaces of the coronoid, extending downwards onto the anterior mandibular ramus and further to the buccinator line. A buccal approach for the surgical removal of the third molar transects the lowest part of the temporalis tendon to facilitate the removal of the buccal and the distal bone covering the impacted molar. Excessive injury to the large portion of this tendon and the ramal attachment of the muscle may result in trismus.

In addition, the mylohyoid muscle demarcates the floor of the mouth and is important in relation to the lingual nerve. At the posterior attachment of the muscle, which lies in the third molar region the

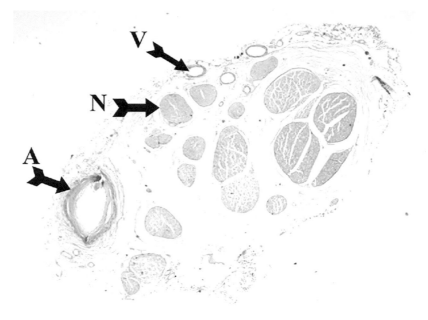

Figure 3.4 Histologic examination of specimen from the right third molar region as seen from behind showing inferior alveolar canal contents. The vein (V), lying superiorly, consists of a number of venules, whereas the artery (A), lying lingually, contains only a single vessel. The nerve (N) itself consists of around 16 fascicles at this point. (Hematoxylin and eosin; original magnification ×40.) (Adapted with permission from Pogrel MA, Dorfman D, Fallah H. Inferior alveolar neurovascular bundle. *J Oral Maxillofac Surg.* 2009 Nov;67(11):2452–4. doi: 10.1016/j.joms.2009.06.013.)

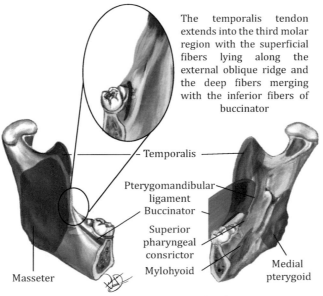

The temporalis tendon extends into the third molar region with the superficial fibers lying along the external oblique ridge and the deep fibers merging with the inferior fibers of buccinator

Temporalis

Pterygomandibular ligament

Buccinator

Superior pharyngeal consrictor

Mylohyoid

Masseter

Medial pterygoid

Muscles and ligaments in the third molar region

Figure 3.5 Musculature and ligamentous structures relevant to the mandibular third molar region. Note the formation of the "pterygomandibular ligament" with its buccal and lingual relation to various anatomical structures.

lingual nerve remains superior to it before it makes an anteromedial turn.

REGIONAL BLOOD VESSELS

The third molar region is mainly supplied by the inferior alveolar and the buccal arteries and drained by their corresponding veins. Other important arteries of the region are the ascending palatine artery, lower masseteric, and facial artery.

a. *Inferior alveolar artery and vein:* Inferior alveolar artery originates from the first segment of the maxillary artery, gives off the mylohyoid branch, and enters the inferior alveolar canal through the mandibular foramen, supplying the mandibular body, posterior teeth, the alveolar and the gingival region. The artery continues anteriorly as two divisions: the incisive artery and the mental artery.

   The vessels are normally located superior to the inferior alveolar nerve in the canal and are therefore the first to be injured, which may occur when the impacted tooth is impinging on the canal or when injudicious removal of the buccal cortical bone injures the artery in a canal placed lateral to the tooth. Injury to the artery during surgical procedures may lead to excessive bleeding.

b. *Buccal artery:* Originating from the second part of the maxillary artery, it supplies the buccinator muscle and the buccal mucosa in the third molar region. It is also responsible for the collateral supply anastomosing with the inferior alveolar artery through the retromolar foramen.

c. *Ascending palatine artery:* It originates from the facial artery and supplies the pharyngeal wall and tonsillar region passing along the anterior faucial pillars. Injury to this artery can occur in the region of the faucial pillar when excessive force is applied while retraction resulting in tearing of the flap or injury with injudicious use of an instrument like an elevator which may cause heavy bleeding.

d. *Facial artery and vein:* After its origin from the external carotid artery, the facial artery passes upward and forward medial to the ramus of the mandible, deep to the submandibular salivary gland, and crosses the inferior border of the mandible just anterior to the masseter muscle, close to the second molar.

Accidental injury to the facial vessels may occur due to slipping of the scalpel during placement of the buccal releasing incision or the intentional extension of the incision in the buccal vestibule (Figure 3.6).

Lymphatics of the third molar region drains in the submandibular and retropharyngeal lymph nodes.

ADJACENT NERVES AND INNERVATION

The inferior alveolar region has innervation form the inferior alveolar nerve, lingual nerve, long buccal nerve. Additionally, the anatomy and the role of the mental and mylohyoid nerves should be considered (Figures 3.7 and 3.8).

A. *Inferior alveolar nerve:* A mixed nerve branching from the posterior division of the mandibular nerve, which descends medial to the lateral pterygoid muscle, lateral and posterior to the lingual nerve, to the region between the sphenomandibular ligament and the medial surface of the mandibular ramus, enters the mandibular canal at the level of the mandibular foramen. It travels along the canal mostly lying inferior and lingual to the roots of the third molar (Figures 3.7 and 3.8). Kim et al. classified the buccolingual location of the mandibular canal into three types [8]:

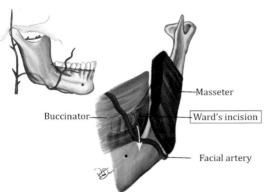

Masseter

Buccinator

Ward's incision

Facial artery

Facial artery passing superiorly along the anterior border of the masseter is at risk of injury if vertical release of Ward's incision slips, extending anterior and buccally

Figure 3.6 Facial artery with its relation to the mandibular angle and the anterior masseteric region.

- Type 1 (70%), where the canal follows the lingual cortical plate at the mandibular ramus and body;
- Type 2 (15%), where the canal follows the middle of the ramus behind the second molar and the lingual plate passing through the second and first molars;
- Type 3 (15%), where the canal follows the middle or the lingual one-third of the mandible from the ramus to the body.

In rare cases, the mandibular nerve may also be present as bifid or trifid branched variations that have varying relationships with the roots of third molars.

The third molar roots can lie in different relations to the inferior alveolar canal

1. Related but not involving the canal
   a. Separated
   b. Superimposed
   c. Adjacent
2. Involved with the canal
   a. Roots buccal to the canal
   b. Roots in line with the canal
   c. Roots lingual to the canal
   d. Canal passing inter-radicular between the roots

When roots are involving the canal, removal of the third molar carries a high risk of injury to the nerve. Even when not in close proximity, injudicious elevation can lead to compression and neuropraxic injury of the nerve.

B. ***Long buccal nerve*:** Also known as the buccinator nerve and is a branch of the anterior division of the mandibular nerve that passes between

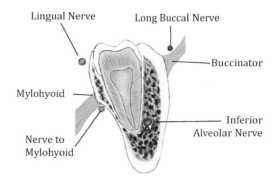

Nerves in relation with mylohyoid and buccinator muslces in the third molar region

Figure 3.7 Nerves and their relation with the mandibular third molar region.

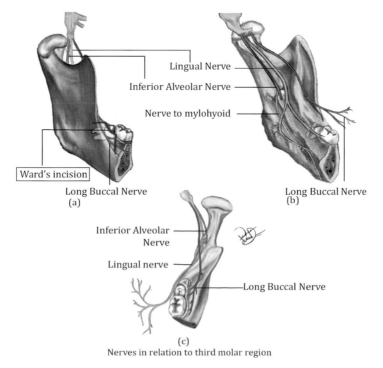

Nerves in relation to third molar region

Figure 3.8 Nerves in relation to the third molar region: (a) Lateral view. (b) Medial view. (c) Superior view.

the two heads of the lateral pterygoid muscle, courses inferiorly along the temporalis muscle, emerging under the anterior border of the masseter continuing in an anterolateral direction. At the occlusal level of the mandibular second or third molar, it crosses in front of the anterior border of the ramus entering the cheek region through the buccinator muscle (Figure 3.8). It supplies sensory innervation to the mucosa of the buccal gingiva and retromolar area in this region (refer Figure 3.8a, b and c).

Branches of the nerve may often be cut at the point of its crossing the ramus while placing the incision. However, the effects of the injury are not easily discernible.

C. **Lingual nerve:** A branch of the posterior division of the mandibular nerve, it passes downwards medial to the lateral pterygoid, descending between the muscle and the ramus in the pterygomandibular space. It runs anterior and medial to the inferior alveolar nerve, continuing deep to the pterygomandibular raphe, inferior to the attachment of the superior constrictor muscle, passing lateral to the base of the tongue, immediately under the oral mucosa below and behind the mandibular third molar either in contact with the lingual cortex or within 3 mm medial to it although some studies have reported a wider placement [9,10].

With respect to the alveolar crest at the third molar region, the nerve can lie below the crest, at the level of the crest and in rare cases above the crest or at the retromolar pad region. Behnia et al. examined 669 nerves from 430 fresh cadavers and reported that in 14.05% of examined sites, the nerve was above the lingual crest, but in 0.15%, the nerve was in the retromolar pad region. In the majority of sites examined (85.80%), the mean horizontal and vertical distances of the nerve to the lingual plate and the lingual crest were 2.06±1.10 mm (range 0.00–3.20 mm) and 3.01 +/–0.42 mm (range 1.70–4.00 mm), respectively. In 22.27% of sites examined, the nerve was in direct contact with the lingual plate of the alveolar process [11] (Figure 3.9).

Miloro et al. assessed the lingual nerve in the third molar region using magnetic resonance imaging and reported that the mean vertical distance in the study patients was 2.75 +/–0.97 mm [range 1.52–4.61] and horizontal distance was 2.53 +/–0.67 mm [range 0.00–4.35] to the lingual crest and lingual plate of the mandible [12] (Figure 3.10).

At the region of the second molar, the lingual nerve makes a medial turn into the

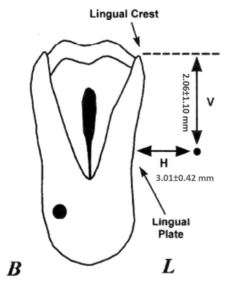

Figure 3.9 Coronal section through the third molar region showing methods of measurement. V, Vertical distance from lingual crest; H, Horizontal distance from the lingual plate; B, Buccal; L, lingual. (Adapted with permission from Behnia H, Kheradvar A, Shahrokhi M. An anatomic study of the lingual nerve in the third molar region. *J Oral Maxillofac Surg.* 2000 Jun;58(6):649–51; discussion 652–3. doi: 10.1016/s0278-2391(00)90159-9.)

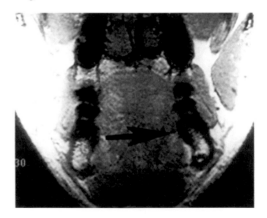

Figure 3.10 Coronal HR-MRI image showing the position of the lingual nerve in the third molar region (arrow). (Adapted with permission from Miloro M, Halkias LE, Slone HW, Chakeres DW. Assessment of the lingual nerve in the third molar region using magnetic resonance imaging. *J Oral Maxillofac Surg.* 1997 Feb;55(2):134–7. doi: 10.1016/s0278-2391(97)90228-7.)

submandibular region and transverses to form the terminal branches (Figure 3.8c).

Injury to the lingual nerve is more prone in lingually inclined impacted third molar. The lingual nerve is also seen to be more cranially placed if there is a shorter distance between the third molar and the ascending ramus. Ample anatomical variations in the relationship of the lingual nerve to the alveolar crest make the prediction of injury unreliable but it can be commonly avoided by keeping dissection and manipulation of the lingual tissues to a minimum. The lingual split technique of removing the impacted third molar is also associated with higher incidence of lingual nerve injury.

D. **Nerve to mylohyoid:** It branches from the inferior alveolar nerve before entering the mandibular canal and supplies the mylohyoid muscle and anterior belly of digastric. Injury to the mylohyoid nerve has been reported in case of excessive retraction of the lingual tissues.

ADJACENT TEETH AND PERIODONTIUM

The second molar adjacent to the impacted tooth may often show caries or restorations. Damage can occur to the adjacent teeth or restorations during the removal of the third molar due to injudicious use of force.

The interdental bone between the third and second molar will vary depending on the angulation of the impacted tooth. In the case of horizontal or distoangular impaction, the bone may be minimal or nonexistent. Removal of the impacted tooth along with the interdental bone in such cases may lead to iatrogenic periodontal problems. Where possible, incisions involving the epithelial attachment to the second molar also must be avoided to prevent iatrogenic periodontal complications.

BUCCAL FAT PAD

The buccal fat pad is a structure that may be encountered when removing maxillary impacted third molars. It is most often seen when flap incisions are made too far distal to maxillary second molars. This is usually not encountered with mandibular third molar surgeries.

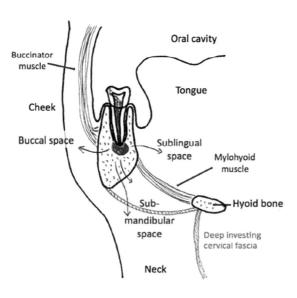

Figure 3.11 Coronal section of right mandible showing potential paths of spread of infection from a carious wisdom tooth. (Adapted with permission from Morosan M, et al. *Anaesthesia and Common Oral and Maxillo-Facial Emergencies.* Elsevier. doi: 10.1093/bjaceaccp/mks031.)

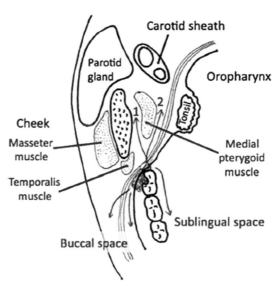

Figure 3.12 Axial section of right mandible showing potential paths of spread of infection from a carious wisdom tooth. (Adapted with permission from Morosan M, et al. *Anaesthesia and Common Oral and Maxillo-Facial Emergencies.* Elsevier. doi: 10.1093/bjaceaccp/mks031.)

SPACES INVOLVED WITH THE MANDIBULAR THIRD MOLARS

Accidental displacement of the lower third molar or its roots is a complication with the removal of the impacted tooth. Displacement commonly occurs in one of the following spaces.

a. Sublingual space
b. Submandibular space
c. Pterygomandibular space

The understanding of the anatomic proximity of the fascial spaces to the mandibular third molar is also vital for understanding the pathways for the spread of infection [13] (Figures 3.11 and 3.12).

REFERENCES

1. Suazo Galdames I. Región del tercer molar inferior. *Int J Morphol*. 2012 Sep;30(3):970–8.
2. Gupta S, Khan TA, Attarde H, Narula J. Surgical anatomy of mandibular third molar. *Austin J Surg*. 2019;6(13):1194.
3. Malamed SF. *Handbook of Local Anesthesia*. Elsevier Health Sciences, New York, United States of America 2004.
4. Sicher H, DuBrull EL. *Oral Anatomy*. St. Louis, MO: Mosby, 1970, pp. 179–81.
5. Sharma A, Deep A, Siwach A, Singh M, Bhargava A, Siwach R. Assessment and evaluation of anatomic variations of retromolar pad: A cross sectional study. *J Clin Diagn Res*. 2016;10(5):ZC143–5. doi: 10.7860/JCDR/2016/19551.7880.
6. Varghese G. Management of impacted third molars. In: Bonanthaya K, Panneerselvam E, Manuel S, Kumar VV, Rai A (eds) *Oral and Maxillofacial Surgery for the Clinician*. Singapore: Springer, 2021. doi: 10.1007/978-981-15-1346-6_14.
7. Pogrel MA, Dorfman D, Fallah H. The anatomic structure of the inferior alveolar neurovascular bundle in the third molar region. *J Oral Maxillofac Surg*. 2009 Nov;67(11):2452–4. doi: 10.1016/j.joms.2009.06.013.
8. Kim ST, Hu KS, Song WC, Kang MK, Park HD, Kim HJ. Location of the mandibular canal and the topography of its neurovascular structures. *J Craniofac Surg*. 2009 May;20(3):936–9.
9. Kieser J, Kieser D, Hauman T. The course and distribution of the inferior alveolar nerve in the edentulous mandible. *J Craniofac Surg*. 2005 Jan;16(1):6–9.
10. Al-Amery SM, Nambiar P, Naidu M, Ngeow WC. Variation in lingual nerve course: A human cadaveric study. *PLoS One*. 2016 Sep;11(9):e0162773.
11. Behnia H, Kheradvar A, Shahrokhi M. An anatomic study of the lingual nerve in the third molar region. *J Oral Maxillofac Surg*. 2000 Jun;58(6):649–51; discussion 652–3. doi: 10.1016/s0278-2391(00)90159-9.
12. Miloro M, Halkias LE, Slone HW, Chakeres DW. Assessment of the lingual nerve in the third molar region using magnetic resonance imaging. *J Oral Maxillofac Surg*. 1997 Feb;55(2):134–7. doi: 10.1016/s0278-2391(97)90228-7.
13. Morosan M, et al. Anaesthesia and common oral and maxillo-facial emergencies. *Br J Anaesth*. 2012 Oct;12(5), 257–62. doi: 10.1093/bjaceaccp/mks031.

4

Indications and contraindications for surgical extraction of the mandibular third molars

PREETI G. BHARGAVA, VIVIANNE IBRAHIM SHEHATA SOBH, AND DARPAN BHARGAVA

The term impaction originates from the Latin word *impactus* (Durbeck, 1945), and it refers to a state where one object is held by another. In the context of the dental sciences, Blum (1923) and Durbeck (1945) defined impaction as arrested tooth eruption caused by a clinically or radiographically detectable physical barrier in the eruption path or by a tooth being malpositioned [1]. Impacted tooth is a tooth that fails to erupt and will not assume its anticipated anatomical position beyond its chronological (expected) age of eruption. Recurrent pericoronitis, pericoronitis infections leading to space infection, follicular cystic alteration related to an unerupted third molar, acute or chronic irreversible pulpitis as a sequela of deep caries of the third molar, any periodontal or pulpal disease affecting adjacent second molar, prophylactic removal for prosthetic and orthodontic purpose or reconstructive surgery and the third molar impinging the inferior alveolar nerve causing chronic facial pain are some common indications for lower third molar removal. A surgeon must be aware of the risks and benefits associated with the third molar surgical removal and should be justified to execute or avoid the procedure for specific contraindications.

DEFINITION

Impacted tooth may be defined as the "one that fails to erupt and will not eventually assume its anatomical arch relationship beyond the chronological eruption date". The impacted teeth, in general, may be unerupted or partially erupted. It should be understood that a tooth may be labelled impacted only when its root formation is complete, and it fails to erupt in the expected anatomical position [2].

> A tooth which is completely or partially unerupted and is positioned against another tooth, bone, or soft tissue so that its further eruption is unlikely, described according to its anatomic position.
>
> *(From Committee on Hospital Oral Surgery Service: Oral Surgery Glossary, Chicago, American Society of Oral Surgeons, 1971.) [3]*

CAUSES FOR THIRD MOLAR IMPACTION

There is evidence of decrease in the jaw size as the process of evolution due to the changing habits of diet in humans and the consumption of soft and processed food. With this decrease in the size of the jaw, the space in the dental arch remains insufficient for the eruption of third molars, as they develop and erupt late during the course of life [4].

DOI: 10.1201/9781003324034-4

During normal development, the lower third molar begins to form in a horizontal angulation, and as the tooth develops and the jaw grows, the angulation changes from horizontal to mesioangular and finally to a vertical position. Failure of rotation is the most common cause of lower third molars becoming impacted.

Chronology of third molars is such that, it may get impacted due to *lack of space* in the dental arch due to *obstruction* (by the dense mandibular bone at the angle, existing pathology like odontome or a tooth already erupted) leading to non-eruption or partial eruption. Also, failure to rotate from horizontal to vertical position justifies the cause for third molar impaction. Development of the third molar begins in a horizontal direction. With the growing jaw and development of the tooth, it rotates from mesioangular to the vertical direction coinciding with the occlusal table. Age is also a predominant factor in the predictability of impacted third molars. The incidence for maximally encountering impacted or partially erupted third molars is between 20 and 25 years of age followed by the 37 and older age group [5].

THEORIES OF TOOTH IMPACTION (DURBECK, 1945)

1. ***Orthodontic theory*:** Jaws develop in the downward and forward directions. Growth of the jaw and movement of teeth occurs in the forward direction, any interference with such a movement will cause an impaction (smaller jaw leading to decreased space). A dense bone formation at the time of third molar eruption decreases the movement of the teeth in the forward direction.
2. ***Phylogenic theory*:** Nature tries to eliminate the disused organs, i.e., use makes the organ develop better, but disuse causes slow regression of an organ. More-functional masticatory force leads to better development of the jaw. Due to changing nutritional habits and consumption of processed food, the need for exerting extreme forces with jaws has been practically eliminated. For this reason, during the course of the evolution, the mandible and maxilla have decreased in size leaving insufficient room for the third molars.
3. ***Mendelian theory*:** Heredity may be considered a noted cause. The hereditary transmission of small jaws from one parent and large teeth from the other parent will result in insufficient space for the eruption of the third molar. This may be an important etiological factor in the occurrence of impaction of lower third molars. The MSX1 and AXIN2 genes have been found to have an association and may be considered as components of the genetic background, characterized by variable expressivity. They have been associated with tooth impaction in circumstances where specific environmental factors coexist and depending on the presence of other modulating genetic factors, additionally increasing the risk.
4. ***Pathological theory*:** Osteosclerosis in the lower third molar region is supposedly considered to be one of the factors in impaction. Chronic infections affecting an individual may bring the condensation of osseous tissue further preventing the growth and development of the jaws.
5. ***Endocrinal theory*:** This theory is based on the assumption that an increase or decrease in the growth hormone secretion causes an imbalance in the endocrinal activity and may affect the size of the jaws resulting in the impaction of third molars [6].

The other rare syndromes and disorders that may include tooth impaction as presenting clinical feature are: cleidocranial dysostosis, hemifacial microsomia, mucopolysaccharidoses, Cretinism, Gardner's syndrome, Down syndrome, Aarskog syndrome, Zimmermann–Laband syndrome, and Noonan's syndrome [7].

INDICATIONS FOR EXTRACTION OF MANDIBULAR THIRD MOLARS

According to the recommendations of the National Institutes of Health (NIH), both impacted and erupted mandibular third molars with evidence of follicular enlargement should be removed electively and the associated soft tissue should be submitted for microscopic examination. Impacted teeth with pericoronitis should also be extracted electively because of their known potential for repetitive infection and morbidity. Furthermore, third molars with non-restorable carious lesions nd third molars contributing to the resorption of adjacent teeth should also be extracted [8,9]. According to National Health Service (NHS) in Great Britain, "*Surgical removal of impacted third molars should be limited to patients with evidence of pathology.*" NHS further defines pathology as:

> Nonrestorable caries, non-treatable pulpal and/or periapical pathology, cellulitis, abscess and osteomyelitis, internal/external resorption of the tooth or adjacent teeth, fracture of tooth, disease of follicle including cyst/tumour, tooth/teeth impeding surgery or reconstructive jaw surgery, and when a tooth is involved in or within the field of tumour resections. [10]

Recurrent pericoronitis

Pericoronitis refers to an infection of the soft tissues covering an impacted or partially erupted tooth usually caused by oral flora. The infection gets aggravated when the host defence is unable to defend against the micro-organisms involved or the host defence is compromised. Pericoronitis can also occur as a sequalae to recurrent trauma from the upper third molar resulting in an inflamed operculum (soft tissue covering the occlusal surface of partially erupted mandibular molar). Another factor that is responsible for this infection is the accumulation of food debris under the operculum leading to bacterial colonization and infection. Commonly associated bacteria with pericoronitis include *Porphyromonas, Fusobacterium*, and *Peptostreptococcus* [11]. Pericoronitis sometimes results in serious space infection involving the pterygomandibular, submandibular, and buccal space and can spread rapidly to the lateral neck. These patients present with trismus, fever, malaise, and facial swelling. In cases having complicated fascial space infection due to pericoronitis, surgical extraction under parenteral antibiotic coverage and careful monitoring should be done. Uncomplicated recurrent pericoronitis is also a clear indication for the removal of the impacted tooth.

Caries

Caries in partially or completely erupted molars can often be encountered involving mostly the occlusal or mesioproximal surfaces as the third molar region lacks adequate cleaning due to its obscured position. Unrestorable caries due to inaccessibility and to reduce the risk of periapical and fascial space infection, extraction of the third molar is advisable [12].

Periodontal disease

Incidence of distal pocket with respect to the second molar is commonly associated with partially or completely erupted third molars as a result of food impaction and inadequate oral hygiene. Radiographic evaluation helps in assessing the adequacy of space for the third molar and the amount of bone adjacent to the distal root of the second molar. Early advanced isolated periodontitis affecting only the distal aspect of the second molar with normal sulcular depth of the tooth in the oral cavity is often an indication for an impacted third molar. Recent literature shows young individuals with otherwise good periodontal health clinically demonstrate periodontal pocketing, attachment loss, inflammatory and pathogenic inflammatory markers distal to second molars in the presence of third molars [13,14]. Extracting the third molars is an effective way of pocket elimination and tissue preservation distal to the second molar.

Obscure facial pain

Vague pain or paraesthesia in the lower facial region that cannot be explained or attributed to any cause. Although the reason remains unclear, the possibility of the effects of the impacted tooth (commonly during the course of its development) on the inferior dental nerve or the adjacent tooth may be considered. In such a case, it is must to inform the patient that removal of the impacted tooth may or may not relieve the pain.

Previous attempted extraction

In case of a history of failed previous attempts of third molar removal, the particular cause of failure and difficulty level should be assessed before planning for the surgical removal.

Prosthetic considerations

On clinical suspicion, a prior radiographic evaluation of the third molar region should be done before the rehabilitation of an edentulous jaw for any retained or impacted tooth, and removal of the same should be planned. The teeth below the prosthesis may pose a problem of exposure as the ridge resorbs with the pressure of the prosthesis on the jaw bone on function.

Orthodontic reasons

In patients anticipated to have marked disproportion between the tooth material and the jaw size, prophylactic removal of the third molar may be considered to prevent its effect on the periodontium of the second molar or on the tooth itself. In the opinion of a few orthodontists, the imbrication of the lower incisors may be a possibility as a result of ineffectual attempts of the third molar to erupt. However, this concept remains controversial. When the distalization of the molars for orthodontic treatment is planned, this can be considered the reason for the prophylactic removal of third molars [15].

Preparation for orthognathic surgery

Patients who are candidates for orthognathic surgery and have the third molars present should be planned for early removal of third molars at the potential osteotomy sites. Sagittal split osteotomies at the ramus-angle region of the mandible can be predictably performed when third molars are not present at the osteotomy site or are prophylactically removed at least 6–12 months before the surgery. Delay in the removal of the third molar, especially in mandibular advancement surgery, reduces the quality and thickness of the lingual cortex at the disto-proximal segment where fixation screws need to be inserted. Reliable fixation of the osteotomized segments is aided when there is adequate sound bone available to secure screws for the bone plate osteosynthesis [16,17].

Presence of pathological lesion

Most developmental odontogenic cyst arise from the follicular tissues of the unerupted tooth. The impacted third molars that are related to follicular cystic alteration should be considered for removal. The follicular tissues may also lead to the development of an odontogenic tumour or rarely malignancy. In case of malignant lesions, the related

tooth should be removed prior to irradiation of the targeted area. Incidence of commonly encountered pathologies associated with the mandibular impacted third molars is as follows: Dentigerous cyst (28%), odontogenic keratocyst (3%), odontoma (0.7%), ameloblastoma (0.5%), carcinoma (0.23%), calcifying odontogenic cyst (0.23%), and myxoma (0.04%).

Trauma

An impacted tooth in the line of fracture should be considered for removal if it is a potential cause for infection. The consideration to retain the tooth may depend on the clinician's decision based on the fact that the tooth may aid in the anatomical reduction of the fracture. For such teeth, future removal may be planned if indicated [18].

Partially or completely erupted third molars causing chronic tissue injury such as chronic check biting and ulceration should be considered for removal.

Prevention of jaw fracture

Impacted molars in the mandible occupy the ramus-angle space that is otherwise filled with bone. This weakens the mandible and renders the jaw more susceptible to fracture at the site of impaction at the mandibular angle region. Athletes playing contact sports should be considered for the prophylactic removal of the third molar to prevent jaw fracture. An impacted third molar presents an area of lowered resistance to fracture in the mandible and is, therefore, a common site for fracture. It increases the risk of angle fracture to almost 2.8-fold [19].

Professional, social and economic factors

Financial factors involved in the prophylactic third molar removal surgery and time constraints for the patient should be considered by the operator for the procedure.

Focal infection theory

Marciani has stated that the systemic or organ health remote from the oral cavity unfavourably affected by dentoalveolar inflammatory conditions o longer can be dismissed as a resurrection of the centuries-old "focal infection" theory.

The consequences of peri-coronal infection related to the mandibular third molars and the connection of the periodontal diseases with the role of oral inflammation in flair-ups at pregnancy, preterm births, kidney disease, and heart disease must be sought as consideration for pre-emptive removal of the "foci of infection" [16].

Consideration for removal should be given for patients planned or treated for head and neck cancers with anticipated "tooth in line for radiation" or post-radiation xerostomia that may affect oral health. Such patients would pose difficulty for extraction procedures due to the reduction in the oral-opening post-surgery and/or radiation.

CONTRAINDICATIONS FOR EXTRACTION FOR MANDIBULAR THIRD MOLARS

Various systemic diseases preventing minor oral surgery and the socio-economic status of the patient may be restraining factors for the removal of the third molar and remain the probable major contraindications. An erupted, symptomless, disease-free third molar or an unerupted, disease-free, symptomless third molar fully covered with hard and soft tissue can be considered for being retained provided the patient can be regularly followed up [20]. Contraindications to anaesthetic medication(s) are also a deterrent to the surgical execution of the third molar removal. Patients on intravenous therapy with antiresorptive agents, i.e., bisphosphonates and denosumab are at a greater risk of medication-related osteonecrosis of the jaw (MRONJ) that leads to surgical insult and bacterial invasion of the bone during surgery. Chemotherapy and ionizing radiation to eradicate malignant cells also interfere with haematopoiesis and host defence mechanism leading to haemorrhage and infection. Patients on these active therapies are contraindications for elective third molar surgery. Another important factor that is against the removal of the third molar is instigating potential damage to the adjacent structures, most commonly the inferior alveolar nerve. Studies have shown that with growing age (more than 30 years of age), the risk of damaging the nerve increases (0.5%–5%) [21]. The root formation for the mandibular third molars is completed by approximate age of 21 years, removal before this age reduces the risk of nerve injury [22]. Radiographic evaluation discloses the proximity of the nerve to the apex of the roots and in cases with close approximation with a high risk of trauma to the nerve, the tooth should be retained or alternative procedures like coronectomy should be given consideration [23].

REFERENCES

1. Durbeck WE. *The Impacted Lower Third Molar.* Great Britain: Dental Items of Interest Publishing Company, 1945.
2. Srinivasan B. *Textbook of Oral Maxillofacial Surgery,* 2nd ed. Elsevier (A Division of Reed Elsevier India Pvt. Limited), 2003. ISBN: 8181470184, 9788181470188.
3. Harry Archer W. *Oral & Maxillofacial Surgery,* Vol. 1, 5th ed. Philadelphia: W.B. Saunders Company. ISBN: 0-7216-1362-4.
4. Dimitroulis G. *Illustrated Lecture Notes in Oral & Maxillofacial Surgery.* Chicago: Quintessence Pub, 2008.
5. Hupp JR, Ellis III E, Tucker MR. *Contemporary Oral and Maxillofacial Surgery,* 7th ed. Philadelphia: Elsevier, 2019, pp. 161–166.
6. Satwik A, Naveed N. Third molar impaction: Review. *Research J Pharm Tech.* 2014;7(12):1498–1500.
7. Bayar GR, Ortakoglu K, Sencimen M. Multiple impacted teeth: Report of 3 cases. *Eur J Dent.* 2008;2(1):73–78.
8. Removal of third molars. Sponsored by the National Institute of Dental Research, November 28–30, 1979. *Natl Inst Health Consens Dev Conf Summ.* 1979;2:65–68.
9. Juodzbalys G, Daugela P. Mandibular third molar impaction: Review of literature and a proposal of a classification. *J Oral Maxillofac Res.* 2013 Jul;4(2):e1. doi: 10.5037/jomr.2013.4201.
10. National Institute for Clinical Excellence. *Guidance on the Extraction of Wisdom Teeth.* Available at: http://www.nice.org.uk/pdf/wisdomteethguidance.pdf. Accessed 3 October 2005.
11. Peltroche-Llacsahuanga H, Reichhart E, Schmitt W, Lütticken R, Haase G. Investigation of infectious organisms causing pericoronitis of the mandibular third molar. *J Oral Maxillofac Surg.* 2000 Jun;58(6):611–616.

12. Marques J, Montserrat-Bosch M, Figueiredo R, Vilchez-Pérez MA, Valmaseda-Castellón E, Gay-Escoda C. Impacted lower third molars and distal caries in the mandibular second molar: Is prophylactic removal of lower third molars justified? *J Clin Exp Dent.* 2017;9(6):e794–e798. doi: 10.4317/jced.53919.

13. Stella P, Falci S, Oliveira de Medeiros LE, Douglas-de-Oliveira DW, Gonçalves PF, Flecha OD, Dos Santos C. Impact of mandibular third molar extraction in the second molar periodontal status: A prospective study. *J Ind Soc Periodontol.* 2017;21(4):285–290.

14. Ye ZX, Qian WH, Wu YB, Yang C. Pathologies associated with the mandibular third molar impaction. *Sci Progr.* 2021;104(2):1–10.

15. Lindauer SJ, Laskin DM, Tüfekçi E, Taylor RS, Cushing BJ, Best AM. Orthodontists' and surgeons' opinions on the role of third molars as a cause of dental crowding. *Am J Orthod Dentofacial Orthop.* 2007;132(1):43–48.

16. Marciani RD. Third molar removal: An overview of indications, imaging, evaluation, and assessment of risk. *Oral Maxillofac Surg Clin North Am.* 2007 Feb;19(1):1–13, doi: 10.1016/j.coms.2006.11.007.

17. Steinbacher DM, Kontaxis KL. Does simultaneous third molar extraction increase intraoperative and perioperative complications in orthognathic surgery? *J Craniofac Surg.* 2016 Jun;27(4): 923–926. doi: 10.1097/SCS.0000000000002648.

18. Balaji P, Balaji SM. Fate of third molar in line of mandibular angle fracture – Retrospective study. *Ind J Dent Res.* 2015 May–Jun;26(3):262–6. doi: 10.4103/0970-9290.162875.

19. Soós B, Janovics K, Tóth Á, Di Nardo MD, Szalma J. Association between third molar impaction status and angle or condylar fractures of the mandible: A retrospective analysis. *J Oral Maxillofac Surg.* 2020 Jul;78(7):1162.e1–1162.e8.

20. Ventä I. Current care guidelines for third molar teeth. *J Oral Maxillofac Surg.* 2015 May;73(5):804–805.

21. Osborn TP, Frederickson G Jr, Small IA, Torgerson TS. A prospective study of complications related to mandibular third molar surgery. *J Oral Maxillofac Surg.* 1985 Oct;43(10):767–769.

22. Bagheri SC, Khan HA. Extraction versus nonextraction management of third molars. *Oral Maxillofac Surg Clin North Am.* 2007 Feb;19(1):15–21.

23. Renton T, Hankins M, Sproate C, McGurk M. A randomised controlled clinical trial to compare the incidence of injury to the inferior alveolar nerve as a result of coronectomy and removal of mandibular third molars. *Br J Oral Maxillofac Surg.* 2005 Feb;43(1):7–12.

5

Classification for impacted mandibular third molars

PUNEET WADHWANI, SAPNA TANDON, DARPAN BHARGAVA,
AND PRAMOD KUMAR GANDRA

INTRODUCTION

In early 1954, Mead defined impacted tooth as "A tooth that is prevented from erupting into position because of malposition, lack of space or impediments" [1]. Later, Peterson defined it as "A tooth that fails to erupt into oral cavity within its expected developmental time period & can no longer reasonably be expected to do so" [2]. Anderson et al. (1997) defined impacted tooth as "Cessation of the eruption of a tooth caused by a clinically or radiographically detectable physical barrier in the eruption path or by an ectopic position of the tooth" [1–4].

According to a study by Passi et al. (2018), prevalence of impacted mandibular third molar is 26.04% and mesioangular impaction (49.2% when compared with other impaction types) is the most common type [2,4]. The reported range of incidence of a tooth to get impacted is from 6.9% to 76.6% [5]. The most common of all teeth to get impacted are third molars, especially in the mandible [6]. They are among the most commonly impacted teeth next to the maxillary canine and mandibular second premolar [7,8].

To aid in and accurately perform the surgery, the spatial positioning and relation of the mandibular third molar with surrounding vital anatomical structures should be assessed. This assessment may be assisted by categorizing the mandibular third molars by classifying them. There are numerous classification systems published in the literature; each classification has its advantages and a few shortcomings. The important classification systems are discussed [9–11].

CLASSIFICATION SYSTEMS FOR IMPACTED MANDIBULAR THIRD MOLAR

The available classification systems for the mandibular third molar can be grouped under two broad categories:

A. Core classification systems mandating competence (are the basis for understanding the various clinical presentations and aid in the surgical execution of the transalveolar extraction)
   1. Winter's classification
   2. Pell and Gregory's system
   3. Rood's criteria
   4. Maglione's system (for cone-beam computed tomographic images)
B. Additional classification systems requiring familiarity
   1. Tetsch and Wagner
   2. Asanami and Kasazaki
   3. Patil S
   4. Yuasa et al.
   5. Juodzbalys and Daug
1. Classification proposed by Winter (1926) [1,2,5] (Figure 5.1)

DOI: 10.1201/9781003324034-5

Based on angulation (the angle formed with the long axis of the adjacent mandibular second molar):

A. Mesioangular
B. Distoangular
C. Bucco-version
D. Linguo-version
E. Vertical
F. Inverted
G. Horizontal

2. Classification proposed by Pell and Gregory (1933) [1,2,5] (Figure 5.2)

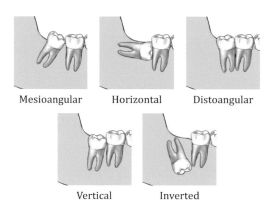

Mesioangular   Horizontal   Distoangular

Vertical   Inverted

Winter's Classification
(Classification based on angulation of tooth)

Figure 5.1 Winter's classification: Based on angulation.

Based on relationship of the occlusal plane of the impacted tooth to that of the second molar

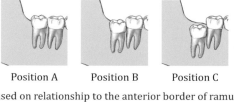

Position A   Position B   Position C

Based on relationship to the anterior border of ramus

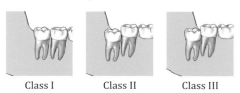

Class I   Class II   Class III

Pell and Gregory Classification

Figure 5.2 Classification as proposed by Pell and Gregory (1933).

Based on depth (assessed by the bone covering the tooth and relation to the adjacent molar):

- **Position A** – the highest cusp of the impacted molar is above the occlusal plane of the second mandibular molar
- **Position B** – the highest cusp of the impacted molar is between the occlusal plane and the cervical line of the second mandibular molar
- **Position C** – the highest cusp of the impacted molar is below the cervical line of the second mandibular molar

Based on the availability of space (assessed by space present between the second mandibular molar and anterior border of the ramus of mandible):

- **Class I** – the mesiodistal width of crown is less than the space available between the distal surface of the second mandibular molar and the anterior border of ramus
- **Class II** – the mesiodistal width of crown is slightly more than the space available between the distal surface of the second mandibular molar and the anterior border of ramus
- **Class III** – the mesiodistal width of crown is more than the space available between the distal surface of the second mandibular molar and the anterior border of ramus

3. Classification based on the tissue covering the third molar [3] (Figure 5.3)

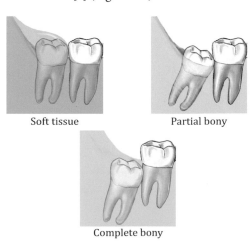

Soft tissue   Partial bony

Complete bony

Based on coverage of tissues

Figure 5.3 Classification based on tissue coverage over the impacted third molar.

a. Soft tissue
b. Partial bony
c. Complete bony impaction
4. Classification proposed by Tetsch and Wagner (1985) [2]

   Based on the form of impaction (assessed by the angle formed between the long axis of impacted tooth and the occlusal plane)
   a. *Vertical impaction* – the impacted tooth is at 90° to the occlusal plane
   b. *Horizontal impaction* – the impacted teeth are aligned parallel at a 0° to the occlusal plane
   c. *Sagittal impaction* –
      – **Mesioangular** – the occlusal surface of impacted teeth is facing the second molar tooth
      – **Distoangular** – the occlusal surface of impacted teeth is facing the anterior border of the ramus of mandible

d. *Cross-impaction* –
   – **Bucco-version** – the occlusal surface of impacted teeth is facing the buccal cortex
   – **Linguoversion** – the occlusal surface of impacted teeth is facing the lingual cortex
e. *Oblique impaction* – the angulation of the impacted teeth to the occlusal plane is between 0° and 90°
   – Mesioangular
   – Distoangular
   – Linguoangular
   – Buccoangular
f. *Displacement impaction* – impacted third molar is displacing the second molar tooth
5. Inferior alveolar canal approximation indicators as proposed by Rood and Shehab (1990) [9] (Figure 5.4)

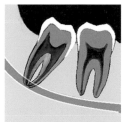
Darkening of root tip

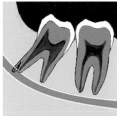
Dark and bifid apex of root

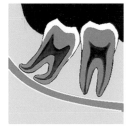
Deflection of the root

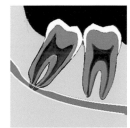
Narrowing of the root

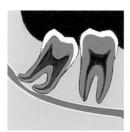
Narrowing of the canal

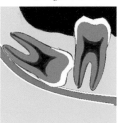
Interruption of the white line of the canal

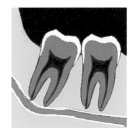
Diversion of canal

Figure 5.4 Classification based on seven radiological diagnostic signs as reviewed from literature and proposed by Rood and Shehab (1990).

Based on the relationship between the third molar and mandibular canal as seen on radiographs

  a. Darkening of root
  b. Dark and bifid apex of root
  c. Narrowing of the canal
  d. Deflection of root
  e. Interruption of the white line of the canal
  f. Narrowing of root
  g. Diversion of canal

6. Classification proposed by Asanami and Kasazaki (1990) [2]

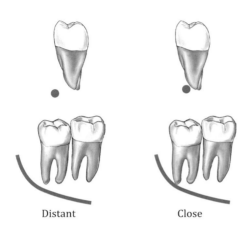

Distant   Close

Based on proximity to the mandibular canal

Figure 5.5 Proximity of the roots to the mandibular canal.

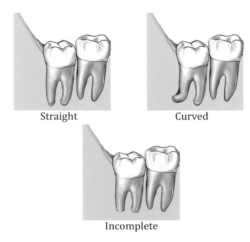

Straight   Curved

Incomplete

Based on root curvature

Figure 5.6 Root curvature of the mandibular third molars.

Based on the degree of impaction – depending on the angulation of tooth in the vertical and horizontal direction.

In the *vertical direction*, it is determined by the degree of impaction as

  a. Minor impaction
  b. Average impaction
  c. Deep impaction

In the *horizontal direction*, it is determined by the degree of inclination of the third molar to the long axis of the second molar tooth as

  a. Vertical position
  b. Distal inclination
  c. Anterior inclination
  d. Horizontal position
  e. Horizontal lingual position
  f. Lingual inclination
  g. Horizontal buccal position
  h. Buccal inclination
  i. Inverted position

7. Classification proposed by Patil (2015) [8]

Based on the association with a pathology

Class I – No associated pathology

Class II – Only clinical signs and symptoms

Class III – Class II plus noninflammatory radiologic changes

Class IV – Class III plus mild inflammatory radiological changes

Class V – Class IV plus severe inflammatory radiological changes (osteomyelitis)

Class VI – Class V plus radiological signs of cysts or benign tumours

Class VII – Class VI plus malignant radiological signs of tumours

8. Classification proposed by Yuasa et al. (2002) [2]

Based on proximity to the mandibular canal (Figure 5.5)

  a. Distant
  b. Close

Based on root curvature (Figure 5.6)

  a. Straight
  b. Curved
  c. Incomplete

Based on the width of root (Figure 5.7)

  a. Thin
  b. Bulbous
  c. Thick/multiple roots
  d. Incomplete

Based on the number of roots (Figure 5.8)

a. Single
b. Multiple
c. Incomplete

Based on periodontal membrane space
(Figure 5.9)

a. Present
b. Partly present
c. Not present

9. Classification proposed by Juodzbalys and Daugela (2013) [8]

Based on anatomical and radiological findings (Table 5.1)

10. Classification proposed by Maglione et al. (2015) [3] (Figures 5.10 and 5.11)

Classification of impacted mandibular third molars based on cone-beam CT (CBCT) images [depending on the relation of tooth to the inferior alveolar canal; IAC]

Class 0 – No relation

Class 1 – the IAC runs apically or buccally

   1A – space between tooth and IAC is more than 2 mm

   1B – space between tooth and IAC is less than 2 mm but not touching the tooth

Class 2 – the IAC runs lingually

   2A – space between tooth and IAC is more than 2 mm

   2B – space between tooth and IAC is less than 2 mm but not touching the tooth

Class 3 – the IAC runs apically or buccally touching the impacted tooth

   3A – IAC is in contact with the tooth with the preserved outline of the IAC

   3B – IAC is in contact with the tooth without the preserved outline of the IAC

Class 4 – the IAC runs lingually touching the impacted tooth

   4A – IAC is in contact with the tooth with the preserved outline of the IAC

   4B – IAC is in contact with the tooth without the preserved outline of the IAC

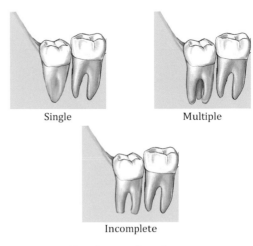

Single   Multiple

Incomplete

Based on number of roots

Figure 5.8 Assessment of the number of the root(s) of the mandibular third molars.

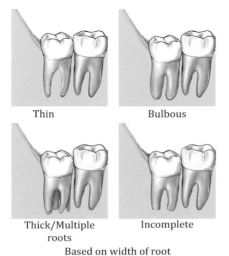

Thin   Bulbous

Thick/Multiple roots   Incomplete

Based on width of root

Figure 5.7 Assessment of the width of the roots of the mandibular third molars.

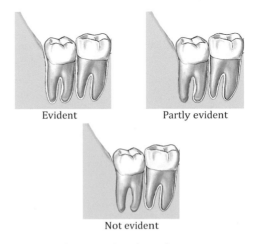

Evident   Partly evident

Not evident

Based on periodontal membrane space

Figure 5.9 Periodontal membrane space with respect to mandibular third molars.

Table 5.1 Classification proposed by Juodzbalys G and Daugela P

Position of mandibular third molar	Risk degree of presumptive intervention (score)			
	Conventional (0)	Simple (1)	Moderate (2)	Complicated (3)
Mesio-distal position in relation to the second molar (M) and the mandibular ramus (R)				
Relation to the second molar (M)	Crown directed at or above the equator of the second molar	Crown directed below the equator to the coronal third of the second molar root	Crown/roots directed to the middle third of the second molar root	Crown/roots directed to the apical third of the second molar root
Relation to the mandibular ramus (R)	Sufficient space in dental arch	Partially impacted in the ramus	Completely impacted in the ramus	Completely impacted in the ramus in a distoangular or horizontal position
Apicocoronal position in relation to the alveolar crest (A) and the mandibular canal (C) [IAN injury risk]				
Relation to the adjacent alveolar crest (from the uppermost point of the tooth) (A)	Tooth is completely erupted	Partially impacted, but the widest part of the crown (equator) is above the bone	Partially impacted, but the widest part of the crown (equator) is below the bone	Completely encased in the bone
Relation to the mandibular canal (from the lowest point of the tooth) (C)	≥3 mm to the mandibular canal	Contacting or penetrating the mandibular canal, wall of the mandibular canal may be identified	Contacting or penetrating the mandibular canal, wall of the mandibular canal is unidentified	Roots surrounding the mandibular canal
Buccolingual position in relation to the mandibular lingual and buccal walls-B (LN injury risk)				
Relation to mandibular lingual and buccal wall (B)	Closer to the buccal wall	In the middle between the lingual and buccal wall	Closer to the lingual wall	Closer to the lingual wall, when the tooth is partially impacted or completely encased in the bone. (A2 or A3.)
Spatial position-S				
Spatial position (S)	Vertical (90°)	Mesioangular ≤60°	Distoangular ≥120°	Horizontal (0°) or inverted (270°)

Note: IAN, inferior alveolar nerve; LN, lingual nerve.

Class 5 – the IAC runs between the roots of the impacted third molar without touching it

  5A – space between the tooth root and IAC is more than 2 mm

  5B – space between the tooth root and IAC is more than 2 mm

Class 6 – the IAC runs between the roots of the impacted third molar touching it

  6A – IAC is in contact with the tooth with the preserved outline of the IAC

  6B – IAC is in contact with the tooth without the preserved outline of the IAC

Class 7 – the IAC is seen between the fused roots of the third molar

Class	Subtype	Scheme of relationship between tooth and Inferior Alveolar Nerve (IAN)
Class 0 The mandibular canal is not visible on the image (plexiform canal)		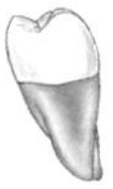
Class 1 The mandibular canal runs apically or buccally with respect to the tooth but without touching it (the cortical limitations of the canal are not interrupted)	1A: IAN–tooth distance is greater than 2 mm	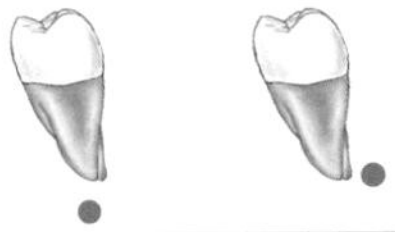
	1A: IAN– tooth distance is less than 2 mm	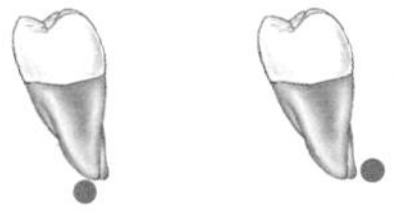
Class 2 The mandibular canal runs lingually with respect to the tooth but without touching it (the cortical limitations of the canal are not interrupted)	2A: IAN–tooth distance is greater than 2 mm	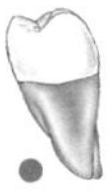
	2A: IAN–tooth distance is less than 2 mm	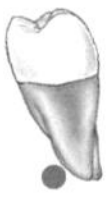
Class 3 The mandibular canal runs apical or buccal to the tooth touching it	3A: In the point of contact the mandibular canal shows a preserved diameter	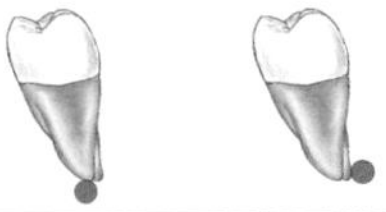
	3B: In the point of contact the mandibular canal shows a smaller calibre and/or an interruption of cortication	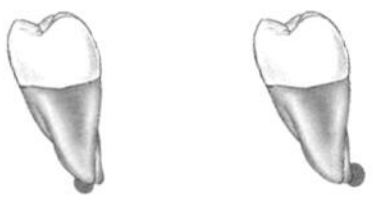
Class 4 The mandibular canal runs lingual to the tooth touching it	4A: In the point of contact the mandibular canal shows a preserved diameter	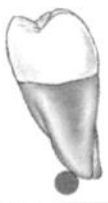
	4B: In the point of contact the mandibular canal shows a smaller calibre and/or an interruption of cortication	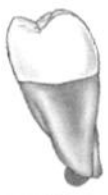

CBCT Radiological classification for the mandibular third molars

Figure 5.10 Classes 0–4. (Adapted from: Maglione M, Costantinides F, Bazzocchi G. Classification of impacted mandibular third molars on cone-beam CT images. *J Clin Exp Dent.* 2015 Apr 1;7(2):e224–e231. doi: 10.4317/jced.51984.)

Class	Subtype	Scheme of relationship between tooth and Inferior Alveolar Nerve (IAN)
Class 5 The mandibular canal runs apically or buccally with respect to the tooth but without touching it (the cortical limitations of the canal are not interrupted)	5A: IAN–tooth distance is greater than 2 mm	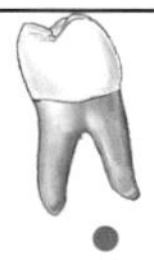
	5A: IAN–tooth distance is less than 2 mm	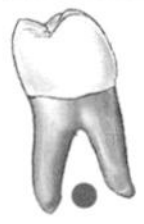
Class 6 The mandibular canal runs lingually with respect to the tooth but without touching it (the cortical limitations of the canal are not interrupted)	6A: In the point of contact the mandibular canal shows a preserved diameter	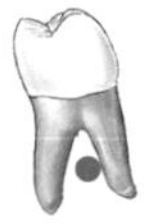
	6B: In the point of contact the mandibular canal shows a smaller calibre and/or an interruption of cortication	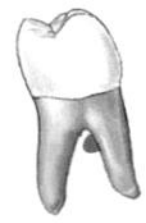
Class 7 The mandibular canal runs apical or buccal to the tooth touching it		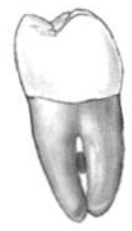

Figure 5.11 Classes 5–7. (Adapted from: Maglione M, Costantinides F, Bazzocchi G. Classification of impacted mandibular third molars on cone-beam CT images. *J Clin Exp Dent*. 2015 Apr 1;7(2):e224–e231. doi: 10.4317/jced.51984.)

Table 5.2 Pederson difficulty index for the surgical removal of mandibular third molars

Spatial relationship (S)

Mesioangular	1
Horizontal/transverse	2
Vertical	3
Distoangular	4

Depth (D)

Level A	1
Level B	2
Level C	3

Ramus relationship/space available (R)

Class 1	1
Class 2	2
Class 3	3

Table 5.3 Difficulty scores utilizing Pederson difficulty index criteria

Difficulty (S + D + R)

Very difficult	7–10
Moderately difficult	5–6
Slightly difficult	3–4

DIFFICULTY INDEX

Prediction and assessment of the surgical difficulty can be evaluated utilizing common and widely accepted indices proposed by McGregor and Pederson.

1. Pederson difficulty index (1988)
   Based on Winter's and Pell & Gregory's classification system (Tables 5.2 and 5.3) [10]
2. WHARFE assessment as proposed by McGregor (1985) (Figure 5.12, Table 5.4) [10]

Table 5.4 Scoring details for the WHARFE assessment (McGregor, 1985)

Category	Score
Winters classification (W)	
Horizontal	2
Distoangular	2
Mesioangular	1
Vertical	0
Height of mandible (H)	
1–30	0
30–34	1
35–39	2
Angulation of second molar (degrees) (A)	
1°–59°	0
60°–69°	1
70°–79°	2
80°–89°	3
90° +	4
Root shape and development (R)	
Less than 1/3rd complete	2
1/3rd–2/3rd complete	1
Complex (more than 2/3rd complete)	3
Unfavourable curvature (more than 2/3rd complete)	2
Favourable curvature (more than 2/3rd complete)	1
Follicle size (F)	
Normal	0
Possibly enlarged	−1
Enlarged	−2
Impaction relieved	−3
Exit path (E)	
Space available	0
Distal cusp covered	1
Mesial cusp covered	2
All covered	3
Total	**33[a]**

[a] More the cumulative score, more would be the difficulty for the surgical extraction. The score indicates the total score that would be captured for an individual case. The maximum score that can be captured is 14

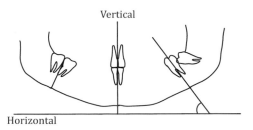

Figure 5.12 Reference lines for radiographic measurements for WHARFE assessment. The height of the mandible is measured from the distal profile of the amelocemental junction of the second molar to the nearest point on the lower border of the mandible. The angle of the second molar is that made by its long axis with long axis with a fiducial horizontal line.

REFERENCES

1. Yilmaz S, Adisen Z, Misirlioglu M, Yorubulut S. Assessment of third molar impaction pattern and associated clinical symptoms in a central anatolian Turkish population. *Med Princ Pract.* 2016;25:169–175. doi: 10.1159/000442416.

2. Jaron A, Trybek G. The pattern of mandibular third molar impaction and assessment of surgery difficulty: A retrospective study of radiographs in east Baltic population. *Int J Environ Res Public Health.* 2021;18:6016.

3. Maglione M, Costantinides F, Bazzocchi G. Classification of impacted mandibular third molars on cone-beam CT images. *J Clin Exp Dent.* 2015;7(2):e224–e231. doi: 10.4317/jced.51984.

4. Divya T, Themozhi MS. Third molar impaction – A review. *J Pharm Sci Res.* 2014;6(11):363–367.

5. Eshghpour M, Nezadi1 A, Moradi Z, Shamsabadi RM, Rezaei NM, Nejat A. Pattern of mandibular third molar impaction: A cross-sectional study in northeast of Iran. *Nigerian J Clin Pract.* 2014;17(6):63–77.

6. Yassaei S, Wlia FO, Nik ZE. Pattern of third molar impaction: Correlation with malocclusion and facial growth. *OHDM.* 2014;13(4):1096–1099.

7. Alfadil L, Almajed E. Prevalence of impacted third molars and the reason for extraction in Saudi Arabias. *Saudi Dent J.* 2020;32:262–268.

8. Juodzbalys G, Daugela P. Mandibular third molar impaction: Review of literature and a proposal of a classification. *J Oral Maxillofac Res.* 2013;4(2):e1. doi: 10.5037/jomr.2013.4201.

9. Yussa H, Kawai T, Sugiura M. Classification of surgical difficulty in extracting impacted third molar. *Br J Oral Maxillofac Surg.* 2002;40:2–31.

10. Latt MM, Chewpreecha P, Wongsirichat N. Prediction of difficulty in impacted lower third molars extraction: Review literature. *Dent J.* 2015;35:281–290.

11. Haddad Z, Khorasani M, Bakhshi M, Tofangchiha M, Shalli Z. Radiographic position of impacted mandibular third molars and their association with pathological conditions. *Int J Dent.* 2021;2021:1–11.

6

Basics of radiology for impacted mandibular third molars

SONAM KHURANA, PRASHANT JAJU, AND DARPAN BHARGAVA

INTRODUCTION

During the evolution of the human race, food habits have changed and preference is towards a softer diet with the availability of processed food. The softer diet has led to less attrition and reduced mesial migration of the teeth leading to the reduced arch space available for third molar eruption along with the effects of the evolution. Other causes for tooth impaction include limited skeletal growth, genetic inheritance, and variation in the third molar calcification pattern.[1] Due to various complications associated with the third molar impaction, thorough treatment planning is necessary. The factors considered for treatment planning include tooth angulation, tooth development, proximity with the adjacent tooth, cortex, inferior alveolar canal, and depth relative to the occlusal plane.[2,3] Different two-dimensional (2D) and three-dimensional (3D) imaging modalities are used for the pretreatment evaluation of impacted teeth. The clinician should use imaging wisely based on the recommendations in the National Commission on Radiation Protection and Measurements (NCRP 177) guidelines.[4] An imaging protocol should be developed that addresses the use of cone-beam computed tomography (CBCT) only for a specific clinical question not managed by the 2D modality. This chapter describes the utility of different imaging modalities to help clinicians in their day-to-day practice for the evaluation of mandibular third molars.

CONVENTIONAL INTRAORAL PERIAPICAL RADIOGRAPH

Conventional periapical radiographs are widely available and remain the preferred modality for screening impacted third molars. It provides an image with the best spatial resolution. However, it is not easy to know the precise anatomical relationship due to the superimposition. Another disadvantage is dimensional distortion due to incorrect horizontal and vertical angulation during acquisition. Intraoral films/sensor placement may induce gagging in some patients with hyperactive pharyngeal reflexes. Some relaxing exercises and topical local anaesthetic agents are helpful in such cases.[5]

TUBE SHIFT INTRAORAL RADIOGRAPHIC TECHNIQUE

The technique is based upon Clark's rule, which states that the radiographic position of two objects changes when the acquisition projection angle of the image changes. The acronym SLOB used for tube shift techniques is "Same Lingual Opposite Buccal". The tube shift technique works well with both horizontal and vertical angulation change. Horizontal angulation can help to locate the buccolingual position of the impacted third molar. In contrast, vertical angulation can help to find the buccolingual position of the inferior alveolar canal in relation to the third molar.

DOI: 10.1201/9781003324034-6

For example, for horizontal angulation change, the impacted third molar is superimposed over the distal root of the second molar on the first radiograph. Another radiograph is acquired from mesial beam angulation, and the tooth moves distally; indicating that the tooth is localized buccally.[5]

For vertical angulation change, directing the beam 20° upward projects the image of the buccal object above that of the lingual object. For example, if the upward angulation causes the image of the mesio-buccal root apex to appear above the mesio-lingual root, it suggests that the mandibular canal lies to the lingual side of the tooth root. If the inferior border of the mandibular canal appears above the apexes of all the roots, the mandibular canal lies to the buccal side of the root apices. Suppose the inferior border of the mandibular canal lies above the apices of the mesio-lingual and distal roots. In that case, it suggests that the canal lies to the buccal side of the apexes of the mesio-lingual and distal roots. In addition, dilacerated roots or multiple curved roots can be better observed because of the improved capacity for interpretation.[6]

PANORAMIC RADIOGRAPHS

Panoramic radiograph or orthopantomograms (OPG) has the advantage of complete demonstration of the dentition. A panoramic radiograph helps in the overall assessment of the third molar. Panoramic radiograph gives a broader overview of the orientation, root morphology, relation with inferior alveolar canal, effect on adjacent teeth, and any associated pathology (Figure 6.1).

However, due to the two dimensionalities in some cases, it is essential to supplement with CBCT for better pretreatment evaluation.[7]

Rood and Shaeb,[8] in their literature review gathered seven radiographic associations between lower third molars and the inferior alveolar canal based on the findings on periapical (IOPAR) and OPG, described under:

Four signs noted on the root are:

1. ***Darkening of the root***: Due to the impingement of the inferior alveolar canal over the root surface.
2. ***Deflected roots***: Due to abrupt root deviation on buccal/lingual or mesial/distal sides when the root reaches the canal.
3. ***Narrowing of root***: Due to the involvement of the greatest diameter of the root by the canal, it appears as deep grooving or perforation of the root.
4. ***Dark or bifid root***: Due to crossing the canal at the apex, identified by the double periodontal ligament space of the bifid apex.

Three signs noted on the canal are:

1. ***Interruption of the white line(s)***: The white lines are referred to as superior and inferior cortices of the canal. The interruption of one or both lines is considered a "danger sign" depicting a direct relationship between the root and inferior alveolar canal. If the interruption is associated with the narrowing of the canal, it could be due to root perforation.

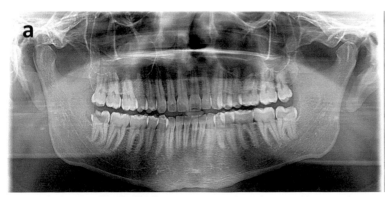
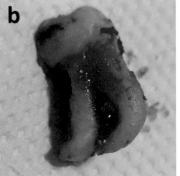

Figure 6.1 Panoramic radiograph, demonstrating dilacerated roots of tooth #48 (a). Elevation in toto was feasible due to the disto-coronal bone loss as a result of recurrent pericoronitis. Note the bulbous and dilacerated roots (b).

(a)

Class	Subtype	Scheme of relationship between tooth and Inferior Alveolar Nerve (IAN)
Class 0 The mandibular canal is not visible on the image (plexiform canal)		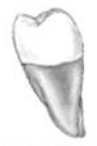
Class 1 The mandibular canal runs apically or buccally with respect to the tooth but without touching it (the cortical limitations of the canal are not interrupted)	1A: IAN–tooth distance is greater than 2 mm	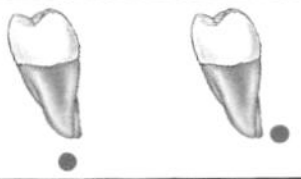
	1A: IAN–tooth distance is less than 2 mm	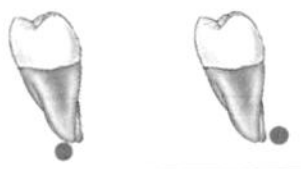
Class 2 The mandibular canal runs lingually with respect to the tooth but without touching it (the cortical limitations of the canal are not interrupted)	2A: IAN–tooth distance is greater than 2 mm	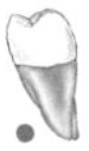
	2A: IAN–tooth distance is less than 2 mm	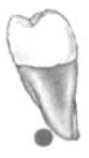
Class 3 The mandibular canal runs apical or buccal to the tooth touching it	3A: In the point of contact the mandibular canal shows a preserved diameter	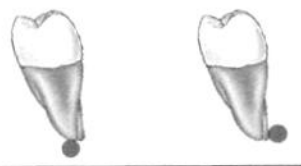
	3B: In the point of contact the mandibular canal shows a smaller caliber and/or a interruption of cortication	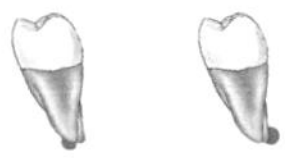
Class 4 The mandibular canal runs lingual to the tooth touching it	4A: In the point of contact the mandibular canal shows a preserved diameter	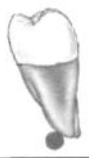
	4B: In the point of contact the mandibular canal shows a smaller calibre and/or an interruption of cortication	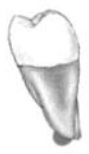

CBCT Radiological classification for the mandibular third molars

(b)

Class	Subtype	Scheme of relationship between tooth and Inferior Alveolar Nerve (IAN)
Class 5 The mandibular canal runs apically or buccally with respect to the tooth but without touching it (the cortical limitations of the canal are not interrupted)	5A: IAN–tooth distance is greater than 2 mm	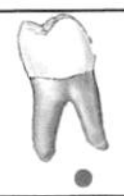
	5A: IAN–tooth distance is less than 2 mm	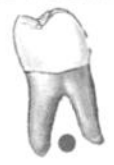
Class 6 The mandibular canal runs lingually with respect to the tooth but without touching it (the cortical limitations of the canal are not interrupted)	6A: In the point of contact the mandibular canal shows a preserved diameter	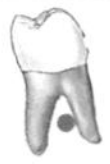
	6B: In the point of contact the mandibular canal shows a smaller calibre and/or an interruption of cortication	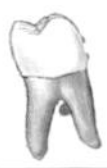
Class 7 The mandibular canal runs apical or buccal to the tooth touching it		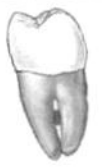

Figure 6.2 CBCT radiological classification for mandibular third molars schematically demonstrating the section of a right third molar and its relationship with the mandibular canal in a buccolingual section for each classification types and subtypes. (a) Class 0–4. (b) Class 5–7.

2. ***Diversion of the inferior alveolar canal***: Due to the displacement of the canal when it crosses the tooth.

3. ***Narrowing of the inferior alveolar canal***: Due to a reduction in the canal diameter when it crosses the tooth. It could be due to inferior displacement of the upper border of the canal or due to displacement of both superior and inferior borders, indicating partial or complete encirclement of the canal around the root.[6]

2D images obtained from intraoral radiographs and panoramic radiographs do not provide information on the depth of the anatomical structures studied. On 2D imaging, if the suspicion for tooth-root canal close approximation is detected, a three-dimensional imaging modality may be ordered to aid in documentation, patient counselling, surgical planning, and procedure execution.

CONE-BEAM COMPUTED TOMOGRAPHY

CBCT is the advanced maxillofacial imaging modality that can assess all three anatomical planes – axial, coronal, and sagittal. Compared with the multislice CT (MDCT), CBCT provide acceptable spatial resolution using a smaller voxel size at a lower radiation dose. CBCT should always be used as an adjunct rather than a replacement of 2D imaging.[4]

CBCT precisely assesses the anatomy, position and pathology associated with the third molar. CBCT can aid in detecting the absence of cortication of the mandibular canal that is in contact with the tooth root, which is a risk indicator for IAN injury during third molar surgery.[4] Classification of impacted mandibular third molars based on CBCT has been proposed by Maglione et al.[9] (Figure 6.2a and b)

Examples of cone-beam computed tomographic scans for the evaluation of the impacted mandibular third molars are demonstrated in Figures 6.3–6.5.

MAGNETIC RESONANCE IMAGING

Magnetic resonance imaging has superior soft tissue contrast and allows the assessment of intracanal neurovascular tissue and its proximity to the third molars. Although MRI does not use ionizing radiation, its use for routine third molar evaluation is limited owing to the high cost.[10]

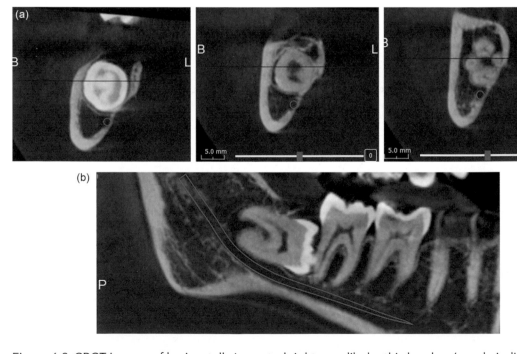

Figure 6.3 CBCT images of horizontally impacted right mandibular third molars (purple indicator denotes inferior alveolar canal). (a) Sagittal view. (b) Cross-sectional images at coronal, middle third, and apical third levels. Note the canal approximation.

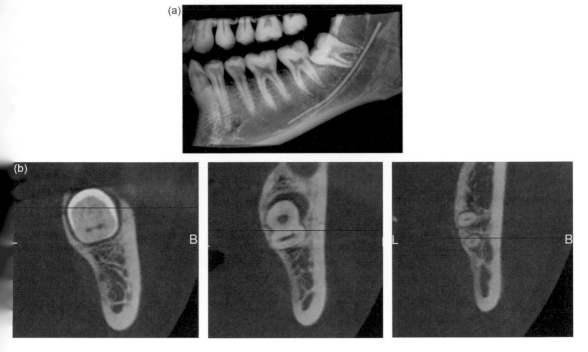

Figure 6.4 CBCT imaging of a mesioangular impacted left mandibular third molar on CBCT (Purple indicator denotes inferior alveolar canal). (a) Maximum intensity projection (MIP) image of the impacted mandibular third molar. (b) Cross-sectional images at coronal, middle, and apical third levels.

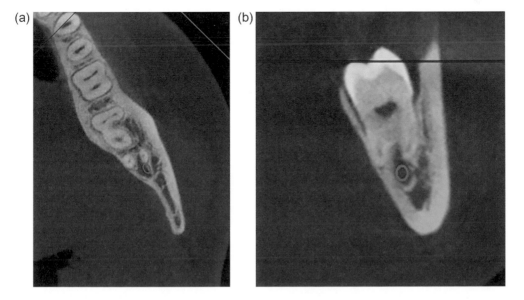

Figure 6.5 (a) CBCT axial image demonstrating the mandibular canal passing through the bifurcation region. (b) CBCT coronal image showing the mandibular canal passing through the bifurcation region.

CONCLUSION

CBCT is an excellent diagnostic method for selected situations in oral and maxillofacial surgery, including the evaluation of mandibular third molars. Intraoral periapical or panoramic radiography may be sufficient in most cases for planning and removal of mandibular third molars; CBCT may be indicated when one or more signs of close contact between the tooth/root and the mandibular canal is detected.

REFERENCES

1. Hattab FN, Alhaija ESJA. Radiographic evaluation of mandibular third molar eruption space. *Oral Surg Oral Med Oral Pathol Oral Radiol Endod*. 1999;88:285–91. doi: 10.1016/S1079-2104(99)70029-6.

2. Peterson LJ, Ellis III E, Hupp JR, Tuker MR. Principles of management of impacted teeth. In *Contemporary Oral and Maxillofacial Surgery*, 3rd ed. St. Louis, MO: Elsevier, 1998.

3. Öhman A, Kivijärvi K, Blombäck U, Flygare L. Preoperative radiographic evaluation of lower third molars with computed tomography. *Dentomaxillofac Radiol*. 2006;35:30–5.

4. *NCRP Report No. 177: Radiation Protection in Dentistry and Oral and Maxillofacial Imaging*. Bethesda: National Council on Radiation Protection and Measurement, 2019. Available at: https://ncrponline.org/shop/reports/report-no–177.

5. Mallya SM, Lam EWN. *White and Pharoah's Oral Radiology: Principles and Interpretation*, 8th ed. St. Louis, MO: Elsevier, 2019.

6. Richards AG. Roentgenographic localization of the mandibular canal. *J Oral Surg (Chic)*. 1952 Oct;10(4):325–9.

7. Tassoker M. Diversion of the mandibular canal: Is it the best predictor of inferior alveolar nerve damage during mandibular third molar surgery on panoramic radiographs? *Imaging Sci Dent*. 2019;49:213–8. doi: 10.5624/isd.2019.49.3.213.

8. Rood JP, Shehab BA. The radiological prediction of inferior alveolar nerve injury during third molar surgery. *Br J Oral Maxillofac Surg*. 1990;28:20–5.

9. Maglione M, Costantinides F, Bazzocchi G. Classification of impacted mandibular third molars on cone-beam CT images. *J Clin Exp Dent*. 2015 Apr;7(2):e224–31. doi: 10.4317/jced.51984.

10. Al-Haj Husain A, Stadlinger B, Winklhofer S, Müller M, Piccirelli M, Valdec S. Mandibular third molar surgery: Intraosseous localization of the inferior alveolar nerve using 3D double-echo steady-state MRI (3D-DESS). *Diagnostics (Basel)*. 2021 Jul;11(7):1245. doi: 10.3390/diagnostics11071245.

7

Clinical and radiographic assessment for impacted mandibular third molars

DARPAN BHARGAVA

Text is based on the principles and teachings from:

1. **Geoffrey L. Howe**: Minor Oral Surgery; Wright, 1966
2. **A. J. MacGregor**: The Impacted Lower Wisdom Tooth; Oxford University Press, 1985

CLINICAL ASSESSMENT

Thorough clinical and radiological evaluation remains a vital aspect of the treatment planning for the mandibular third molar surgery. Age (increase in difficulty for extraction with age) and sex (incidence of increase of sclerotic bone in males with age/consider the incidence of post-menopausal osteoporosis in females) of the patient with a thorough case history including the detailed systemic and local evaluation should be recorded. (Refer case history format for transalveolar mandibular third molar surgery in Chapter 17.) Patients with smaller mouth (microstomia) would pose more difficulty for the procedure due to the difficult access intra-orally in the third molar region. Patients with larger mouth opening will be easier candidates. During the clinical examination, it is of importance that the operator palpates the external oblique ridge and assesses its relation to the mandibular third molar, where feasible. When the ridge is situated behind the tooth, access is good whereas if the ridge is alongside or in front of the third molar access is poor with the anticipated increase in difficulty during extraction. In case of completely or partially erupted third molars, note the condition of the pericoronal tissues and evidence of caries.

In general, commonly enlisted patient factors predicting increased difficulty of mandibular third molar removal include: obesity, dense bone, large tongue, dilacerated roots, strong gag reflex, unfavourable position of the inferior alveolar canal, advanced age, fractious patient, apical root of lower third molar in cortical bone, uneven anaesthetic, atrophic mandible and factors contributing to limited surgical access (e.g., microstomia, large tongue in an obese patient with a distoangular impaction, etc.) [1–3].

RADIOGRAPHIC ASSESSMENT

The radiographs of choice include:

1. Intra-oral periapical radiograph (IOPAR)
2. Orthopantomogram/panoramic radiograph (OPG)
3. Cone-beam computed tomography (CBCT)

    Where these specialized radiographic techniques are not available, a lateral oblique view of the mandible (which can be taken using general radiology setup on an X-ray film used for extra-oral facial radiographs) may be utilized with due limitations of this technique.

Intra-oral periapical radiographs for assessment of mandibular third molars

PATIENT POSITIONING FOR THE RADIOGRAPH

Patient should be seated in such a way that the occlusal plane of the mandibular teeth is horizontal and remains parallel to the floor with his mouth open. The upper portion of the IOPAR film should be held using a film holder or a straight haemostat and should be inserted on the lingual side of the mandibular teeth with its anterior edge in line with the medial surface of the first molar. The X-ray tube should be positioned in such a way so that the central ray remains parallel to the occlusal surface of the second molar and is directed towards the distal cusp of the second molar, passing at the right angles to the film. In a correctly taken IOPAR, the lingual and the buccal cusps of the second mandibular molar tooth should appear superimposed on each other in the vertical and horizontal planes. An ideal IOPAR should demonstrate the typical "enamel cap appearance" of the second molar and the absence of interproximal (contact point) overlap of the teeth (Figures 7.1 and 7.2).

INTERPRETATION OF THE IOPAR FOR MANDIBULAR THIRD MOLAR SURGERY [1,2] (TABLE 7.1)

1. ***Access:*** Difficulty of the access to the surgical site may be assessed by evaluating the radiopaque line casted by the external oblique ridge, if the line remains vertical, anticipated access would be poor whereas if the line is horizontal, access would be good for the surgery (Figure 7.3).

2. ***Position and depth:*** Position and depth of the impacted mandibular third molar may be described based on the imaginary descriptive lines described by George Winter. The lines are commonly referred to as "WAR" lines. For better understanding, the lines are denoted with distinctive colours; W: White, A: Amber, R: Red and hence are termed *Winter's WAR lines* (Figure 7.4).

   Based on the assessment of the long axis of the impacted tooth, the tooth may be considered as horizontal, vertical, mesioangular (medially inclined) or distoangular (distally inclined). It should be noted that, considering the path of exit of the tooth, theoretically, the application of the elevator is on the mesial

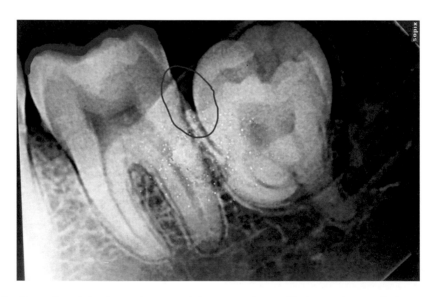

Figure 7.1 The lingual and the buccal cusps of the second mandibular molar tooth demonstrate reasonable superimposition on each other in the vertical and horizontal planes. An ideal IOPAR should demonstrate typical "enamel cap appearance". Note that there is no interproximal superimposition between the second and third molar tooth.

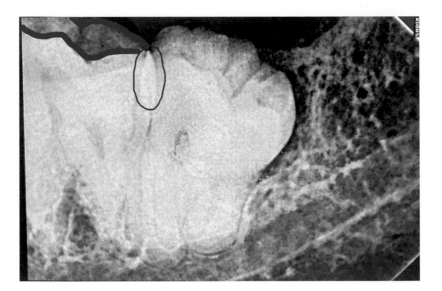

Figure 7.2 Note the lingual and the buccal cusps of the second mandibular molar tooth, without superimposition. The interproximal (contact point) overlap of the teeth is also present.

Table 7.1 Considerations for evaluating and interpretation of the intra-oral periapical radiograph (IOPAR) for mandibular third molar surgery

1	Access
2	Position and depth
3	Root pattern of an impacted mandibular third molar
4	Crown shape
5	Texture of the investing bone
6	Root pattern and position of the second molar
7	Localization and identification of the inferior alveolar canal

aspect of the tooth (at the cementoenamel junction) *except* in cases of distoangular impactions where the application of the elevator is expected to be on the distal aspect of the impacted tooth.

White line: A line is drawn along the occlusal surfaces of the erupted mandibular molars and extended posteriorly over the third molar region. The relationship of the occlusal surface of the impacted tooth to those of the erupted molars may be estimated in reference to the white line

Amber line: It is drawn from the surface of the bone lying distal to the mandibular third molar, to the crest of the interdental septum (inter-radicular crestal bone) between the first and second molars. The Amber line indicates the amount of the alveolar bone enclosing the tooth. When the soft tissues are reflected only the portion of the tooth shown on the film to be lying above and in front of the amber line will be visible the remaining tooth will be enclosed within the bone.

Red line: The red line is used to assess the depth at which the impacted tooth lies within the mandible. It is a perpendicular drawn from the "amber" line to an imaginary point of application for an elevator which is usually the cementoenamel junction (CEJ) on the mesial surface of the impacted tooth, except in cases of a distoangular impaction where the point of application for an elevator is distal to the impacted tooth. If the length of the red line is more than 5 mm, anticipate

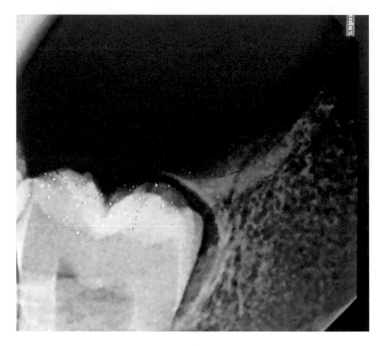

Figure 7.3 Note the position of the external oblique ridge in relation to the impacted mandibular third molar.

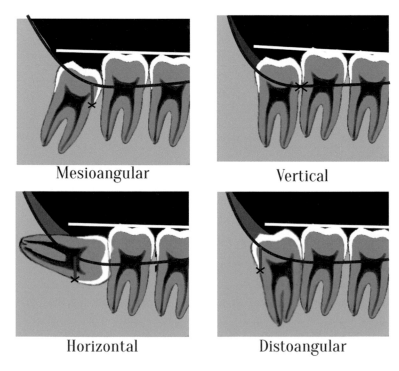

Mesioangular

Vertical

Horizontal

Distoangular

WAR lines indicating degree of difficulty of removal

Figure 7.4 Winter's WAR lines (Winter, 1926).

difficult extraction. For every additional 1 mm beyond 5 mm, the difficulty becomes three times (3×)

Clinical tips:

a. When a vertical impaction is present the anterio-posterior width of the coronal end of the interdental septum (inter-radicular bone) between the 2nd and 3rd molar is similar to that of the septum (inter-radicular bone) between the 1st and 2nd molars. In cases with distoangular impaction, the coronal end of the inter-radicular septum between the second and third molar teeth is much narrower than in between the first and second molar teeth.

b. To distinguish vertical impactions from distoangular impactions, the occlusal surface of the impacted tooth is compared to the white line. The occlusal surface of the vertically impacted tooth is parallel to the white line and that of a distoangular impaction, the occlusion surface of the tooth and the white line are seen to converge as if to meet in front of the impacted third molar tooth.

3. **Root pattern of an impacted mandibular third molar:** The root pattern of the impacted mandibular third molars should be scrutinized meticulously on a radiograph. The possibility of hypercementosis/bulbous roots or conflicting lines of withdrawal (including the dilacerated roots) may indicate the need for tooth sectioning. Root pattern is a dictator for the clinical decision for deciding the "line of withdrawal" or "the path of exit" and the appropriate "point of application" of the elevator (Figure 7.5).

4. **Crown shape:** The shape of the crown is relatively a lesser contributor to the difficulty in the removal of the impacted tooth. Usually, teeth with large square crowns and prominent cusps are more difficult to remove than teeth with small conical crowns and flat cusps. The crown and the cusp shape are particularly significant and should be assessed accurately when the line of withdrawal of the third molar is completely obstructed by the presence of a part of the second molar tooth. The cusp(s) of the third molar may be seen superimposed on to the distal surface of the second molar in a standard radiograph (Figure 7.6). In such situations, the application of force on the mesial surface of the impacted tooth may damage the supporting structures of the second molar, or the second

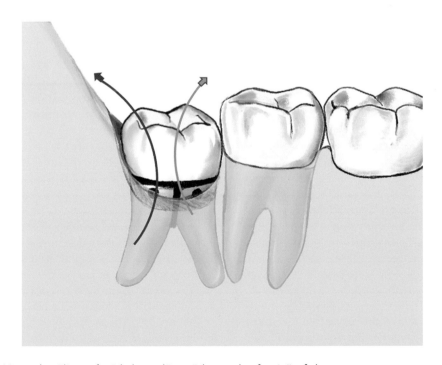

Figure 7.5 Note the "line of withdrawal" or "the path of exit" of the roots.

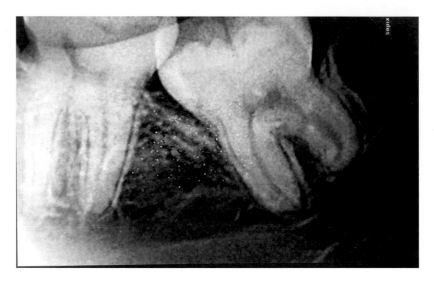

Figure 7.6 The cusp of the third molar superimposed onto the distal surface of the second molar.

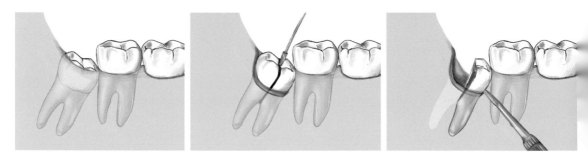

Figure 7.7 The application of force on the mesial surface of the impacted tooth may damage the supporting structures of the second molar or the second molar itself. To avoid complications, the crown of the impacted tooth should be sectioned before removal.

molar itself. To avoid complications, the crown of the impacted tooth should be sectioned before removal (Figure 7.7). At rare instances, the impacted tooth itself would have caused damage to the periodontal support of the second molar or in extreme cases the root of the second molar, which will warrant periodontal and/or endodontic intervention to salvage the second molar tooth. (Refer Chapter 11.)

5. **_Texture of the investing bone_**: The texture of the investing bone varies among individuals and also with age. In general, the bone has a tendency to become more sclerosed and less elastic with advancing age. The texture of the bone can be determined using routine standard radiographs, only if strict standardization protocols of exposure and developing techniques are practiced, which at most instances is not practical. In general, the texture of the investing bone may be grossly assessed by noting the size of the cancellous spaces and the density of bone structure enclosing them in a standard intra-oral periapical radiographic image. If the spaces are too large and the bone structure is fine then the bone is typically elastic, whereas if the spaces are small and bone shadows are dense, the bone should be anticipated to be sclerotic.

6. **_Root pattern and position of the second molar_**: Root pattern and position of the second molar are contributors to the anticipated difficulty for the extraction of the third molar. The "distal tilt" of the long axis of the second molar may contribute towards enhanced difficulty (Figure 7.8). The second molars with conical roots are at a risk of dislodgment during elevator application on the mesial aspect of the impacted tooth.

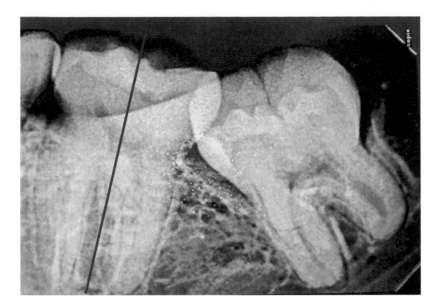

Figure 7.8 "Distal tilt" of the long axis of the second molar.

7. ***Localization and identification of the inferior alveolar canal:*** Inferior dental canal can be identified in relation to the roots of the mandibular third molar on imaging utilizing standard radiographs. The condensed bone forming the roof and floor of the canal is represented by two parallel lines of radio opacity. Overlap or interruption of continuity of one or both the lines may be noted as they cross the tooth root. Overlap of roots with the canal at most instances appears due to the radiographic superimposition (Figure 7.9) nonetheless on occasions a grooving or perforation of the root of the mandibular third molar may be present (Figure 7.10). Grooves indented by the inferior alveolar canal are usually situated on the lingual surface of the roots. Rood and Shehab (1990), evaluated radiological diagnostic signs based on the periapical views and orthopantomogram as predictors of likely injury to inferior alveolar nerve. They reviewed literature to identify seven signs indicative of a close relationship between the mandibular third molar tooth and the inferior alveolar canal. Four of these signs are seen on the root of the tooth and the other three are changes in the appearance of the inferior alveolar canal. The positional relationship between the root of the mandibular third molar and the inferior alveolar nerve may produce the following noted radiographic signs: Darkening of the root(s), deflected roots, narrowing of the root, dark and bifid root (Figure 7.11), interruption of the white line(s), diversion of the inferior alveolar canal, narrowing of the inferior alveolar canal. As reported by Rood and Shehab, the most significant sign related to nerve injury was the diversion of the inferior alveolar

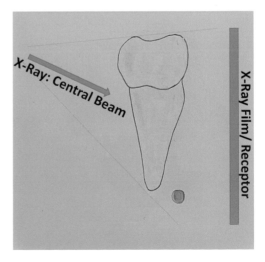

Figure 7.9 Overlap of roots with the canal in most instances appears due to the radiographic superimposition. Note the direction and tilt of the central X-ray beam at the time of exposure that results in root and canal superimposition.

(a) (b) (c)

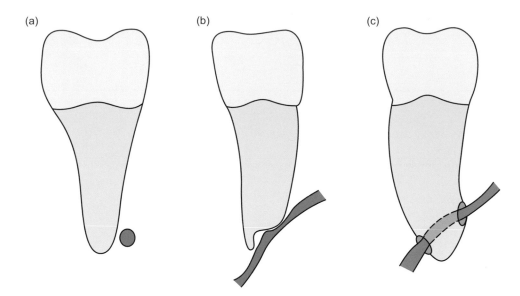

Figure 7.10 At occasions a grooving or perforation of the root of the mandibular third molar may be present. (a) Canal approximation. (b) Root indentation or grooving. (c) Perforation of the root.

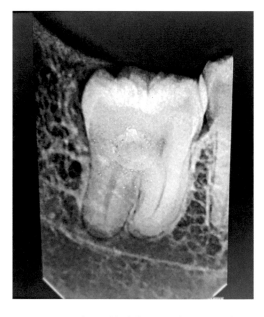

Figure 7.11 Dark and bifid (mesial) root with interruption of the superior white line.

canal followed by darkening of the root and interruption of the white line (Figure 7.12). In cases with sign(s) related to nerve injury on preliminary screening radiograph, a more definitive assessment utilizing the cone-beam computed tomography may be indicated [4]. Inferior alveolar nerve injury is a potential complication associated with the removal of the third molar which can lead to lower labial sensory impairment. The incidence of injury to the inferior alveolar nerve as reported by various studies is variable, 0.26%–8.4% [5].

SUMMARY OF DIFFICULTY ASSESSMENT INDICES

WAR lines/Winter's lines (Figure 7.4, Table 7.2)

A method of assessing the angulation and extent of impaction of mandibular third molars was first described by Winter (1926).

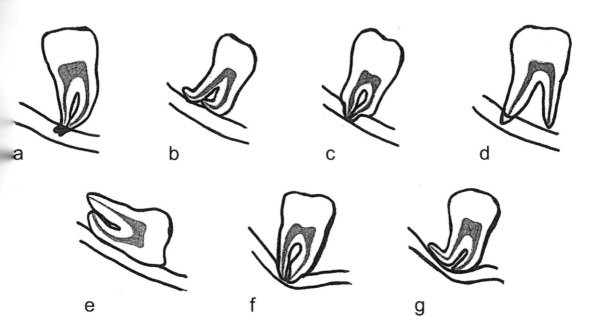

Figure 7.12 Radiographic classification of the relationship between mandibular third molar roots and inferior alveolar nerve (IAN) canal, Rood and Shehab (1990): (a) Root darkening. (b) Root deflection. (c) Root narrowing. (d) Dark and bifid root apex. (e) Interruption of IAN canal white line. (f) IAN canal diversion. (g) IAN canal narrowing. (Modified from: Rood JP, Shehab BA. The radiological prediction of inferior alveolar nerve injury during third molar surgery. *Br J Oral Maxillofac Surg.* 1990;28(1):20–5.)

Table 7.2 WAR lines (Winter, 1926)

White line	It is drawn along the occlusal surfaces of the mandibular molars and extended posteriorly over the third molar region.
	This line is used to assess the axial inclination of the impacted tooth.
Amber line	This line is drawn from the surface of the bone lying distally to the third molar to the crest of the interdental septum between the first and second mandibular molars.
	It indicates the amount of alveolar bone enclosing the impacted tooth.
Red line	The third or "red" line is used to measure the depth at which the impacted tooth lies within the mandible.
	It is a perpendicular drawn from the "amber" line to an imaginary point of application for an elevator which is usually the cementoenamel (CE) junction on the mesial surface of the impacted tooth. (Distal for distoangular.)
	If the length of the red line is more than 5 mm, anticipate difficult extraction. For every additional 1 mm beyond 5 mm, difficulty becomes 3×.

Pell and Gregory class and position assessment (1933) (Figure 7.13, Table 7.3)

WHARFE assessment by McGregor (1985) (Figure 7.14, Table 7.4)

Based on relationship of the occlusal plane of the impacted tooth to that of the second molar

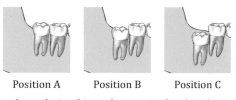

Position A   Position B   Position C

Based on relationship to the anterior border of ramus

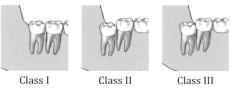

Class I   Class II   Class III

Pell and Gregory Classification

Figure 7.13 Pell and Gregory class and position assessment. (Best utilize the panoramic radiograph for this assessment, to visualize the anterior ramus.)

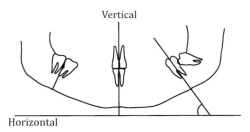

Figure 7.14 Reference lines for radiographic measurements for WHARFE assessment. The height of the mandible is measured from the distal profile of the amelocemental junction of the 2nd molar to the nearest point on the lower border of the mandible. The angle of the 2nd molar is that made by its long axis with long axis with a fiducial horizontal line. (Utilize the panoramic radiograph for this assessment.)

Table 7.3 Pell and Gregory's classification system (1933)

Relationship of impacted mandibular third molar to ramus of mandible and second molar

Class I	Sufficient amount of space available between the anterior border of ascending ramus and the distal surface of the second molar for the accommodation of the third molar
Class II	The space available between the anterior border of ramus and the distal side of the second molar is less than the mesio-distal width of the crown of the third molar
Class III	The third molar is totally embedded in the bone from the ascending ramus because of absolute lack of space

According to depth

Position A	The highest portion of the tooth is on a level with or above the occlusal plane
Position B	The highest position is below the occlusal plane, but above the cervical level of the second molar
Position C	The highest position is below the cervical line of the second molar

Table 7.4 WHARFE surgical difficulty assessment for mandibular third molars (McGregor, 1985)

Category	Score
Winters classification (W)	
Horizontal	2
Distoangular	2
Mesioangular	1
Vertical	0
Height of mandible (H)	
1–30	0
30–34	1
35–39	2
Angulation of second molar (degrees) (A)	
1°–59°	0
60°–69°	1
70°–79°	2
80°–89°	3
90° +	4
Root shape and development (R)	
Less than 1/3rd complete	2
1/3rd–2/3rd complete	1
Complex (more than 2/3rd complete)	3
Unfavourable curvature (more than 2/3rd complete)	2
Favourable curvature (more than 2/3rd complete)	1
Follicle size (F)	
Normal	0
Possibly enlarged	−1
Enlarged	−2
Impaction relieved	−3
Exit path (E)	
Space available	0
Distal cusp covered	1
Mesial cusp covered	2
All covered	3
Total	**33[a]**

[a] More the cumulative score, more would be the difficulty for the surgical extraction. The score indicates the total score that would be captured for an individual case. The maximum score that can be captured is 14

Pederson's difficulty index (Table 7.5)

Table 7.5 Pederson's surgical difficulty index for mandibular third molars (Pederson, 1988)

Classification	Difficulty index
Angulation (A)	
Mesioangular	1
Horizontal/transverse	2
Vertical	3
Distoangular	4
Depth (D)	
Level A	1
Level B	2
Level C	3
Ramus relationship (R)	
Class I	1
Class II	2
Class III	3
Difficulty level (score) (A+D+R)	
Very difficult	7–10
Moderately difficult	5–7
Minimally difficult	3–4

REFERENCES

1. Howe GL. *Minor Oral Surgery*. England: Wright, 1966.
2. MacGregor AJ. *The Impacted Lower Wisdom Tooth*. Oxfordshire: Oxford University Press, 1985.
3. Marciani RD. Third molar removal: An overview of indications, imaging, evaluation, and assessment of risk. *Oral Maxillofac Surg Clin North Am*. 2007 Feb;19(1):1–13. doi: 10.1016/j.coms.2006.11.007.
4. Rood JP, Shehab BA. The radiological prediction of inferior alveolar nerve injury during third molar surgery. *Br J Oral Maxillofac Surg*. 1990 Feb;28(1):20–5. doi: 10.1016/0266-4356(90)90005-6.
5. Kim HJ, Jo YJ, Choi JS, Kim HJ, Kim J, Moon SY. Anatomical risk factors of inferior alveolar nerve injury association with surgical extraction of mandibular third molar in Korean population. *Appl Sci*. 2021;11:816. doi: 10.3390/app11020816.

8

Armamentarium for transalveolar extraction of third molars

ELAVENIL PANNEERSELVAM, SASIKALA BALASUBRAMANIAM, AND ARUN VIGNESH

INTRODUCTION

Armamentarium plays a very important role in determining the surgical outcome of the mandibular third molar surgery. The appropriate choice of instruments and proper instrumentation ensure the safe and efficient execution of surgical procedures. Effective application of instruments improves the surgeon's comfort of working as well as reduces intraoperative time. This chapter deals with the various instruments used in performing a third molar surgery, their classification, indications for usage and principles of instrumentation. A short note on the preoperative preparation of instruments and their sterilization has also been provided.

CLASSIFICATION OF INSTRUMENTS

The instruments may be classified based on many factors as mentioned below:

Re-usability of instruments

Surgical equipment may be categorized into two major types based on re-usability as disposable and non-disposable instruments. Most of the instruments are metallic and autoclavable. Hence, they may be used multiple times. Examples of disposable instruments include suction tips, disposable scalpel, syringes and suture materials with needle.

Materials used for manufacturing

The instruments are classified based on the material used as

1. Stainless steel instruments
2. Tungsten carbide instruments
3. Plastic instruments

Stainless steel instruments are the most popular because of the ease of handling and lesser cost involved. Tungsten carbide instruments are harder and have substantial corrosion resistance. They demonstrate good working efficiency and durability. They usually can be identified by a golden handle and are relatively expensive.

Types of tissues to be handled

The tissues handled also dictate the category of instruments namely

1. Soft tissue instruments
2. Hard tissue instruments

Area of instrumentation

Some instruments are exclusive to individual arches in which they are used and may be named as

1. Maxillary instruments
2. Mandibular instruments

DOI: 10.1201/9781003324034-8

Based on the instruments required for each surgical step

The classification of instruments[1]

i. Instruments for diagnosis
Mouth mirror, Straight probe, Explorer, Tweezers/Pliers

ii. Instruments for isolation and preparation of surgical site
Swab Holder/Rampley's Sponge Holder, Towel Clip

iii. Instruments used to maintain mouth opening
Mouth Prop/Bite Blocks (rubber or metal), Heister jaw stretcher, Fergusson's mouth gag

iv. Instruments for the administration of local anaesthesia
Syringes and Cartridge

v. Instruments for clear surgical site
Stainless steel bowl, Irrigation syringe, Suction tip

vi. Instruments for placing incision
Scalpel, Bard parker (BP) Handle, Metzenbaum scissors, Colorado probe.

vii. Instruments for reflection
Periosteal elevators (Molt's no. 9), Howarth periosteal elevator, Moons Probe.

viii. Instruments for retraction
Austin retractor, Tongue depressor, Bowdler–Henry retractor.

ix. Instruments for bone removal
Carbide burs for use with motorized instruments (Round burs no. #4, #8; fissure burs no. 701, 702 and 703), Handpiece (Straight and Contra angle), Chisel, Mallet, Rongeurs and Bone File.

x. Instruments for teeth removal
Elevators, Periotome, Luxators, Forceps

xi. Instruments for socket management
Curette, Allis tissue holding forceps, Mitchell's trimmer

xii. Instruments and materials for haemostasis and wound closure
Electrocautery, Haemostatic Packs (Surgicel, Gel Foam), Toothed and non-toothed forceps, Needle holder, Suture needle and material, and Suture cutting scissors

INSTRUMENTS FOR DIAGNOSIS

a. **Mouth mirror** (Figure 8.1)
It is the primary instrument to be used for the initial screening of impacted third molar. The mouth mirror helps in (1) clinical assessment of the angulation and position of complete/partially erupted third molars in relation to the second molar as well as the status of the soft tissue covering the impacted tooth by enabling reflection of cheek (2) evaluation of the lingual mucoperiosteum and (3) better visualization of the dental sockets and fractured roots using reflected illumination. As compared to a flat-faced mirror, a concave mouth mirror presents a magnified and more illuminated image.

b. **Straight probe** (Figure 8.2)
Usually, the straight probe has a handle and a pointed working end bent at right angles to the long axis of the handle. The blunt-ended probe (periodontal probe) is useful in assessing the distal periodontal pocket depth of the second molar, to assess the thickness of soft tissue covering the impacted third molar and to check the anaesthesia achieved following administration of the local anaesthetic solution

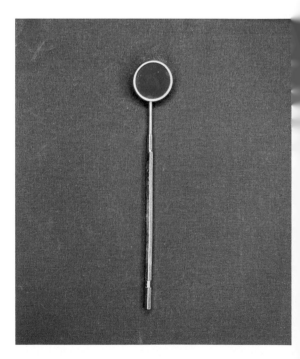

Figure 8.1 Mouth mirror.

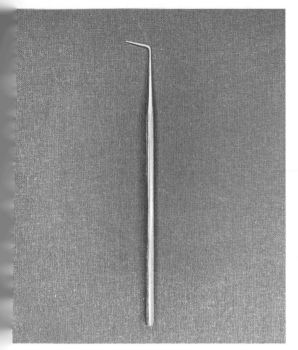

Figure 8.2 Straight probe.

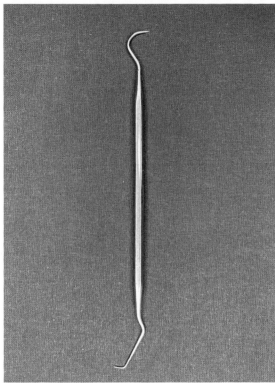

Figure 8.3 Explorer.

(Moon's probe). This may also be used to check the adequacy of bone removal (depth and continuity of guttering) before the elevation of an impacted tooth.

c. **Explorer** (Figure 8.3)

It consists of a sharp curved working end which is used to locate and evaluate dental caries of the second and third molars, especially in the interproximal regions. The explorer is effective in identifying the furcation of the third molar during tooth sectioning. It is also helpful to lift up submerged sutures behind the second molar and facilitate cutting with scissors.

d. **Tweezers/cotton pliers** (Figure 8.4)

Tweezers are used to hold cotton and gauze for mopping the surgical site to clear saliva/blood. It is also useful to place any dressing over the surgical site and pick up tiny fragments of bone or tooth.

INSTRUMENTS FOR PREPARATION OF THE SURGICAL SITE

a. **Swab holder** (Figure 8.5)

Sponge holder (Rampley's) is an instrument used to hold gauze which may be dipped in an antiseptic solution for scrubbing the surgical site. The looped and serrated tips ensure a firm grasp of a sufficient amount of gauze while facilitating the squeezing of the excess antiseptic solution. The long handles help in scrubbing the extra-oral facial skin as well as reaching the deeper, intraoral third molar region for preparation of the surgical site. It incorporates a ratchet that helps in self-retained clamping for ease of scrubbing.

b. **Towel clip** (Figure 8.6)

This instrument helps to hold the sterile towel that is draped around the patient in the proper position, without slipping. It is of two types; Mayo-Backhaus (Figure 8.6a) and Schaedel (Figure 8.6b) type. Both are self-retaining; Mayo-Backhaus works on the ratchet mechanism while Schaedel follows the cross-action principle. The clips are also used to secure the suction tube and motor cables. Towel clips can also be classified as atraumatic (Figure 8.6c) and traumatic. Atraumatic clips

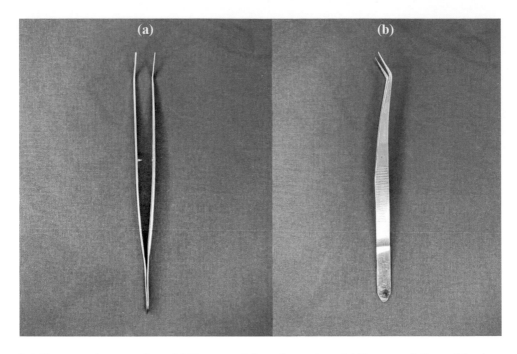

Figure 8.4 Tweezers/cotton pliers. (a) Tweezers/pliers, front view. (b) Tweezers/pliers, side view.

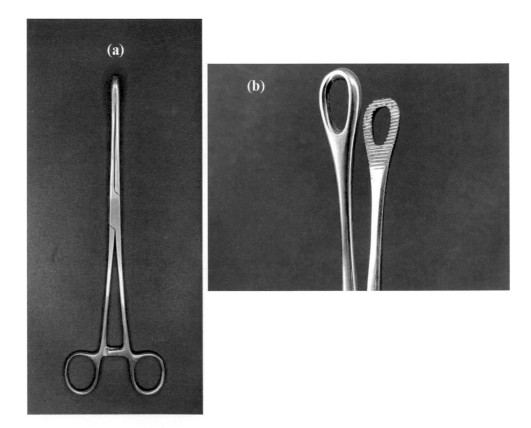

Figure 8.5 Swab holder. (a) Swab holder, full view. (b) Enlarged view of the working end.

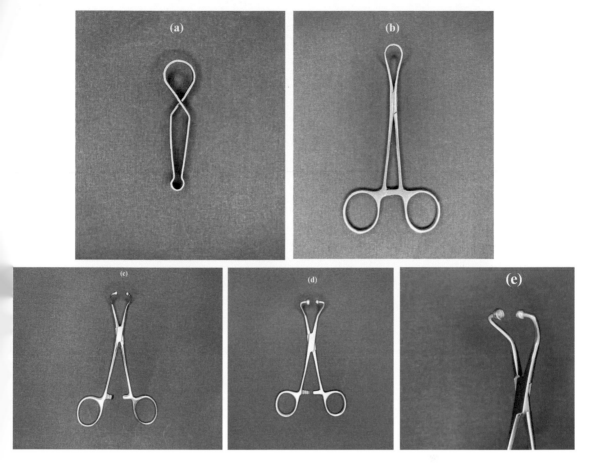

Figure 8.6 Towel clip. (a) Mayo-Backhaus. (b) Schaedel. (c) Atraumatic towel clip with ball ends, full view. (d) Atraumatic towel clip with ball and socket end, full view. (e) Enlarged view of working end demonstrating ball (right) and socket (left) ends.

have a ball or ball and socket arrangement (Figure 8.6d and e) on the working tips which prevent the tips from piercing deeper into the linen.

INSTRUMENTS USED TO MAINTAIN MOUTH OPENING

a. ***Bite block/mouth prop*** (Figure 8.7)

It is a rubber or metal bite block available in three or four different sizes connected by a chain. The blocks are positioned between the upper and lower molar teeth to keep the mouth open during the surgical procedure. It consists of a vertical block with concave serrated surfaces above and below for resting the teeth. It is usually positioned on the side opposite the surgical field.

b. ***Doyen's mouth gag*** (Figure 8.8)

This instrument is also called Molt's mouth gag. It is a self-retaining gag which is very useful for procedures which require mouth opening for a longer duration. The locking system and finger rings make instrumentation easier. The blades are curved and wider making it more convenient to rest on the molars.

c. ***Heister jaw stretcher*** (Figure 8.9)

This instrument has two flat blades, a handle and key for opening the blades. It is used to forcibly open the mouth in the presence of restricted mouth opening. This is especially useful in managing post-operative trismus.

d. ***Fergusson mouth gag*** (Figure 8.10)

It is also used to forcibly open the mouth in a patient with restricted mouth opening. It has two flat blades with serrations and can be kept

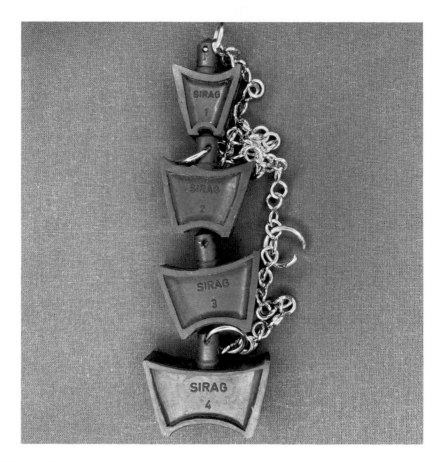

Figure 8.7 Bite block/mouth prop.

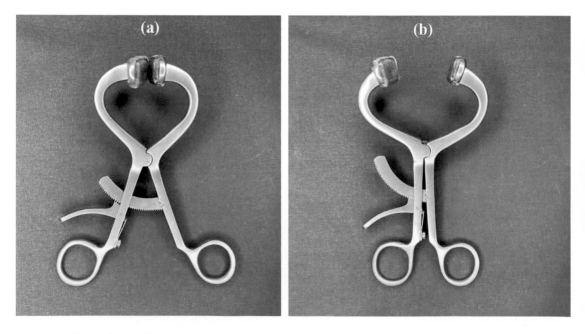

Figure 8.8 Doyen's mouth gag. (a) Doyen's mouth gag close. (b) Doyen's mouth gag open.

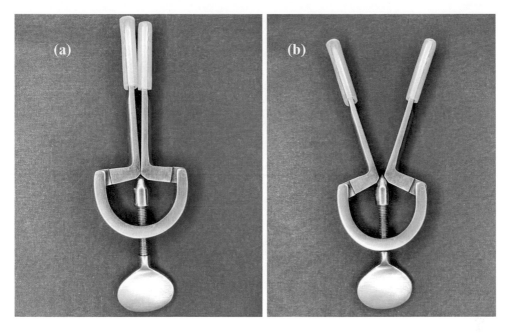

Figure 8.9 Heister jaw stretcher. (a) Heister jaw stretcher close. (b) Heister jaw stretcher open.

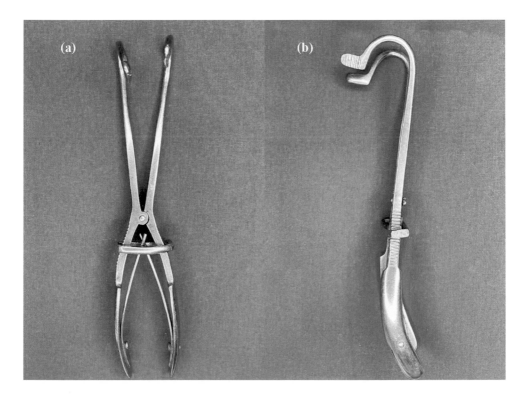

Figure 8.10 Fergusson mouth gag. (a) Fergusson mouth gag front view. (b) Fergusson mouth gag side view.

in an open position by using the catch present in the handle. The long and curved handles help in convenient positioning of the blades and ensure good control of the instrument extra-orally.

INSTRUMENTS FOR ADMINISTRATION OF LOCAL ANAESTHESIA

a. *Syringes*

Syringes may be of either disposable (Figure 8.11) or non-disposable, cartridge type (Figure 8.12). Disposable syringes are made of plastic and hence light weighted. They may be of luer slip (non-luer lock) (Figure 8.11a) or luer lock (Figure 8.11b) type. Luer-lock syringes permit the needle to be locked onto the syringe and hence prevent needle displacement when the injection pressure is high during the administration of the local anaesthetic (LA) solution. Cartridge Syringes (Figure 8.12a) are made of metal and are popular because they use disposable needles (Figure 8.12b) and

pre-determined volumes of LA solutions, by using cartridges (Figure 8.12c). This prevents cross-contamination due to the re-loading of LA solutions from multi-use/multi-vial LA bottles. Further, cartridge syringes permit easy aspiration because of the thumb ring design. "Self-aspirating" cartridge syringes are also available. A self-aspirating syringe has a small bump/disc on the plunger tip instead of the harpoon. It does not require pulling of the plunger behind to initiate aspiration. Instead, it relies on the elastic recoil of the silicone diaphragm of the carpule to produce negative pressure when given a mild push and relaxed.[2]

b. *Needles*

Needles are of different gauges and lengths.
- *Gauge* refers to the diameter of the needle. The lesser the gauge, the more the diameter of the needle. Needles of smaller diameter elicit less pain on injection. 24–27 gauge are the most commonly used needles for

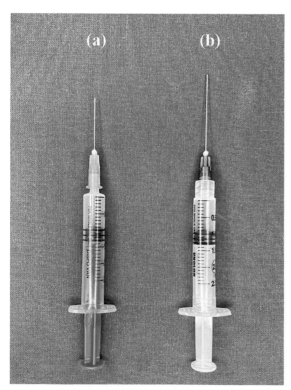

Figure 8.11 Disposable syringe. (a) Non-luer-lock syringe. (b) Luer-lock syringe.

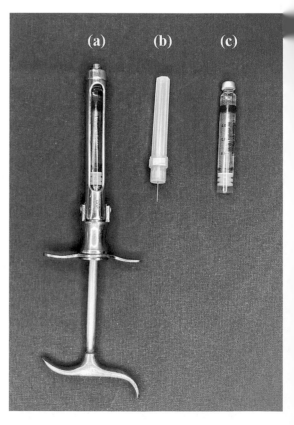

Figure 8.12 Cartridge syringe. (a) Non-disposable cartridge syringe, loaded. (b) Disposable needle. (c) Cartridge.

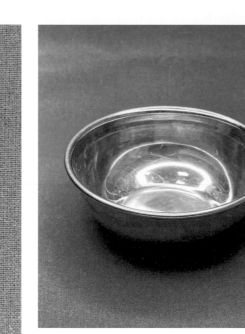

Figure 8.13 Needle length. (a) Short. (b) Long.

both block and infiltration. Typically, cartridge syringes use thin needles.

- *Length* (Figure 8.13) of the needle is chosen based on the type of technique used for LA administration; extra short 12 mm needle is used for intra-ligamentary injection. Short 20–25 mm needle, for infiltration and long 30–35 mm needle for regional nerve blocks. For inferior alveolar nerve block, 25–27 gauge, long needle is recommended.

INSTRUMENTS FOR CLEAR SURGICAL SITE

a. *Stainless steel bowl* (Figure 8.14)

Bowls constitute receptacles for storing irrigation fluid such as saline. Irrigation is needed to minimize the heat produced by bur during bone removal and also to clear the bur of clogged bone debris.

b. *Irrigation syringe* (Figure 8.15)

This is the wide bore syringe (usually 10 mL) with an 18 gauge needle which is used for irrigation during bone removal. Blunt irrigation tips may be used, where available.

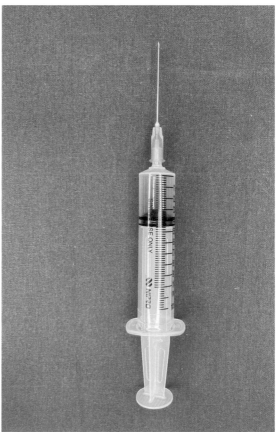

Figure 8.14 Stainless steel bowl.

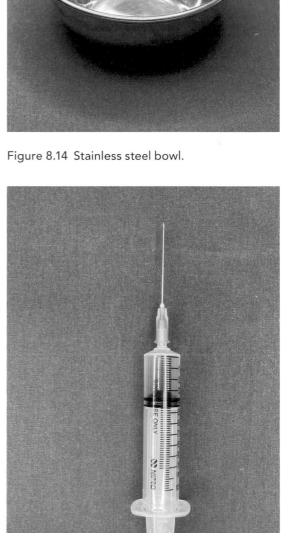

Figure 8.15 Irrigation syringe (10 mL).

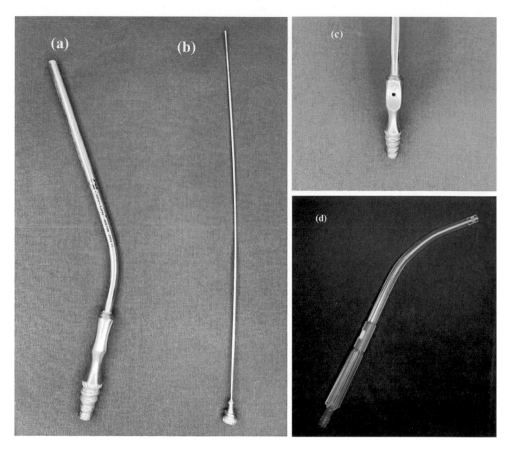

Figure 8.16 Suction tip. (a) Frazier metal suction tip. (b) Stylet. (c) Relief hole. (d) Yankauer suction tip.

c. **Suction tip** (Figure 8.16)

Suction tips are available as disposable and non-disposable types made of plastic and metal, respectively. They are used to suction the blood, oral secretions, irrigating fluids, etc.

Frazier Metal Suction tip (Figure 8.16a) is a thin instrument, ideally curved to reach the third molar region without hindering surgical access and visibility of the surgical site. The stylet (Figure 8.16b) that comes along is used to clean the cannula and maintain patency. The suction tip has a relief hole (Figure 8.16c) on the thumb rest which acts as a control valve. Suction pressure can be modified by either closing or opening the hole. For achieving stronger suction, the relief hole is closed. Standard number 4 and 5 suction tips are the commonly used sizes.

Yankauer Suction tip (Figure 8.16d) is broader and made of firm plastic or metal.

d. **Surgical aspirator** (Figure 8.17)

This instrument is smooth and ergonomically curved to suction the intraoral fluids. They are available in metal (Figure 8.17a) and plastic (Figure 8.17b), in multiple sizes.

INSTRUMENTS FOR PLACING INCISION

a. **Scalpel** (Figure 8.18)

It consists of two parts: handle and blade.
- *BP handle* (Figure 8.18a) is available in various sizes as number 3, 4, and 7. Handle number 3 is used for receiving blades numbered 11, 12, and 15 and handle number 7 is used for receiving blade number 15. It is also available as reusable (metal) and single-use disposable (plastic) handles with a fixed blade.
- *BP blade* (Figure 8.18b) is also available in different sizes and shapes. Number 15 is

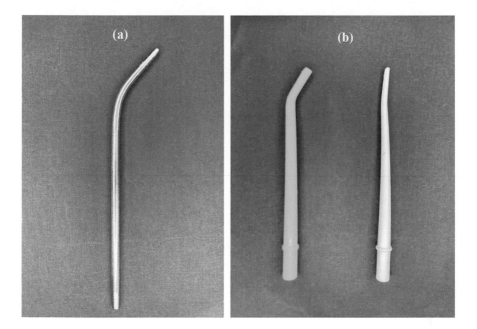

Figure 8.17 Aspirator. (a) Metal. (b) Plastic.

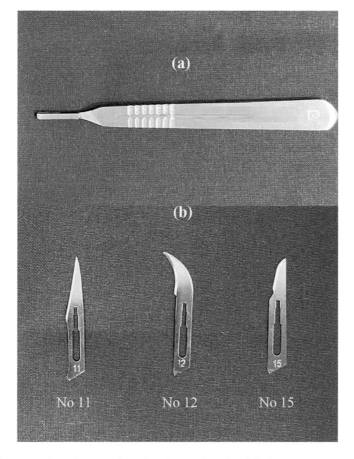

Figure 8.18 Scalpel. (a) Bard Parker (BP) handle. (b) Bard Parker blade.

used for placing incision for exposure of the impacted third molar. Number 12 blade is crescent-shaped and used for making an incision along the crevice of teeth. It is also used to excise the pericoronal tissue (operculectomy), in select cases.[3] Number 15 is used for making the anterior release incision and posterior extension along tuberosity and retro-molar region. Scalpel should be held in pen grasp between thumb, index and middle finger and should have proper finger rest for making good incision. Safety scalpels with retractable blades or sheaths are available which help in preventing blade injuries. Scalpel blade removers also minimize injury during the removal and disposal of blades. Where scalpel blade removers are not available, haemostats may be used for blade fitment and removal.

b. **Metzenbaum scissors** (Figure 8.19)

These heavy tissue-dissecting scissors have flatter and slightly curved blades with blunt tips. It may be used to complete the distal part of the incision after elevating a tent of muco-periosteal tissue distal to the mandibular third molar. The curved blades create the ideal angulation necessary for the distal release incision.

c. **Electrosurgery scalpel** (Figure 8.20)

Electrosurgery uses high-frequency alternating current for incising tissues with minimal

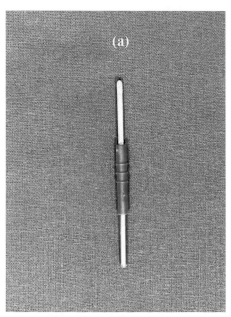

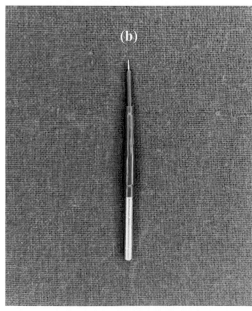

Figure 8.20 Electrosurgery scalpel. (a) Conventional electrosurgical tip. (b) Colorado microdissection needle.

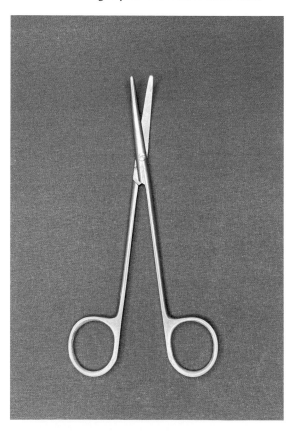

Figure 8.19 Metzenbaum scissors.

cutting time. Conventional electrosurgical tip (Figure 8.20a) is bigger and hence associated with more lateral heat and tissue damage. *Colorado microdissection needle* (Figure 8.20b) is a special type of electrosurgical scalpel that has a delicate tungsten tip which ensures precise incision with minimal pressure and less dissipation of heat to the adjacent tissues that reduces tissue necrosis. Its coagulant action creates a bloodless, clean surgical field and minimizes surgical time. The resultant wound healing and patient comfort have been found comparable to cold scalpel. As compared to scalpel, the disadvantage cited in the literature is offensive odour during the procedure due to the fumes generated by tissue coagulation. This may be warded off by using high-pressure suction equipment and applying perfumed Vaseline on the perioral area. Electrocautery which uses a direct current to heat the working tip may be used for operculectomy.

INSTRUMENTS FOR REFLECTION

a. ***Molt's no. 9 periosteal elevator*** (Figure 8.21a)
   Molt's elevator consists of two working ends connected by handle. The pointed end (Rugine end, Figure 8.21b) is used for reflecting the interdental papilla in a prying motion. The broader end (raspatory end, Figure 8.21c) is rounded and blunt and is used in push stroke to reflect the mucoperiosteum from the bone. Periosteal elevator may also be used to protect the lingual nerve during bone guttering.

b. ***Howarth periosteal elevator*** (Figure 8.22)
   Howarth elevator displays two ends; one end is blunt and broad termed raspatory end while the other is sharp and curved, called rugine. It is used to reflect mucoperiosteum by push stroke.

c. ***Moon's probe*** (Figure 8.23)
   Moon's probe consists of a thin blade which helps in effective reflection of attached gingiva from the tooth. This may also be used to check anaesthesia.

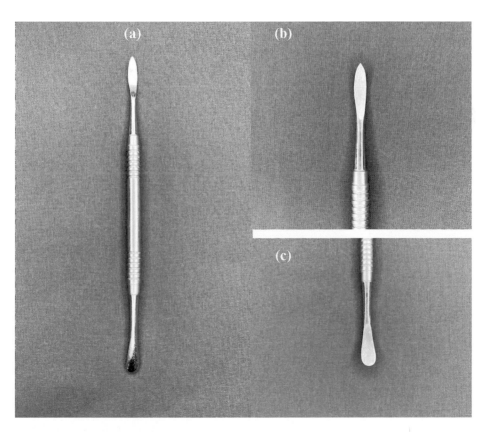

Figure 8.21 Molt's no. 9 periosteal elevator. (a) Molt's no. 9 periosteal elevator, full view. (b) Rugine end. (c) Raspatory end.

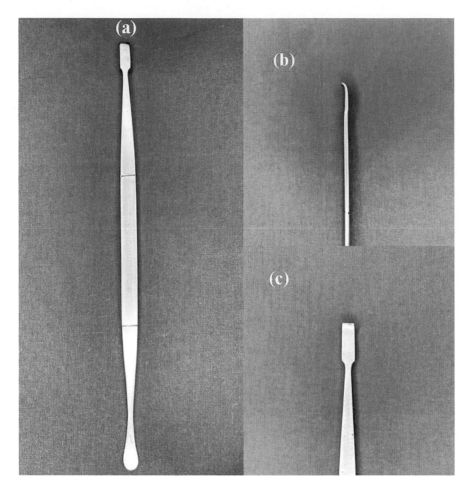

Figure 8.22 Howarth periosteal elevator. (a) Howarth periosteal elevator, full view. (b) Enlarged view of rugine end, lateral view. (c) Enlarged view of rugine end, frontal view.

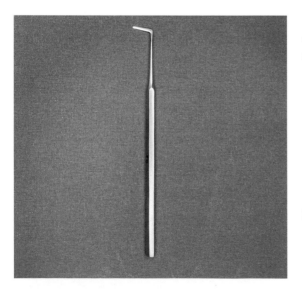

Figure 8.23 Moon's probe.

INSTRUMENTS FOR RETRACTION

a. **Austin retractor** (Figure 8.24)

It is a L-shaped retractor with one end rounded and the other, forked. It is the most commonly used instrument for retracting the mucoperiosteal flap for third molar surgery. For firm retraction, the forked end must be positioned intra-orally, to rest on the bone. Austin's retractor with an in-built suction tip is also available. This reduces the number of instruments within the oral cavity during the procedure.

b. **Tongue depressor** (Figure 8.25)

As the name implies, it is used for retracting the tongue during the surgical procedure and also for inspecting the lingual aspect of the third molar region. It is a L-shaped instrument with one end of the blade broad and the

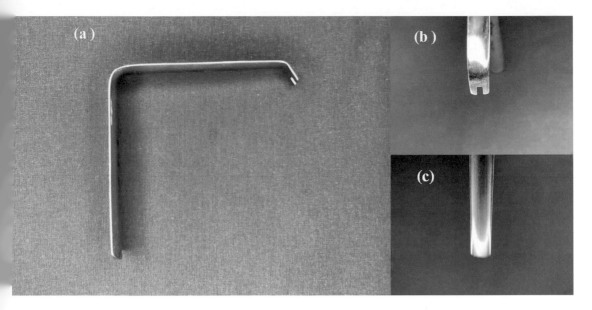

Figure 8.24 Austin retractor. (a) Austin retractor, full view. (b) Enlarged view of forked end. (c) Enlarged view of rounded end.

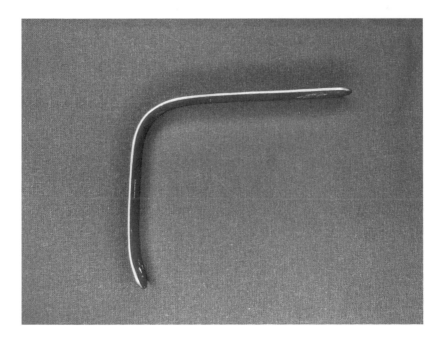

Figure 8.25 Tongue depressor.

other end narrow and slightly curved. The edges of the instrument are well rounded to help in the atraumatic retraction of tissues.

c. **Bowdler–Henry** (Figure 8.26)

It is a L-shaped instrument with a long handle and a curved, serrated tip which helps in achieving a firm and steady grip on the bone. Its long handle ensures easy and better retraction of the mucoperiosteal flap during surgical removal of mandibular impacted teeth.

d. **Laster's maxillary third molar and cheek retractor** (Figure 8.27)

This retractor combines the design of the Howarth raspatory periosteal elevator and

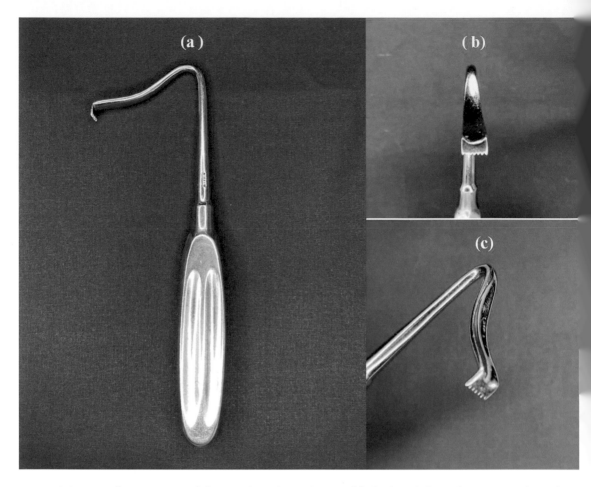

Figure 8.26 Bowdler–Henry. (a) full view. (b) Enlarged view of forked end, frontal view. (c) Enlarged view of forked end, oblique view.

cheek retractor. The tip of the instrument fits snugly behind the tuberosity to provide good retraction of soft tissues in the upper third molar region. It has a polished concave retracting surface which helps in the reflection of light into the operatory site to improve visibility and accessibility. Further, it allows comfortable usage of suction tips and chisel along this concave surface. This instrument is of limited use for mandibular surgery.

INSTRUMENTS FOR BONE REMOVAL AND ODONTOTOMY

a. **Surgical bur** (Figure 8.28)

Burs are the most popular instruments used for quick and efficient bone removal to facilitate surgical removal of third molars. A bur consists of a shank, neck and head and is made of either stainless steel or tungsten carbide. Tungsten carbide burs demonstrate better cutting efficiency. Round burs and fissure burs are most efficient for bone removal and tooth sectioning in third molar surgery.

- *Fissure burs* have a cylindrical head which may be tapered or straight. The flutes of the bur are either plain or cross-cut. Cross-cut burs have increased cutting efficiency, reduced friction and less chances for clogging. The most commonly used type of fissure burs is the *Tapered fissure cross-cut* burs, which are numbered 701, 702, and 703 (Figure 8.28a–c). They are used for the removal of bone, buccal and distal to the impacted third molar by guttering method. The space created by bur

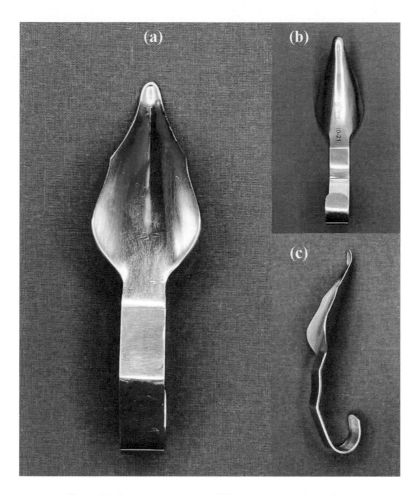

Figure 8.27 Laster's maxillary third molar retractor. (a) Laster's maxillary third molar retractor, full view. (b) Posterior view. (c) Profile view.

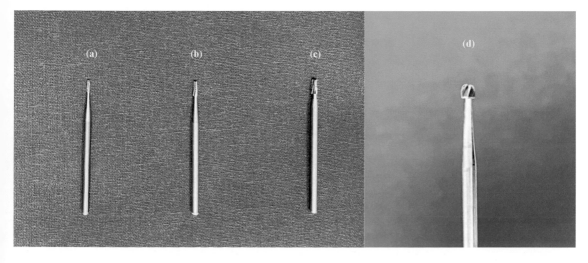

Figure 8.28 Surgical bur-tapered fissure. (a) Surgical bur-tapered fissure 701. (b) Surgical bur-tapered fissure 702. (c) Surgical bur-tapered fissure 703. (d) Surgical bur-round head.

helps in positioning the elevators as well as to create space for tooth movement. Burs also help in creating a point of application on the impacted tooth for using elevators and tooth sectioning (tooth splitting) procedures.

- *Round burs* (Figure 8.28d) (standard number HP 6), are used to remove the bone overlying a completely buried tooth and uncover the crown. It is also used in the postage-stamp method and lateral trepanation technique (for removal of incompletely formed impacted third molar) where holes are placed on the buccal plate.
- 1702 and 1703 are unique surgical burs which are tapered and round ended with cross cuts. These offer the advantages of both a round bur and a fissure bur.
- During the process of bone removal, bur must be continuously irrigated with normal or cold saline to prevent overheating which may lead to potential thermal necrosis of bone and also to prevent clogging of flutes which may reduce cutting efficiency.

b. **Surgical handpiece** (Figure 8.29)

The handpiece is a hand-held rotary device powered by an electric motor (micromotor/physio-dispenser) or compressed air (airotor) and is used to drive a surgical bur for bone removal. The two essential factors important for rotary bone removal are (1) drive speed which signifies the speed at which the surgical bur is rotated by the motor and is quantified in revolutions per minute (rpm) and (2) drive torque which is the force required by motor to make the bur rotate and is measured in newton-centimetres (N-cm). Handpieces are generally classified according to their drive speed as high-speed (>100,000 rpm) and low-speed (<50,000 rpm) or based on their angulation into straight and contra angle.

Low-speed handpieces are powered by electrical motors [micromotor (Figure 8.29a)] while *high-speed handpieces* are powered by compressed air through air turbines [airotor (Figure 8.29b)]. Electric motors produce lower drive speeds with significantly higher torque and are hence more commonly used for wisdom tooth surgery, while high-speed handpieces generate very less torque and may be used for sectioning of teeth purely for their speed. Some common complications associated with the use of high-speed air turbines for bone removal include increased chances for thermal necrosis and iatrogenic air emphysema due to the pressurized air dissecting through the submucosal tissue planes. The use of air turbines is generally discouraged for surgical extraction of the mandibular third molar surgery.

Straight handpieces are those where the working head is non-angulated in relation to the handpiece and are used more commonly in routine surgical practice, while contra-angle handpieces are those where

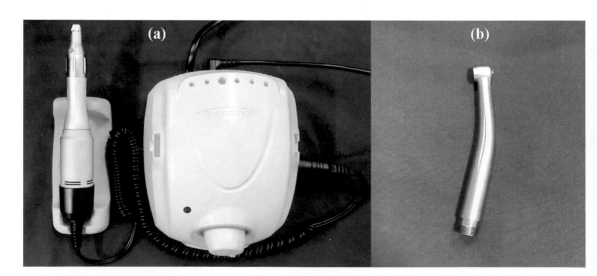

Figure 8.29 Surgical handpiece. (a) Micromotor with handpiece. (b) Airotor handpiece.

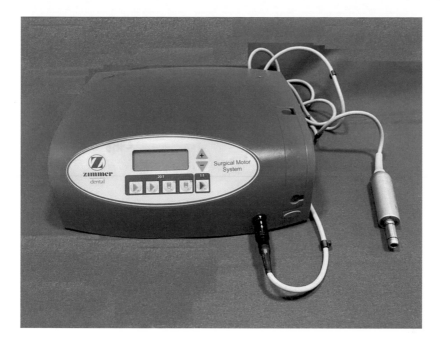

Figure 8.30 Physio-dispenser.

the working head is positioned at varying angulations (45° and 90°) in relation to the handpiece shaft and may be useful in accessing distal bone as well as for easy sectioning of impacted teeth (odontotomy).[4]

c. **Physio-dispenser** (Figure 8.30)

Physio-dispenser is also a preferred equipment in today's practice for bone removal in third molar surgery. It is an electric motor which is specifically designed for performing bone drilling while minimizing bone damage. They incorporate the following features: (1) an electric motor with variable speed (10–40,000 rpm) which aids in bone drilling efficiently with low heat generation and flexible torque settings (5–80 N-cm) which enables to drive the drill efficiently even at very low drive speeds, and (2) a motorized irrigation system which aids in continuous irrigation of the surgical field for reducing bone injury and efficient removal of the bone debris during drilling (ideally utilizing a peristaltic pump).[5]

d. **Chisel** (Figure 8.31)

Gardner Chisel is a uni-bevelled, hand-held instrument which is used for the removal of bone. It consists of a handle, shank and blade. Working blade is available in 5, 6, 10, and 15 mm sizes. Thin blade is used for making

the point of application whereas a larger one is used for bone removal. While positioning the chisel, the bevel must face towards the bone to be removed. Disadvantages of chisel technique include fracture of the mandible due to delivery of injudicious force and unpleasant vibrations perceived by the patient.[6] This may still find its utilization where the lingual split bone technique is planned.[7]

e. **Mallet** (Figure 8.32)

Mallet is used along with chisel to remove bone around the impacted teeth. *Gardner's* Mallet (Figure 8.32a) has a working head which is positioned along the long axis of the handle. It is completely metallic and should ideally weigh 280 g. *Mead's* mallet (Figure 8.32b) has a horizontal working end which is at right angle to the handle. It weighs 212 g approximately and is available in metal and Teflon. Teflon-coated mallet produces less noise and shock. It is used in a free swinging motion. The advantage of using chisel and mallet over bur is the minimal post-operative discomfort. But the noise and vibrations produced by the hand instruments are less tolerated by the patients.

f. **Rongeurs** (Figure 8.33)

Rongeurs has two sharp blades which cut bone when the handles are compressed

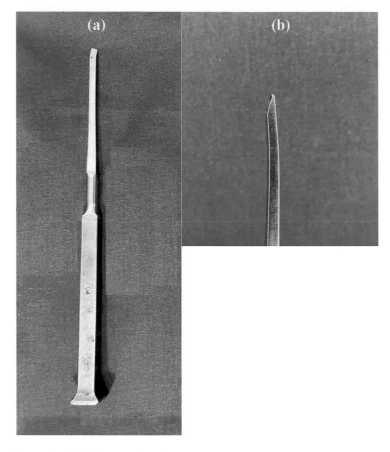

Figure 8.31 Chisel. (a) Chisel, full view. (b) Enlarged working end demonstrating the bevel.

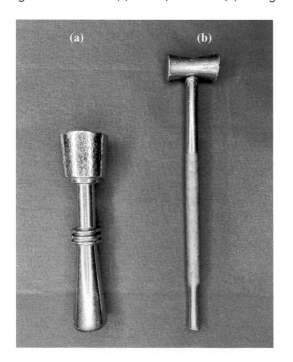

Figure 8.32 Mallet. (a) Gardner. (b) Mead.

together. It is available in two designs (1) side cutting forceps and (2) side and end-cutting forceps. The leaf spring design incorporated into the Rongeurs allows the reopening of the blades automatically. *Jansen* Rongeurs (Figure 8.33a) features straight/curved jaws and double spring plier handles with compound action-joint which is effective in removing a large volume of bone rapidly as well as smoothly. *Blumenthal* Rongeurs (Figure 8.33b) has curved jaws and double spring plier handle and is indicated for cutting inter-septal bone.

g. ***Bone file*** (Figure 8.34)

Miller Colburn bone file is a double-ended instrument with blade, handle and shank. The blade is available in various forms such as curved, spherical and oval with serrations. It should be used in pull stroke to smoothen the bone whereas push stroke leads to burnishing of bone. It is mainly indicated for smoothening of sharp bony margins following the removal of impacted teeth.

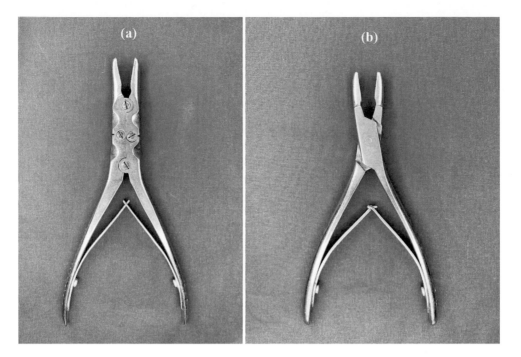

Figure 8.33 Rongeurs. (a) Jansen Rongeurs. (b) Blumenthal Rongeurs.

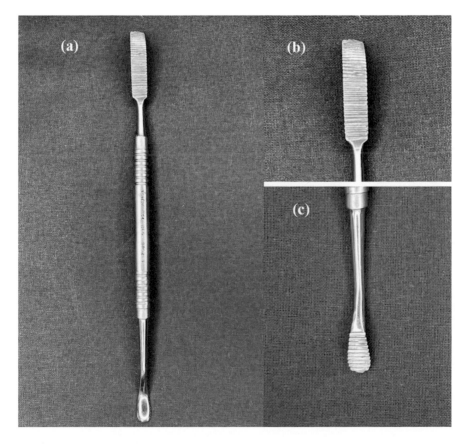

Figure 8.34 Bone file. (a) Bone file, full view. (b and c) Enlarged working end.

INSTRUMENTS FOR TOOTH DELIVERY

a. **Elevators**
   i. *Straight* (Figure 8.35a and b) and *Coupland* (Figure 8.36a–c) elevators possess the following parts; blade, shank and handle. In straight elevator, the blade is pointed with one side serrated and the other convex, whereas in a Coupland elevator, the blade/working tip is concave on one side and convex on the other. Straight and Coupland elevator should be applied at 45° to the long axis of the tooth and bone is used as fulcrum. It works under the principle of first-order lever and wedge. The point of application for all types of impacted teeth is at the cementoenamel junction of the mesial surface of the teeth except the distoangular teeth which are at the cementoenamel junction of the distal surface of the teeth.
   ii. *Winter Cryer* (straight pattern) (Figure 8.37a and b) – It is a paired instrument, designed as right and left sides. It consists of a curved and angulated blade and is usually used to remove the maxillary third molar with a mesiobuccal point of application at the cementoenamel junction. The elevator is applied at 45° to the long axis of the tooth with concavity facing the tooth. It works on both wedge and wheel and axle principles. Cryer is also used to remove the roots/root tips of impacted mandibular teeth.
   iii. *Winter Cryer* (crossbar pattern) (Figure 8.38a and b) – It is a paired instrument with a triangular blade. It is used to remove mandibular roots when the other root has been already removed. This also works under the wheel and axle principle.
   iv. *Apexo elevator* (Figure 8.39a and b) – It is available as mesial and distal instruments with an angulated, thin and sharp blade and works under the wedge principle. Apical third of the root can be removed with this instrument.

   In general, Extreme care must be taken while using the elevators. It is important to provide counter pressure during the

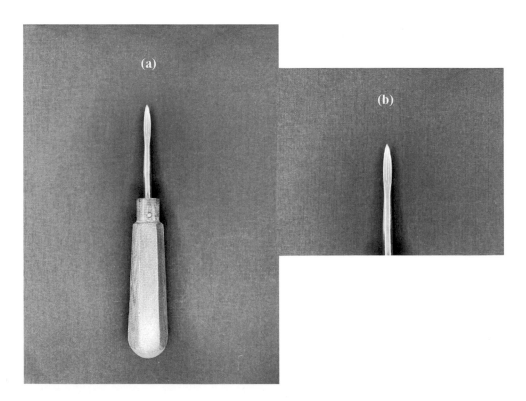

Figure 8.35 Straight elevator. (a) Straight elevator, full view. (b) Enlarged view of working end.

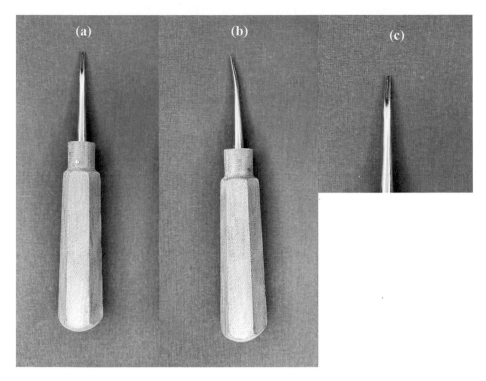

Figure 8.36 Couplands elevator. (a) Coupland elevator, full view. (b) Coupland elevator, profile view. (c) Enlarged view of working end.

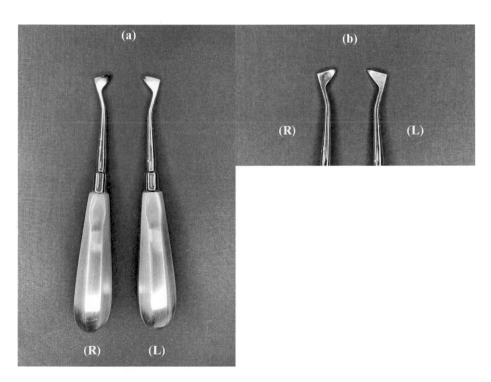

Figure 8.37 Winter Cryer (straight pattern). (a) Winter Cryer (straight pattern), right and left sided, full view. (b) Enlarged view of working end, right and left sided.

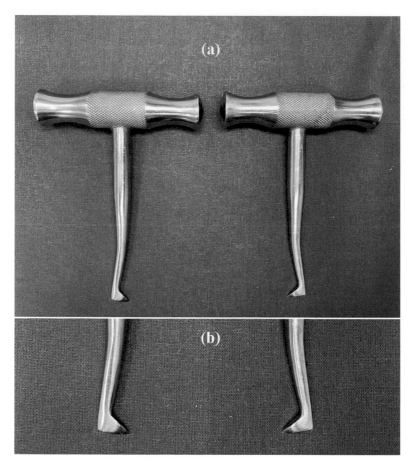

Figure 8.38 Winter Cryer (crossbar pattern). (a) Winter Cryer (crossbar pattern), full view. (b) Enlarged view of working end.

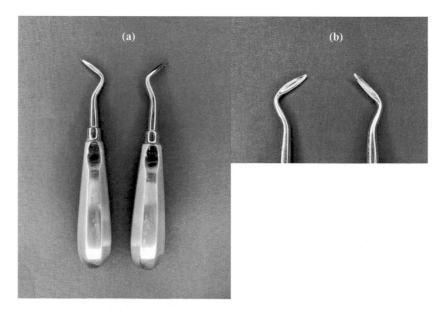

Figure 8.39 Apexo elevator. (a) Apexo elevator, full view. (b) Enlarged view of working ends.

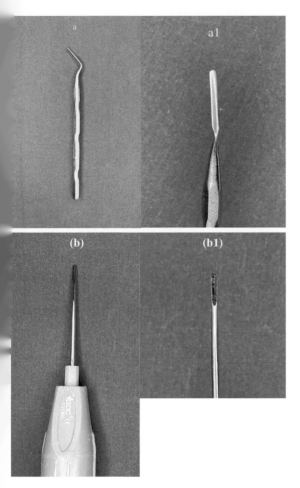

Figure 8.40 Periotome and Luxators. (a) Periotome, full view. (a1) Periotome, profile view. (b) Luxator, full view. (b1) Luxator, enlarged view of working end.

application of elevators to prevent undue transmission of forces to the mandible which may result in angle fracture.

b. *Periotome and Luxators* (Figure 8.40)

These are finer instruments used to luxate the tooth. The instrument is inserted into the periodontal ligament space along the long axis of the tooth and wedged all around the tooth so that the periodontal ligament space is enlarged. Periotome is smaller than luxator. It works under the wedge principle.

c. *Forceps* (Figure 8.41)

- Forceps are used to deliver the molars after luxation and elevation with elevators. Maxillary third molar forceps (Figure 8.41a) have curved handles with a bayonet pattern

to reach the posterior maxillary region in an easy manner. The beaks of the third molar forceps have rounded ends, unlike the conventional upper molar forceps which have one beak sharp and the other rounded. The forceps are not side-specific and can be used for both right and left sides. A more buccal and less palatal movement along with distal rotation is given for the removal of the maxillary third molar.

- *Mandibular third molar forceps* (Figure 8.41b) have a bayonet pattern, with beaks larger than the conventional molar forceps. Both beaks are pointed and are applied below the cementoenamel junction of the tooth. Apical, buccal, and more lingual movement is given to deliver the tooth.

- The *Cowhorn forceps* (Figure 8.41c) may be utilized to remove distoangular mandibular third molar with conical roots by intra-alveolar method. The technique involves the application of forceps interdentally between the second and third molar while keeping the fingers on the occlusal aspect of the second molar to prevent luxation.

INSTRUMENTS FOR SOCKET MANAGEMENT

a. *Curette*

Lucas bone curette (Figure 8.42a) has two shallow scooped ends attached by a handle. It is used to remove granulation tissue from the socket and removal of residual follicular/cystic lining. It is used in pull stroke to scrape the tissues from bone. *Volkmann*'s curette (Figure 8.42b) is available as a single or double-ended instrument with deepened scoop.

b. *Allis tissue holding forceps*

Allis tissue holding forceps (Figure 8.43) have toothed blades with ratchet handles. It is used to grasp delicate tissues that are to be removed e.g., removal of residual dental follicle or de-epithelialization of flap margins.

c. *Mitchell's trimmer* (Figure 8.44)

It is a double-ended instrument with a sharp end and may be used to release and scoop out fibrous attachment around the impacted tooth before bone guttering.

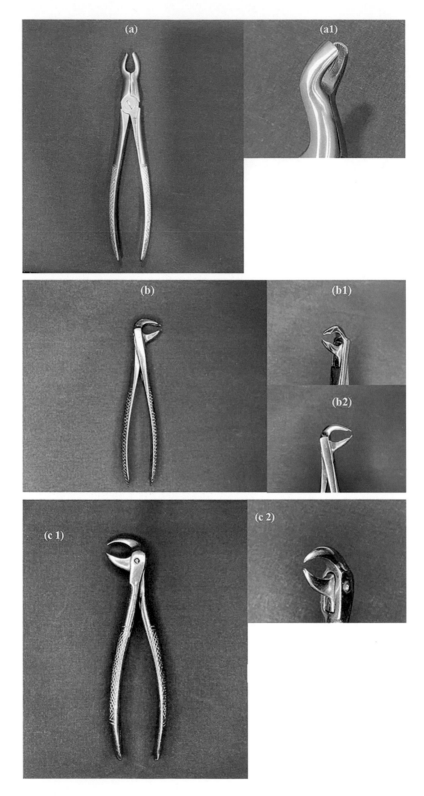

Figure 8.41 Forceps. (a) Maxillary third molar forceps. (a1 and a2) Enlarged view of working end. (b) Mandibular third molar forceps. (b1 and b2) Enlarged view of working end. (c1) Cowhorn forceps, full view. (c2) Cowhorn forceps, enlarged view of working end.

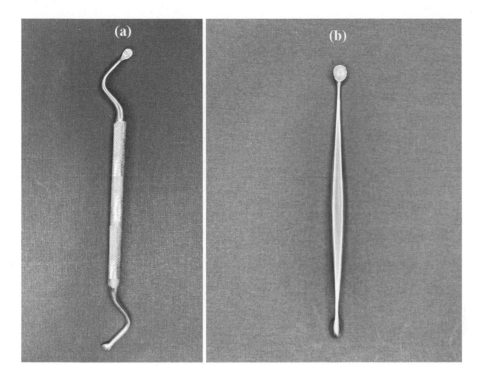

Figure 8.42 Bone curette. (a) Lucas bone curette. (b) Volkmann's curette.

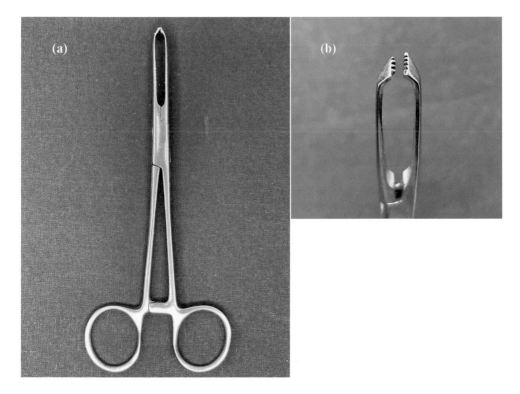

Figure 8.43 Allis tissue holding forceps. (a) Allis tissue holding forceps, full view. (b) Enlarged view of working end.

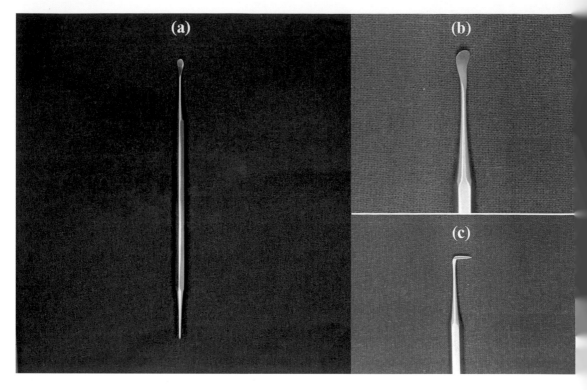

Figure 8.44 Mitchell's trimmer. (a) Mitchell's trimmer, full view. (b and c) Enlarged view of working ends.

INSTRUMENTS AND MATERIALS FOR HAEMOSTASIS AND WOUND CLOSURE

a. *Electrocautery* (Figure 8.45)

Bleeding during third molar surgery may be due to bony or soft tissue causes. Electrocautery can be used to achieve haemostasis by electrocoagulation. Ball-type electrode and unipolar/bipolar electrode are the instruments of choice. Ball electrode and monopolar electrode are useful to arrest bleeding from small bony canals while the bipolar electrode is more useful for achieving haemostasis from soft tissues bleeding.

b. *Burnisher* (Figure 8.46)

Ball Burnisher is available as a single or double-ended instrument with ball-shaped ends. The instrument achieves haemostasis either by mechanical or by thermal action. Mechanical haemostasis is achieved by crushing the surrounding bone and occluding the bleeding canals.[8] Thermal haemostasis is achieved by applying heated burnisher on the bleeding site to facilitate thermocoagulation.

c. *Haemostatic agents*

Local haemostatic agents, such as gelfoam and surgicel, can be used if the bleeding is occurring from soft tissue, whereas for hard tissue bleeding, bone wax can be applied.[9]

- *Surgicel* (Figure 8.47): This is a mesh of regenerated oxidized cellulose. It arrests bleeding by two methods: mechanical and chemical. When placed on the bleeding site, it lowers the local pH and causes denaturation of globulin and albumin. Further, it acts as scaffold for clot formation. It is absorbed slowly by phagocytosis within a period of 4–8 weeks. The disadvantages include delayed healing, nerve injury if applied close to the nerve and granuloma formation.

- *Gelfoam* (Figure 8.48): It is a porous gelatin sponge, which increases in weight and volume up to 40% and 200%, respectively. The increase in size exerts the tamponade effect and also acts as a scaffold for clot formation. It can be applied as dry or moistened with saline or thrombin. It is resorbed in 4–6 weeks by liquefaction and phagocytosis.

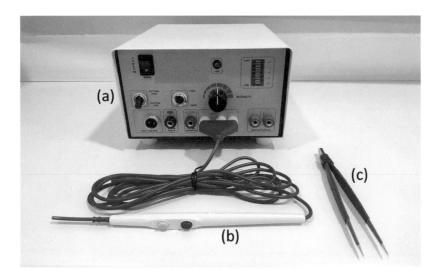

Figure 8.45 Electro surgery. (a) Electrosurgery unit. (b) Monopolar electrode. (c) Bipolar electrode.

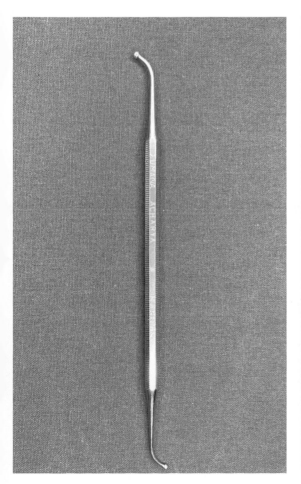

Figure 8.46 Burnisher.

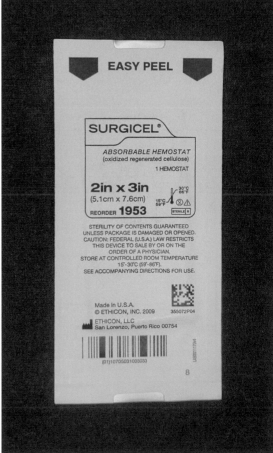

Figure 8.47 Surgicel.

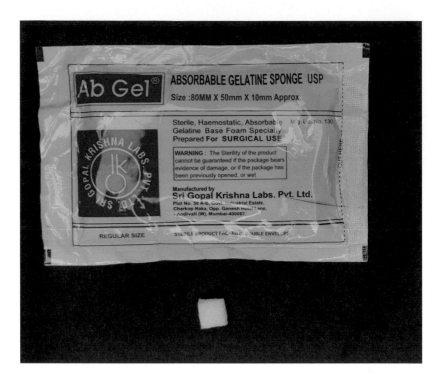

Figure 8.48 Gelfoam.

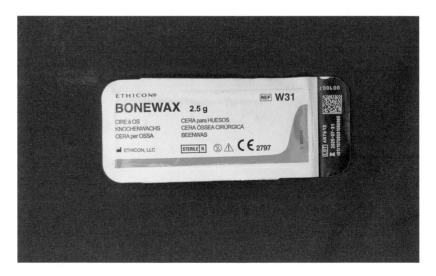

Figure 8.49 Bone wax.

- *Bone wax* (Figure 8.49) It comprises of beeswax, isopropyl palmitate and paraffin. When applied on the bleeding areas on the bone, it achieves haemostasis by occluding the nutrient canals or the vascular canal. Foreign body reaction leading to granuloma formation and infection are the reported disadvantages in the literature.

d. *Needle holder* (Figure 8.50)

Mayo Hegar needle holder consists of beak, shank and handle with ratchet and ring. It is available in many sizes. Unlike the artery forceps, the beaks of the needle holder are short and crosshatched with groove for achieving an adequate grip of the needle. Long straight or angulated needle holders are useful to access

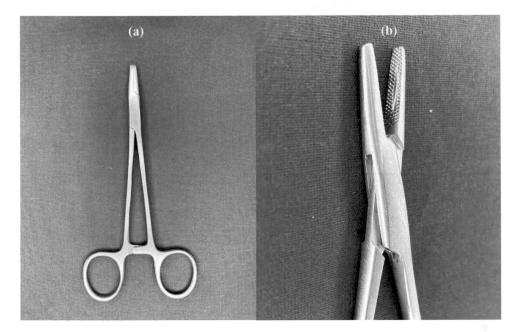

Figure 8.50 Needle holder. (a) Needle holder, full view. (b) Enlarged view of working end demonstrating the vertical slit.

the mandibular and maxillary molar region. Ratchet of the needle holder helps in locking the needle to prevent slippage during suturing.

e. **Needle** (Figure 8.51)

The parts of the needle include the tip, body, and eye. Needles are available in various sizes and shapes; half circle and three eighth circle needles are preferred for intraoral suturing. Atraumatic needles do not have an eye and the suture material is swaged to the needle. The tip of the needle can be either cutting, reverse cutting or round body. In cutting needle, the cutting edge is present on the inner curvature of the needle, whereas the cutting edge is present on the outer curvature in a reverse cutting needle. Reverse cutting needle is ideal for intraoral suturing as it presents less chances of cutting through the tissue. For proper instrumentation, needle must be held at 2/3rd distance from its tip.

f. **Tissue holding forceps** (Figure 8.52)

The parts of Adson tissue holding forceps are handle, shank, jaws, and tip. It is used to hold the mucoperiosteal flap to facilitate suturing. Jaws may be toothed or non-toothed. Toothed forceps offer good grip of the tissues than non-toothed forceps. With non-toothed

forceps, a firm grip of tissues is ensured by the serrations present on the inner surface of the tip. Plain-toothed forceps are used to hold delicate tissue such as non-keratinized mucosa during suturing.

g. **Suture cutting scissors** (Figure 8.53)

Forgesy suture cutting scissors has cutting edges, shank and handle with ring. It is preferred as the long and curved scissors are better suited to reach the posterior region. Ideally, scissors utilized for suture cutting should not be used to cut excess or diseased soft tissue margins of mucoperiosteal flap

h. **Suture material**

Various suture materials are available which are classified based on the diameter, number of filaments and composition of the material. Diameter is mentioned as zeros; as the zero increases, the diameter of the material decreases. The most commonly used suture material for intraoral purposes is 3–0 Silk (non-absorbable) (Figure 8.54) and polyglactin 910 (absorbable)[10] (Figure 8.55). *Silk* is a natural, multifilament material commonly used for intraoral suturing as it has excellent strength and good handling properties. But the disadvantages associated include accumulation

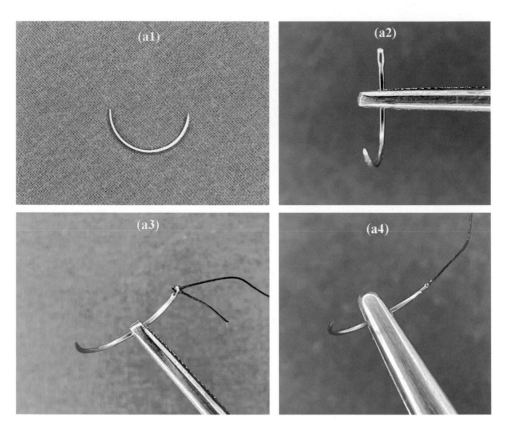

Figure 8.51 Suture needle. (a1) Round body needle, full view. (a2) Round body needle demonstrating eye. (a3) Eyed needle with silk suture. (a4) Eyeless/swaged needle with silk suture.

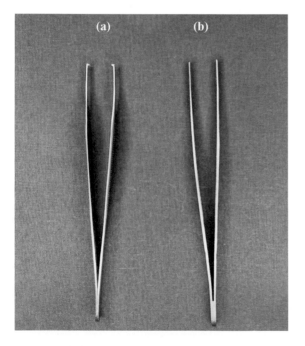

Figure 8.52 Tissue holding forceps. (a) Toothed tissue holding forceps. (b) Non-toothed tissue holding forceps.

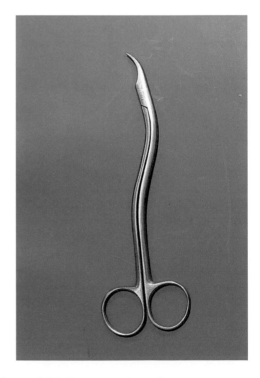

Figure 8.53 Suture cutting scissors.

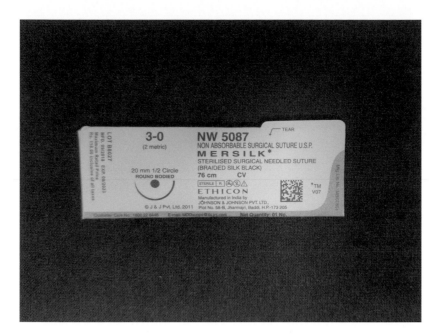

Figure 8.54 Suture material, silk (non-absorbable).

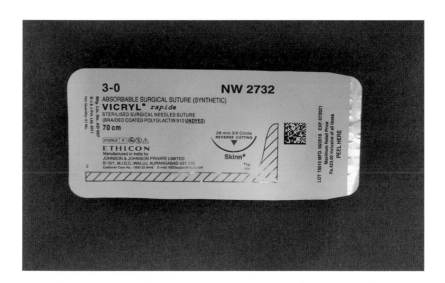

Figure 8.55 Suture material, vicryl (absorbable).

of plaque with resultant bacterial growth. *Polyglactin* 910 is a synthetic, multifilament material, which also has good handling properties. It produces less inflammatory reaction as compared to other absorbable suture material as it absorbs by hydrolysis. Further, no bacterial growth has been associated with polyglactin 910. *Knotless suture* is a special type of

suture material which has barbs incorporated along the long axis. The barbs engaged deep into the tissues and help in approximation without the need for knots.[11]

i. ***Fibrin sealant***

It is a biocompatible adhesive which can be used instead of suturing for closing the wound and requires less time for wound approximation. Fibrin sealant is prepared by mixing four components namely fibrinolysis inhibitor solution, calcium chloride, thrombin and sealer protein. It is delivered by using a specialized Duploject injection which contains thrombin and fibrinogen separately. The prepared solution can be stored for up to 4 hours.[12]

INSTRUMENTS AND MATERIALS FOR POST-OPERATIVE DRESSING

a. **Reso-pac**

It is an adhesive dressing material used to protect the surgical site following removal of impacted third molar. It acts as astringent, antiseptic as well as haemostatic agent. The composition of this material includes extracts of myrahh wood and cellulose. It does not require removal as it disintegrates by itself. It has good handling properties and gives protection to the wound against thermal and mechanical trauma.[13]

b. **Ozone gel**

Ozone gel consists of medical-grade ozone and olive oil which can be applied over the surgical wound to improve wound healing. It is reported to have anti-inflammatory, antimicrobial, anti-hypoxic, analgesic and immunogenic properties which reduce post-operative pain, trismus, and swelling.[14]

INSTRUMENTS FOR STERILIZATION AND STORAGE

Instrument preparation

All instruments must be scrubbed and cleaned well for effective sterilization as blood and mucus would not allow steam to reach microorganism. The instruments can be cleaned by either (1) Manual scrubbing of instruments using water or (2) Ultrasonic vibrations

Sterilization of instruments

- All the instruments must be autoclaved properly before surgical procedure. The various sterilization cycles employed under 15 psi pressure are 121°C for 15 minutes, 126°C for 10 minutes and 134°C for 3 minutes.

- *Sterilization of handpiece:* Handpieces should be sterilized between each patient. The steps involved in sterilization are cleaning, lubrication and autoclaving. Manufacturer's instructions must be meticulously followed for effective sterilization and longevity. The various steps involved are (1) cleaning of the handpiece with external cleaning using disinfectant solution (2) if present, flushing of the waterline attached with handpiece (3) lubricating the handpiece with recommended lubricant, running the handpiece for 30 seconds for uniform distribution and removing excess oil (4) wrapping with either paper-plastic or cloth wrapper (sterilization pouch) and (5) autoclaving. Among the different types of autoclaves such as type N (small), B (medium) and S (big), type B and S ensure complete sterilization.[15]

- *Sterilization of burs*

Surgical burs are best used on a single-use basis. However, the reuse of burs is frequently practised by many. This requires stringent roval of bone debris and sterilization by autoclaving. Repeated sterilization reduces the cutting efficiency.[16]

Monitoring the effectiveness of sterilization

Effectiveness of sterilization may be assessed using two methods; chemical and biological indicators. Chemical indicator shows the processing of instruments or completion of sterilization by change in colour when exposed to temperature of 121°C. Indicator is available in various forms such as tape, disc test pack, tube and pellet. Biological indicators come in different forms as disc, strips and pre-packed vials which consist of heat-resistant spores of *Geobacillus stearothermophilus*. After the sterilization cycle, these indicators are incubated according to manufacturer's instruction along with control indicator to check the growth of microorganism. Unlike the chemical indicator, biological indicator confirms the sterilization of the instruments.

nstrument storage

nstruments should be packed using appropriate cloth, paper pack or metal box before sterilization. They may be maintained in sterile condition for up to 30 days if stored in appropriate aseptic conditions.[17] Although it is recommended to sterilize the instruments before the planned surgical procedure.

ADVANCES

a. *Computer controlled LA delivery system*
   This device automatically regulates the pressure and amount of solution delivered to the site as the flow rate and pressure are important factors for pain perception. Devices available under this category include Wand, Compudent, Control syringe, Quicksleeper, etc. The advantages of this technique over the conventional technique are good tactile perception, precise delivery of solution and less pain, during administration.[18]

b. *LASER*
   Soft tissue diode laser is used with a wavelength ranging from 805 to 910 nm for making incision. Among the various lasers used in oral and maxillofacial surgery, the diode lasers have been found to be compact, inexpensive, portable, and more efficient. Compared to conventional scalpel, laser incision is associated with reduced post-operative pain, swelling and trismus.[19]

   Er:YAG laser is used to remove bone during impacted third molar surgery. It operates at a wavelength of 2,940 nm and provides less post-operative pain. However, instrumentation time is longer as compared to the rotary method.[20]

c. *Piezosurgery*
   It uses ultrasonic micro-vibrations (60–210 µm) with a frequency of 25–30 kHz to cut bone. The advantages are negligible soft tissue damage to vital structures such as inferior alveolar neurovascular bundle and lingual nerve and less post-operative discomfort. Longer surgical time and expense of the equipment are the limitations.[21]

d. *Surgical loupes*
   Surgical loupes have been used for third molar surgery to achieve effective magnification and visualization of surgical site and fractured roots. Light source attached to the loupes provides bright illumination without shadow.

ACKNOWLEDGEMENT

The authors wish to thank the contribution of Dr. Meghana for facilitating and providing the figures for the chapter.

REFERENCES

1. Synan W, Stein K. Management of impacted third molars. *Oral Maxillofac Surg Clin North Am.* 2020 Nov;32(4):519–559.
2. Malamed SF. *Handbook of Local Anesthesia*, 7th ed. St. Louis, MO: Elsevier, 2013, pp. 86–89.
3. Rao HBS, Rai BG, Sinha SS. Comparison of healing process of operculectomy with laser and surgical knife – A clinical study. *Int J Curr Res* 2016;8:25368–25373.
4. Yin L, Wei L, Hong-Jiu L, An Y, You-Yong C. Contra-angle high speed turbine handpiece in the extraction of impacted mandibular third molars. *J Oral Maxillofac Surg.* 2015;25(2):134.
5. Pathak N, Shukla D, Shringarpure K, Goryawala SN. Physiodispenser versus conventional rotary instrument in transalveolar extraction of impacted mandibular third molars – A randomized controlled clinical trial. *Int J Appl Dent Sci.* 2019;5(2):45–50.
6. Vivek M, Ebenezer V, Balakrishnan R. Bur technique and chisel mallet technique in impacted 3rd molar. *Biomed Pharmacol.* 2014;7(1):281–284.
7. Howe GL. *Minor Oral Surgery*, 3rd ed. Mumbai: Varghese Publishing House, 1996, pp. 136–138.
8. Howe GL. *Minor Oral Surgery*, 3rd ed. Mumbai: Varghese Publishing House, 1996, pp. 387–388.
9. Schonauer C, Tessitore E, Barbagallo G, Albanese V, Moraci A. The use of local agents: Bone wax, gelatin, collagen, oxidized cellulose. *Eur Spine J.* 2004;13(Suppl. 1):S89–96.
10. Chandrasekhar H, Sivakumar, Santhosh MP. Comparison of influence of vicryl and silk suture materials on wound healing after third molar surgery – A review. *J Pharm Sci Res.* 2017;9:2426–2428.
11. Ramkumar Ceyar KA, Thulasidoss GP, Cheeman RS, Sagadevan S, Panneerselvam E, Krishna Kumar Raja VB. Effectiveness of knotless

suture as a wound closure agent for impacted third molar – A split mouth randomized controlled clinical trial. *J Craniomaxillofac Surg.* 2020;48(10):1004–1008.

12. Gogulanathan M, Elavenil P, Gnanam A, Raja VB. Evaluation of fibrin sealant as a wound closure agent in mandibular third molar surgery – A prospective, randomized controlled clinical trial. *Int J Oral Maxillofac Surg.* 2015;44(7):871–875.

13. Raghavan SL, Panneerselvam E, Mudigonda SK, Raja KKVB. Protection of an intraoral surgical wound with a new dressing: A randomised controlled clinical trial. *Br J Oral Maxillofac Surg.* 2020;58(7):766–770.

14. Sivalingam VP, Panneerselvam E, Raja KV, Gopi G. Does topical ozone therapy improve patient comfort after surgical removal of impacted mandibular third molar? A randomized controlled trial. *J Oral Maxillofac Surg.* 2017;75(1):51.

15. Sasaki JI, Imazato S. Autoclave sterilization of dental handpieces: A literature review. *J Prosthodont Res.* 2020;64(3):239–242.

16. Al-Jandan BA, Ahmed MG, Al-Khalifa KS, Farooq I. Should surgical burs be used as single-use devices to avoid cross infection? A case-control study. *Med Princ Pract.* 2016;25(2):159–162.

17. Moriya GA, Graziano KU. Sterility maintenance assessment of moist/wet material after steam sterilization and 30-day storage. *Rev Lat Am Enfermagem.* 2010;18:786–791.

18. Kim C, Hwang KG, Park CJ. Local anesthesia for mandibular third molar extraction. *J Dent Anesth Pain Med.* 2018;18(5):287–294.

19. Misir Mo, Sencimen M, Ozkan A, Misir SE. The effects of conventional scalpel versus diode laser incision on postoperative morbidity after impacted third molar extractions. *Dent Oral Maxillofac Res.* 2021;7:4–5.

20. Passi D, Pal US, Mohammad S, Singh RK, Mehrotra D, Singh G, Kumar M, Chellappa AA, Gupta C. Laser vs bur for bone cutting in impacted mandibular third molar surgery: A randomized controlled trial. *J Oral Biol Craniofac Res.* 2013;3(2):57–62.

21. Basheer SA, Govind RJ, Daniel A, Sam G, Adarsh VJ, Rao A. Comparative study of piezoelectric and rotary osteotomy technique for third molar impaction. *J Contemp Dent Pract.* 2017;18(1):60–64.

9

Principles and flaps for mandibular third molar surgery

DARPAN BHARGAVA

INTRODUCTION

The surgical practice of minor oral surgery including exodontia is based on sound principles for the use of instrumentation and the execution of the procedures. A single or a combination of these described criteria, when utilized appropriately with a thorough understanding, induce enhanced surgical outcomes with greater patient satisfaction.

PRINCIPLES OF TOOTH EXTRACTION

Tooth extraction should include the removal of tooth or root as a whole without extensive injury to the investing soft and hard tissues surrounding the tooth. The three principles involved in exodontia are mentioned below [1,2,3,4]:

1. Expansion of the bony socket
2. Use of lever and fulcrum
3. Insertion of wedge and wedges

Expansion of the bony socket: This permits the removal of tooth by using the tooth itself as the dilating instrument. To remove a tooth completely using forceps, the sufficient structure of the tooth should be present, i.e., the crown portion, for the forceps beak to grasp the tooth. The beaks of the forceps should be placed to firmly grasp the tooth with apical pressure in order to expand the surrounding bone. The tooth can dilate the bone and

aid in delivery from the socket only if the bone is adequately elastic. The prescribed bucco-palatal or bucco lingual tractional forces before the tooth extraction aid in bone expansion (Figure 9.1).

Sometimes the extraction is accompanied by micro-fractures of the buccal cortical plate or the inter-radicular bone. These minute fracture fragments have attached periosteum over them. Socket compression with digital pressure post-extraction helps in maintaining the adherence of the

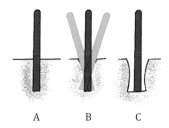

A   B   C

Expansion of the socket

Figure 9.1 Expansion of the elastic bone using the tooth as a post may be understood with this example. The removal of a post embedded in wet mud or clay. (a) Can be easily done by moving the post laterally. (b) To displace the mud or clay to make room for the post removal. (c) Displaced mud or clay, with space around the post. Although in exodontia, the root morphology and the consistency of the enclosing bone will limit or prevent lateral movements. The bucco lingual or bucco-palatal traction mauver aids in expanding the bone.

DOI: 10.1201/9781003324034-9

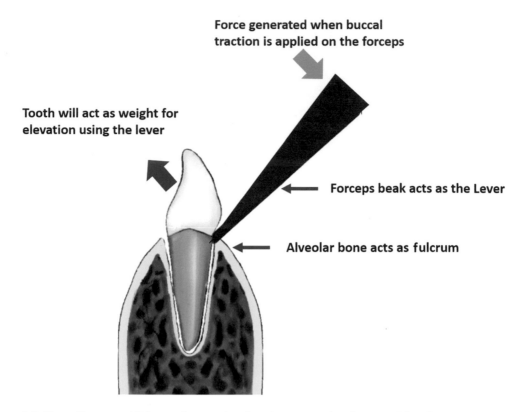

Force generated when buccal traction is applied on the forceps

Tooth will act as weight for elevation using the lever

Forceps beak acts as the Lever

Alveolar bone acts as fulcrum

Figure 9.2 Use of lever and fulcrum for exodontia using extraction forceps. The diagram represents the input force on the forceps handle during buccal/labial traction causing the resultant force that is generated at the beak which acts as the lever utilizing the alveolar bone as fulcrum. Similar effect would be observed on the other beak of the same forceps on the palatal or lingual side when palatal or lingual traction is applied.

periosteal layer to the bony fragment, thus regaining the integrity of the bony socket. Any loose bony fragment detached from its periosteum should be cleaned after tooth removal to avoid delayed wound healing as they may act as the source for infection.

Use of lever and fulcrum: This principle aids to force a tooth or root out of the socket along the path of least resistance. The use of lever utilizing an appropriate fulcrum (usually the alveolar bone) forms the basis for governing the use of elevators and also the forceps to extract a tooth and/or root. The handles represent the power or force, beaks grasping the tooth or the root represents the weight and the bone acts as a fulcrum. Lever principle involves the application of modest force which is transmitted through the handles of the forceps (Figure 9.2).

Insertion of wedge or wedges: Insertion of a wedge between the tooth and the bony wall of socket causes the tooth to rise in its socket. The point at the forceps beak creates a wedging effect aiding in tooth delivery (Figures 9.3 and 9.4).

Dental extraction forceps is the most versatile instrument to remove teeth in routine clinical practice. It is essential to be proficient in using forceps for closed or non-surgical extractions before attempting to master the art of complicated exodontia and the use of elevators for tooth removal. For the extraction of the mandibular third molar with favourable path of exit in a closed manner using forceps, the mesial application of straight elevator often facilitates forceps extraction. This is often attempted in case of vertically erupted third molars having convergent or single root. After the application of the elevator, mandibular third molar forceps or the mandibular molar forceps is applied along the long axis of the tooth firmly grasping at the cemento enamel area, with a rotatory or figure-of-eight motion that expands the socket and aids in extraction. Buccal traction is generally avoided as the buccal cortex is quite thick in this region. Also, the external oblique ridge adds extra strength to the thick buccal

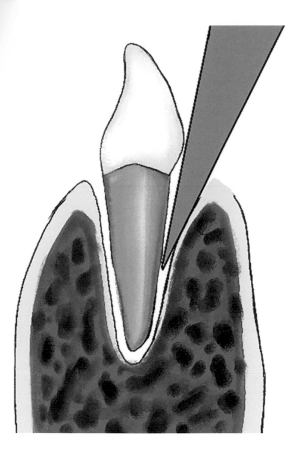

Figure 9.3 Insertion of a wedge in between the alveolar bone and the tooth.

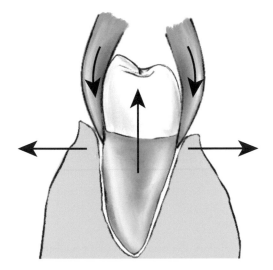

Figure 9.4 The wedging effect of the forceps beaks during exodontia.

cortex. Lingual traction is avoided to prevent fracture of the lingual plate and nerve injury to the adjacent lingual nerve.

USE OF DENTAL ELEVATORS FOR THIRD MOLAR SURGERY

Elevators are applied at a 45° angulation between the alveolar bone and the tooth or root either buccally, mesially or distally taking buccal or distal alveolar bone or interdental bone as a fulcrum to luxate the tooth out of the socket. Impacted third molars do not sustain much occlusal load, do have a wider periodontal ligament space and are generally less adherent to the surrounding bone when compared to the erupted third molars. This aids in easy displacement of the tooth or root using elevators from the socket after removing a sufficient amount of covering bone. One should be cautious in applying the right amount of force in the right direction while using elevators to prevent unwanted damage to the hard and soft tissues surrounding the tooth. The elevator should be grasped and the index finger should be used to take finger rest over the alveolar bone to provide complete control to the operator.

Elevators can be used to luxate and remove impacted, malposed, fractured or carious tooth which cannot be engaged using forceps, remove sectioned or fractured roots engaging the buccal or distal alveolar bone, inter-radicular or interdental bone as fulcrum.

Basic rules for use of elevators

1. Do not use the adjacent tooth as fulcrum unless that tooth also has to be extracted.
2. Do not use buccal plate at the gingival line as fulcrum point except when odontectomy is performed.
3. Avoid using lingual plate as the fulcrum point.
4. The concave or the flat surface of the tip should face the tooth or the root which is to be extracted.
5. Use finger guard, where possible, to prevent injury to the adject tissues in case the elevator slips.
6. Caution should be taken during elevator application and ensure that the tip of the elevator is exerting optimum pressure in the correct direction.

Parts of an elevator

The elevators have the following parts

a. Handle – part of elevator that is continuous from the shank or at the right angle to provide the grip to deliver adequate force.
b. Shank connects the handle with the working blade/tip and transmits the applied force from the handle to the blade.
c. Blade/tip – the working end that engages the area between the bone and the crown/root to transmit the force and gain the desired action.

Types of elevators and their indications

The elevators can be classified based on their use or their form summarized in Table 9.1 and Figure 9.5.

Principles in use of elevators

The work principles as applied to the use of elevators in oral surgery are based on the lever, the wedge, the wheel and axle or a combination of any two or more of the above.

1. **Lever principle:** This is the commonly employed work principle in the use of elevators. The elevator is a lever of first class. In a first-class lever, the fulcrum position is between the effort (E) and the resistance (R). To gain mechanical advantage, the effort arm on one side of the fulcrum must be longer than the resistance arm on the other side of fulcrum (Figure 9.6).

   Formula for Lever: $R \times SA = LA \times E$ (where R: Resistance; E: Effort; SA: Short Arm; LA: Long Arm)

   The standard prototype downward input force of 10 lb acting at the end of the long arm results in output force of 30 lb at the end of the short arm (William Harry Archer, 1975).

Table 9.1 Dental elevators used for exodontia

Elevator	Uses
Straight elevator	Luxate entire tooth (engaging the mesial space between the tooth and the interdental bone)
Coupland elevator	Luxate entire tooth from the buccal gutter where the buccal bone is thick acting as fulcrum to elevate the tooth
Apexo elevators (Standard Hu-Friedy no. 301, Schmeckebier no. 4 and no. 5)	Removal of root separated from the crown at the gingival line
Cryer elevators (right and left[a])	To remove roots broken off halfway at apex engaging the inter-radicular bone from the empty socket of one root (mesial or distal) To elevate lower third molars engaging the furcation area taking the thick buccal bone as fulcrum
Winter's cross bar elevators (right and left[a])	Removal of broken roots which may be apical one-third or apical two third same as Cryer elevators
Root tip elevators/apical fragment ejectors	Removal of apical third of root as in the case of horizontal impaction
Periosteal elevator	To raise mucoperiosteal flap
Elevators can also be classified based on the form and design as follows:	
Based on form	Type/character of elevator
Straight	Wedge type (straight)
Angular	Right and left[a]
Cross bar	Handle at right angle to shank

[a] Right or left *do not* denote the quadrant on which the surgery is proposed. Directions denote the curvature of the tip, working tip is angulated with one convex and another flatter or convex surface. Both the instruments in a set may find its utility in the same quadrant (Figure 9.5).

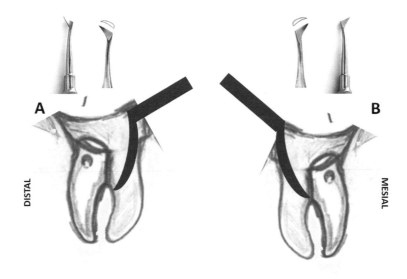

Figure 9.5 Utilization of paired Cryer elevator set for root elevation. In the same dental quadrant. (a) One from the set may be used for distal root elevation. (b) Other from the set may be utilized for mesial root elevation.

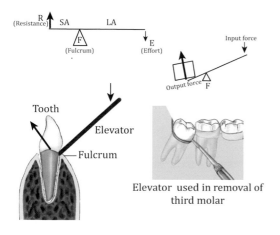

Lever work principle as applied for tooth removal

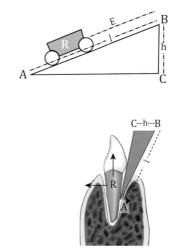

Figure 9.6 Lever principle for the use of dental elevators for exodontia. Note the short resistance arm (SA) and the long effort arm (LA).

Figure 9.7 Wedge principle. Each pound of pressure applied is multiplied by 2.5. (Mechanical advantage is 2.5 times the applied force.)

Mechanical Advantage: Output Force/Input Force = 30 lb/10 lb = 3

2. **Wedge principle:** Some elevators primarily can be used based on the wedge principle such as Apexo elevators. They are also referred to as wedge elevators. These elevators are forced between the tooth root and the investing bony tissue parallel

to the long axis of the root, either by hand pressure or mallet force. Wedges are mostly used in conjunction with lever principle (Figure 9.7).

Wedging principle finds its application with the use of chisel and osteotomes. While using a chisel a movable inclined plane overcomes a

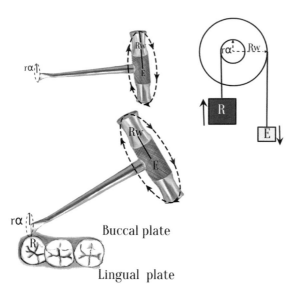

Wheel and axle principle as applied in the use of
cross bar elevator

Figure 9.8 Wheel and axle principle. Note that
each pound of pressure applied to the cross bar
is multiplied 4.6 times.

large resistance at right angles to the applied
effort (tapping with a mallet). The effort is
applied to the plane base and the resistance has
its slant effect on the side at the tip. Osteotomes
are instruments having two inclined planes
placed in a base-to-base manner. The sharper
the angle of wedge, the less effort is required to
overcome a given resistance.

Formula for wedge: $E \times l = R \times h$ (or)
$R/E = l/h$ (where, R: Resistance; E: Effort; l:
Length; h: Height)

Assuming standard prototype: $l = 10\,mm$,
$h = 4\,mm$; Mechanical advantage $l/h = 10/4 = 2.5$
(William Harry Archer, 1975)

Mechanical Advantage: $l/h = 2.5$

3. *Wheel and axle principle*: It is a simple
   machine, a modified form of lever. The effort
   is usually applied to the wheel circumference
   which turns the axle so as to raise the weight.
   The effort arm is Rw and the resistance arm
   is rα (Figure 9.8). It can be used as a sole
   principle to extract tooth, although it may be
   utilized in conjunction with wedge or lever
   principle.

   Formula for Wheel and Axle Principle:
   Effort × Radius of the
   Wheel = Resistance × Radius of Axle

   $R/E = Rw/r\alpha$ (where R: Resistance; E: Effort;
   Rw: Radius of Wheel; rα: Radius of Axle)

Assuming standard prototype: Rw = 42 mm;
rα = 9 mm; Mechanical advantage Rw/
rα = 42/9 = 4.6 (William Harry Archer, 1975)

Mechanical Advantage = 4.6

Each pound of pressure applied to the cross
bar is multiplied 4.6 times. Utilization of the
wheel and axle principle produces the maximum mechanical advantage resulting in the
enhanced forces that are delivered at the working blade of the elevator that may even result in
bone fracture. The cross bar elevator that works
on the wheel and axle principle should be used
with due caution (Figure 9.8).

Two major concerns while using the
elevators are the amount of force generated
on the jaws/tooth and slippage of the instrument. The jaws must be supported to prevent
bone fracture or dislocation during the use
of elevators. The surrounding soft and hard
tissues must be protected from potential damage by accidental slippage. Protection can be
achieved using continuous careful controlled
directional force that is applied to the bone
surrounding the tooth or against the tooth
being luxated.

While extracting the lower third molars
in the fourth quadrant the thumb and the
index fingers should grasp the alveolus and
the rest three fingers are used to support
the mandible from beneath with the non-
dominant hand. In third quadrant, the index
finger and the second finger should grasp the
alveolus and the thumb is placed beneath the
mandible. The instrument is grasped with
the dominant hand.

FLAPS FOR THE MANDIBULAR THIRD MOLAR EXTRACTION

An important step in transalveolar extraction (TAE)
of mandibular third molar extractions is the reflection of the mucoperiosteal flap for a successful,
uneventful procedure right from the start up till the
complete healing of the wound. The surgeon should
handle the soft tissues with all caution when reflecting, retracting and closing the flap. The flaps should
be designed in such a manner that it renders good visibility and accessibility to the area of operation [2,3,4].

Mucoperiosteal flaps for mandibular third
molar surgery are primarily classified as envelope, triangular, and trapezoidal flaps. Although
there are numerous proposed variations and flap

Table 9.2 Classification of flaps

Based on thickness	Based on side of reflection	Based on placing releasing incision
Full thickness	Buccal flap	Envelope flap
Partial thickness[a]	Lingual flap	Two-sided triangular flap
		Three-sided or four-cornered trapezoidal flap
		Semilunar flap

[a] As a conventional practice for the removal of the mandibular third molars, a full thickness mucoperiosteal flap is reflected.

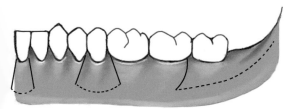

Appropriate flap design

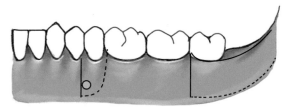

Inappropriately designed flaps

Mandibular mucoperiosteal flap

Figure 9.9 In an appropriately designed flap the base should be broader than the free end to ensure adequate blood supply.

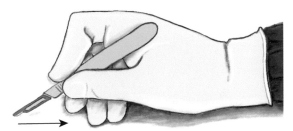

Scapl pen grasp and direction of use

Figure 9.10 Pen grasp and smooth firm stroke while using the no. #15 bard parker blade on a no. #3 handle.

designs, the summary of classification is presented in Table 9.2.

The flap should follow basic principles for its viability and efficacy listed as follows:

1. The base of the flap should be broader than the free end to ensure adequate blood supply (Figure 9.9).
2. Flap should be made according to the requirement of soft tissue reflection for proper visualization. Full thickness flaps are preferred. Partial thickness flaps tend to bleed more. Also, the periosteal coverage over the postsurgical defect aids in bone healing. Accurate and surgically feasible anatomic apposition of the soft tissue should be achieved at the end of the procedure.
3. The incision should lie upon healthy bone whenever possible.
4. Where feasible in the design, a long straight incision is preferred as they heal faster.
5. The incision should be placed firmly through mucosa and periosteum to the bone through a smooth firm stroke.
6. Pen grasp for holding the bard parker blade handle is recommended while placing the incision (Figure 9.10).
7. The soft tissue has to be cut perpendicular to the underlying bone. The mucoperiosteal flap should be reflected from the bone using gentle pressure in order to raise a full thickness flap and prevent tear.
8. Careful reflection and handling of the flap is mandatory to avoid any perforation or button hole (Figure 9.11).

Free end

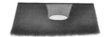

Base

A "button hole" defect in a mandibular flap results in the compromise of the blood supply in the shaded region superior to the defect

Figure 9.11 A button hole defect results in compromised blood supply.

Types of incision for mandibular third molar surgery

There are several types and the modifications of the incision and the flap design are described in the literature (Figure 9.12). Generally, the most common incisions preferred for the mandibular third molar surgery are Ward's incision or the modified Ward's incision (Figure 9.13).

Ward's incision: Standard Ward's incision starts 6 mm anterior and inferiorly to the junction of anterior two-thirds and distal one-third of mandibular second molar at the attached gingival

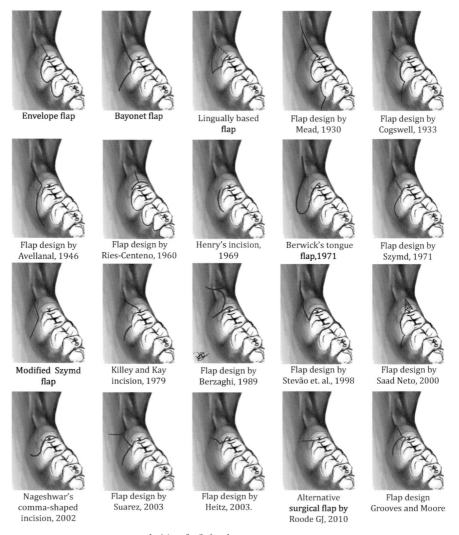

Envelope flap   Bayonet flap   Lingually based flap   Flap design by Mead, 1930   Flap design by Cogswell, 1933

Flap design by Avellanal, 1946   Flap design by Ries-Centeno, 1960   Henry's incision, 1969   Berwick's tongue flap,1971   Flap design by Szymd, 1971

Modified Szymd flap   Killey and Kay incision, 1979   Flap design by Berzaghi, 1989   Flap design by Stevão et. al., 1998   Flap design by Saad Neto, 2000

Nageshwar's comma-shaped incision, 2002   Flap design by Suarez, 2003   Flap design by Heitz, 2003.   Alternative surgical flap by Roode GJ, 2010   Flap design Grooves and Moore

Incisions for 3rd molar surgery

Figure 9.12 Summary of various incisions described for transalveolar extraction of the mandibular third molars.

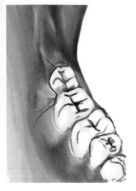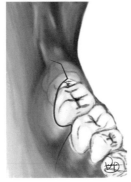

Ward's incision   Modified Ward's

Common incisions for 3rd molar surgery

Figure 9.13 Ward's and modified Ward's incision for transalveolar extraction of the mandibular third molars. In general, modified Ward's incision is employed for situations requiring relatively more exposure of the surgical site.

region with an anterior slant to keep the base of the intended flap broad (without involving the distal papilla of the second molar in the incision, but incorporating it in the flap). The incision is taken upwards to the marginal gingiva of the second molar at the point of distal one-third of the tooth and runs cervically involving distal one-third of the second molar and the third molar if completely erupted or at the midpoint of the third molar in partially or unerupted tooth. The incision from this distal point of the tooth is then taken posteriorly and buccally along the external oblique ridge. The mucoperiosteum is then raised from the anterior portion of the incision, using the sharp end of the periosteal elevator, advancing posteriorly exposing the distal bone to the third molar over the ascending ramus (Figure 9.13).

Modified Ward's incision: For a modified Ward's incision, which is generally indicated for a larger exposure, the incision starts at the mesial aspect of the distal papilla of the first molar (without involving the papilla in the incision, but incorporating it in the flap) (Figure 9.13).

A variety of techniques have been described regarding variations in flap designs for impacted mandibular third molar extraction but trapezoidal and triangular flap remains to be the most common considered flaps in routine clinical practice. The surgical variation between various flap designs is the difference in the extent of surgical site exposure and the post-operative outcome. The operating surgeon should have a thorough knowledge of different types of flaps and should be skilful enough to practice and advocate appropriate techniques in day-to-day practice to execute the procedure uneventfully, as each flap design has its own advantages and disadvantages.

PRINCIPLES OF SUTURING

After removal of the tooth from the socket, sutures may be indicated for approximation of the mucoperiosteal flap for holding the cut edges together to promote healing, control haemorrhage and prevent wound contamination. Usually, 3–0 silk with a swaged reverse cutting or a round body 3/8 circle (22 mm) needle is preferred by most surgeons. The choice of absorbable suture material is polygalactin 910 (copolymer of 90% glycolide and 10% l-lactide) [4].

Principles of suturing should be followed to achieve felicitous closure of the wound [1,2,3,4]:

1. The needle should be grasped with the needle holder at two third of the needle curvature (junction of anterior two-thirds and posterior one-third of the needle), preventing the eye/point or the swaged end (Figure 9.14).
2. The needle should enter perpendicular to the tissue, at an equal depth and distance (minimum 3 mm) on both the flaps to prevent tear of the flap by entering through the smallest point.
3. The needle should pass first from the mobile tissues (buccal flap) to the fixed (attached tissue of the lingual papilla) flap for the ease of rotation of the needle along its curvature.
4. The needle should be passed through the individual flap by grasping the flap with the (toothed) tissue holding forceps one at a time for accurate localization of the second puncture.
5. Sutures should always be placed on the tissues overlying healthy bone (preferably papilla distal to second molars and over posterior extension of the incision line) to support wound edges. The suture distal to the second molar is

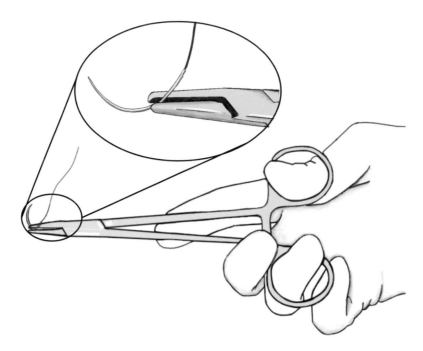

Figure 9.14 Needle grasp with the needle holder. Note the fingers utilized to hold the needle holder. The needle should be grasped more towards the tip of the beaks of the needle holder at the junction of anterior two-thirds and posterior one-third of the needle.

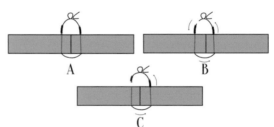

A) Intraoral silk suture is loose and impregnated with detritus in the oral cavity

B) If the suture is cut just below the knot the wound is contaminated as the infected silk is pulled through the tissue

C) This problem can be avoided if suture is pulled and cut as it enters the tissue

Figure 9.15 Knot should be grasped and the thread should be cut where it enters the tissues (A–C).

vital, for the prevention of periodontal pocket distal to the second molar.

6. Sutures should always be tied tight enough to just reapproximate both flaps. Too tight closure of the sutures may cause ischaemia of the margins of the flap resulting in necrosis and wound dehiscence.

7. The knot of the suture should be positioned away from the incision line.

8. Suture removal should be done after 5–7 days postoperatively. Contaminated sutures with debris should be cleaned with a cotton tip applicator soaked in antiseptic solution.

9. While removing the sutures the knot should be grasped and the thread should be cut where it enters the tissues, preventing the contaminated thread from entering the tissue while removal (Figure 9.15).

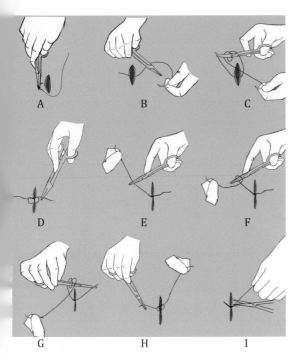

Suturing utilizing instrument to tie the knot:
A, B: The tip of the needle holder is pointed at the needle and passed over the silk twice
C, D: The tip of the short end of the silk is grasped and drawn through the loops
E,F: The needle holder is pointed towards the needle again and passed under the silk once or twice
G: The tip of the short end is then grasped and pulled through the loops, thus completing the knot
H: The loose ends are used to draw the knot to one side of the suture line
I: The suture is cut with scissors

Figure 9.16 Standard simple interrupted suturing technique (steps demonstrated in A–I).

The standard technique recommended for placing the simple interrupted sutures after the mandibular transalveolar extraction of the impacted third molars is summarized in Figure 9.16.

ERGONOMICS

This section provides a brief general overview regarding the patient and the operator positions for dental extraction procedure with variations utilized for the third molar mandibular extractions.

For extracting a tooth from the maxilla, the dental chair should be reclined backwards and

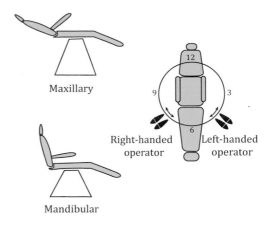

Figure 9.17 Chair positioning for exodontia.

the maxillary occlusal plane should be at 60° to the floor. The height of the chair should be such that the site of the operation is 8 cm (3 in.) below the shoulder level of the operator. In general, to remove a mandibular tooth, the patient should be positioned such that the occlusal plane is parallel to the floor. The height should be adjusted such that the tooth to be extracted is 16 cm (6 in.) below the operator's elbow. The chair should be placed upright and the patient is positioned at 90°. For the surgical or open extraction of the mandibular third molar, the backrest of the chair may be reduced from 90°, to a more comfortable 60° to 80° incline for better visibility and access to the posterior areas of the oral cavity.

For all the maxillary anterior teeth, posterior teeth, and teeth in the third quadrant, a right-handed operator should stand at the 7'o clock position (5'o clock for the left-handed operator). For extracting in the fourth quadrant, the operator should stand in 11'o clock position (2'o clock for the left-handed operator) (Figure 9.17). Although most right-handed operators prefer to operate standing or sitting on the right side of the patient while performing the transalveolar mandibular extractions (left for left-handed operators). On occasions, the left side operator position is preferred by some right-handed surgeons for better visibility and access for the third quadrant impacted mandibular third molar surgery (similarly a right seating or standing left-handed operator position for the fourth quadrant impacted mandibular third molars). Note the operator positions that may be utilized for exodontia in Figure 9.18.

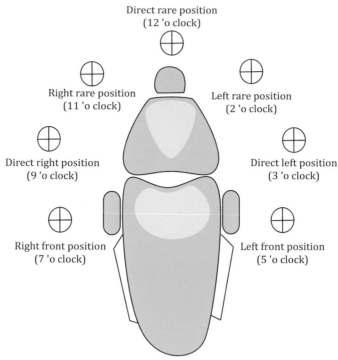

Direct rare position
(12 'o clock)

Right rare position
(11 'o clock)

Left rare position
(2 'o clock)

Direct right position
(9 'o clock)

Direct left position
(3 'o clock)

Right front position
(7 'o clock)

Left front position
(5 'o clock)

Operator positions for tooth extraction

Figure 9.18 Operator positions for exodontia.

It remains the surgeon's preference to operate while sitting on the operating stool or perform the procedure while standing at the prescribed operator position. Appropriate adjustable lighting to illuminate the surgical field and a reasonable surgical suction apparatus is vital for a methodological execution of the procedure in the posterior areas of the oral cavity. The operator's appropriate posture of the back and the neck is vital to limit occupational injury. Following the prescribed principles of ergonomics minimizes musculoskeletal injury to the operator.

REFERENCES

1. Howe GL. *Minor Oral Surgery*. London: Wright, 1966.
2. MacGregor AJ. *The Impacted Lower Wisdom Tooth*. Oxfordshire: Oxford University Press, 1985.
3. Hupp JR, Ellis III E, Tucker ER. *Contemporary Oral and Maxillofacial Surgery*, 7th ed. Philadelphia: Elsevier, 2019.
4. Miloro M, Ghali GE, Larsen PE, Waite PD. *Peterson's Principles of Oral and Maxillofacial Surgery*, 3rd ed. Cham: People's Medical Publishing House, 2011.

10

Surgical techniques for transalveolar extraction of the mandibular third molars

DARPAN BHARGAVA

ASEPSIS AND PATIENT PREPARATION

Transalveolar extraction (TAE) is a technique where the tooth or/and root are surgically separated from its surrounding bone and the soft tissue attachments with the use of appropriate armamentarium. To perform an uneventful surgical extraction, selection of appropriate local anaesthesia (LA) and treatment plan is essential to avoid any potential complication. Various steps should be taken into consideration such as recording the relevant medical history of the patient; clinical and radiological evaluation to assess the surgical difficulty index; selecting an appropriate mucoperiosteal incision and flap; amount of bone removal required; the technique and the instrumentation required to facilitate the delivery of the tooth/root from its socket, wound debridement and wound closure for an uneventful procedure. The patient should be explained about the procedure and the related post-operative complications, so as to ensure smooth rapport during and after the procedure as the "patient co-operation" is an essential factor for oral surgical procedures.

The patient position should be comfortable for both the patient and the operator. A strict aseptic protocol should be followed including sterilization of the surrounding and the instrumentation.

Extra-oral povidone iodine painting and isolation with sterile drapes should be done, before initiating the procedure. Intra-oral preparation is done using chlorhexidine/povidone iodine mouthrinse followed by administration of local anaesthetic injection [1–3].

LOCAL ANAESTHESIA

Achieving an adequate regional anaesthesia is essential to perform a pain-free procedure. LA [Lignocaine Hydrochloride 2%] with adrenaline (1:200,000) is commonly used for tooth extraction procedures, so as to achieve adequate anaesthesia and to minimize bleeding. Inferior Alveolar Nerve Block (IANB) which comprises of the inferior alveolar and lingual block along with the long buccal nerve block should be administered preferably using a 23 G long needle. Approximately 1.5–2 mL of solution should be deposited in the pterygomandibular space and 0.3–0.5 mL for the long buccal nerve block, which will provide desired anaesthesia. Various documented techniques for inferior alveolar nerve anaesthesia that may be utilized for transalveolar extraction of mandibular third molars are summarized in Table 10.1 [1].

Another recently proposed modified LA is the use of twin-mix (TM) solution, which is LA admixed with 4 mg dexamethasone. It can be

DOI: 10.1201/9781003324034-10

Table 10.1 Various documented techniques for inferior alveolar nerve anaesthesia

Conventional inferior alveolar nerve block (direct technique; Halstead block)

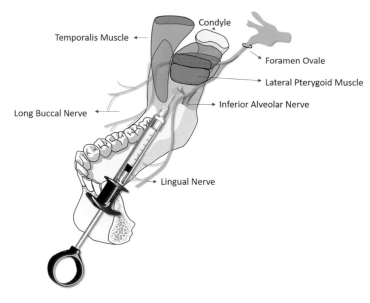

The vital clinical landmarks for this technique are the coronoid notch and pterygomandibular raphe. The insertion point is located ¾ distance down the line drawn from the deepest part of the pterygomandibular raphe to the coronoid notch (lateral to the raphe). The needle must be advanced until the bone is contacted. Aspiration is mandatory preceding to administration of the local anaesthetics.

Figure 10.1 Conventional inferior alveolar nerve block (IANB). (Adapted with permission from Tsukimoto S, Takasugi Y, Aoki R, Kimura M, Konishi T. Inferior alveolar nerve block using the anterior technique to anaesthetize buccal nerve and improve anaesthesia success rates for third molar extraction: A randomized controlled trial and magnetic resonance imaging evaluation. *J Oral Maxillofac Surg.* 2019 Oct;77(10):2004–16.)

Gow–Gates technique

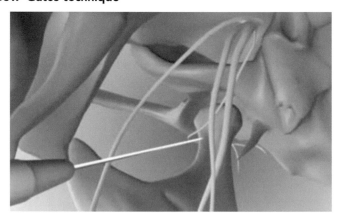

The needle is positioned just inferior to the mesiolingual cusp of the upper second molar and advanced slowly until it makes bony contact at the anteriomedial condylar neck. As the insertion height of this technique is higher from the occlusal plane of the mandible than that of the conventional inferior alveolar nerve block, the Gow–Gates technique anaesthetizes the inferior alveolar, mental, incisor, lingual, mylohyoid, auriculotemporal, and buccal nerves.

Figure 10.2 Final needle placement for the Gow–Gates technique. The needle tip is positioned at the neck of the condyle. (Adapted with permission from Haas DA. Alternative mandibular nerve block techniques: A review of the Gow-Gates and Akinosi-Vazirani closed-mouth mandibular nerve block techniques. *J Am Dent Assoc.* 2011 Sep;142(Suppl. 3):8S–12S. doi: 10.14219/jada. archive.2011.0341.)

(Continued)

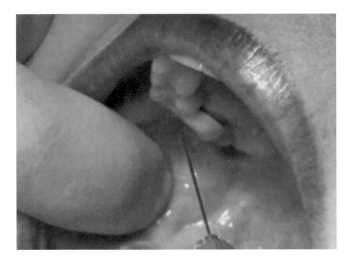

Figure 10.3 Needle insertion point for the Gow–Gates technique. (Adapted with permission from Haas DA. Alternative mandibular nerve block techniques: A review of the Gow-Gates and Akinosi-Vazirani closed-mouth mandibular nerve block techniques. *J Am Dent Assoc.* 2011 Sep;142(Suppl. 3):8S–12S. doi: 10.14219/jada.archive.2011.0341.)

Fischer 1–2–3 technique (indirect technique)

For this technique, the anaesthetic is injected using three different needle positions. To achieve buccal anaesthesia, the needle is first positioned on the midpoint of the thumbnail when the thumb is placed on the external oblique from over the contralateral premolars and inserted to a depth of about 6 mm. Then, the needle is pulled out and moved to the same side so that the needle slides onto the internal oblique ridge. The syringe is maintained parallel to the mandible occlusal plane and the needle is advanced about 8 mm. Then, the syringe is repositioned over the opposite first premolar and the needle is advanced 12–15 mm until the tip makes contact with bone. The needle should be withdrawn a bit for supra-periosteal deposition and aspiration done before the anaesthetic is injected.

(Continued)

Akinosi–Vazirani closed-mouth mandibular nerve block technique

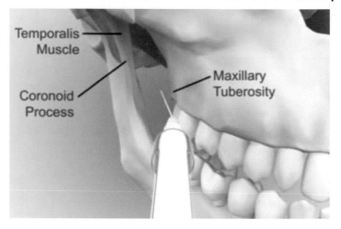

In a closed mouth, needle is positioned parallel to the occlusal plane. The needle is inserted (up to 1 ¼ in.) medial to the ramus while keeping the syringe at the level of muco-gingival junction of maxillary molars and the solution is deposited after multiple aspirations.

Figure 10.4 Bony landmarks for the Akinosi–Vazirani closed-mouth technique insertion. The needle tip position is within the pterygomandibular space. (Adapted with permission from Haas DA. Alternative mandibular nerve block techniques: A review of the Gow-Gates and Akinosi-Vazirani closed-mouth mandibular nerve block techniques. *J Am Dent Assoc.* 2011 Sep;142(Suppl. 3):8S–12S. doi: 10.14219/jada.archive.2011.0341.)

Kurt Thoma technique for mandibular anaesthesia (extra-oral technique)

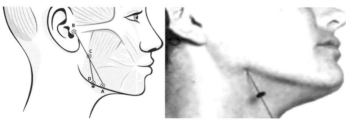

Figure 10.5 Surface marking for the Kurt Thoma technique and demonstration of needle insertion. A: Lowest point on the anterior aspect of the masseter; B: Tragus; C: Midpoint of line AB; D: CD is parallel to the posterior border of ascending ramus; point marked in red (inferior and medial to D) corresponds to the needle insertion point medial to the lower border of the mandible. Point C corresponds to the approximate location of the mandibular foramen and the lingula.

As the patient clenches the teeth, the lowest point on the anterior border of masseter muscle is located. A line is drawn from this point to the tragus of the ear. The midpoint of this line marks externally the mandibular foramen. A line is drawn from this point parallel with posterior border of the mandible up to the lower border. This line is measured and a long 21 gauge (preferably spinal) needle of 6–8 cm length is marked to a similar length using a rubber stopper. The long needle is now inserted into the inner aspect of lower border of the mandible. The needle is gradually inserted parallel along the line marked on the skin of the external surface of the mandible. As the needle approaches the depth indicated by the marker, opposite the point marked on the skin overlying the position of the foramen the solution is slowly injected.

(Continued)

Extra-oral mandibular nerve block (sub-zygomatic approach)

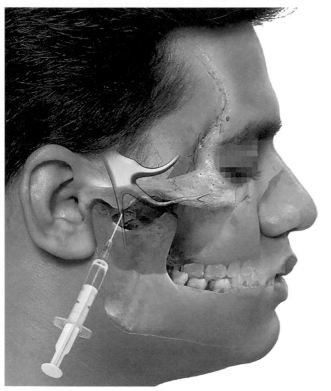

The clinical landmarks include the area below the zygomatic arch anterior to the articular eminence. This corresponds to the region above the midpoint of the sigmoid notch of the mandible. A 25-gauge 90-mm-long spinal needle is preferred for this method; the needle is inserted to a depth of about 45 mm till it contacts the lateral side of the lateral pterygoid plate. Following this, the needle is withdrawn half way and turned posteriorly by 15° to the same depth of 45 mm. This area corresponds to the region just caudal to the foramen ovale through which the mandibular nerve trunk exits the skull base. After negative aspiration, a volume of 2.5–3 mL is injected to anaesthetize the mandibular nerve.

Figure 10.6 Extra-oral technique: Needle insertion for extra-oral mandibular nerve block. (Adapted from John RR. Local anaesthesia in oral and maxillofacial surgery. In: Bonanthaya K, Panneerselvam E, Manuel S, Kumar VV, Rai A (eds) *Oral and Maxillofacial Surgery for the Clinician*. Singapore: Springer, 2021.)

administered as 1.8 mL of 2% lignocaine with 1:200,000 epinephrine admixed with 1 mL of 4 mg dexamethasone solution as an intra-space injection i.e., in pterygomandibular space. Twin-mix solution for mandibular anaesthesia has demonstrated and is clinically proven to reduce post-operative pain, swelling and discomfort significantly. Quality of life-related studies has demonstrated that patients who receive TM solution have better post-operative outcomes as compared to those who receive conventional LA [4,5]. The contraindication to the use of steroids should be considered, while using TM solution as an anaesthetic.

Composition of the standard multi-dose vials of the local anaesthetic solution and twin-mix mandibular anaesthesia solution is summarized in Tables 10.2–10.4. The prescribed maximum recommended dose (MRD) for lignocaine remains: 7 mg/kg body weight (up to a maximum of 500 mg in 24 hours for adults) irrespective of the presence of vasoconstrictor in the solution. The previous recommendations, now not in practice, documents the MRD for lignocaine as 4.4 mg/kg body weight (up to a maximum of 300 mg/24 hours for adults) for solutions without adrenaline (vasoconstrictor) and 6.6 mg/kg body weight for solutions with a vasoconstrictor (up to a maximum of 500 mg in 24 hours for adults). The difference in dosing was considered in connotation with the fact that the vasoconstrictor would restrict the systemic absorption of lignocaine which would theoretically allow higher doses.

According to American Heart Association (AHA) and American Dental Association (ADA) guidelines, there is no contraindication to using

Table 10.2 Standard local anaesthetic solution with vasoconstrictor

2% Lignocaine Hydrochloride and 1:200,000 Adrenaline Injection

Lignocaine hydrochloride	21.3 mg/mL (equivalent to anhydrous lignocaine hydrochloride 20 mg)
Adrenaline bitartrate (vasoconstrictor)	0.009 mg/mL (equivalent to adrenaline 0.005 mg/mL)
Sodium metabisulphite (anti-oxidant for the vasoconstrictor)	0.5 mg/mL[a]
Sodium chloride (for isotonicity)	6.0 mg/mL
Methylparaben (as preservative)	1.0 mg/mL
Water for injection	q.s

Note: The composition may vary for product variants by different manufacturers.
[a] This may be replaced with potassium metabisulphite 1.2 mg/mL.

Table 10.3 Standard local anaesthetic solution without a vasoconstrictor

2% Lignocaine Hydrochloride

Lignocaine hydrochloride	21.3 mg/mL (equivalent to anhydrous lignocaine hydrochloride 20 mg/mL)
Sodium chloride (for isotonicity)	6.0 mg/mL
Methylparaben (as preservative)	1.0 mg/mL
Water for injection	q.s

Table 10.4 Formulation of 2.8 mL twin-mix solution for intra-space pterygomandibular injection

Local anaesthetic (1.8 mL) containing the following:
  Lignocaine hydrochloride IP 21.3 mg/mL (=lignocaine 20 mg/mL)
  Adrenaline (as bitartrate) IP 0.005 mg/mL
  Sodium chloride IP 6.0 mg/mL
  Sodium metabisulphite IP 0.5 mg/mL
  Methyleparaben IP 1.0 mg/mL
  Water for injection IP

Dexamethasone solution for injection (1 mL) containing the following:
  Dexamethasone sodium phosphate IP 4 mg/mL
  Sodium methylparaben IP 0.15% w/v
  Sodium propylparaben IP 0.02% w/v
  Water for injection IP q.s

Source: Adapted from Bhargava D, et al. A prospective randomized double-blind study to assess the latency and efficacy of Twin-mix and 2% lignocaine with 1:200,000 epinephrine in surgical removal of impacted mandibular third molars: A pilot study. *Oral Maxillofac Surg.* 2013;17:275–280. doi: 10.1007/s10006-012-0372-3.

a vasoconstrictor agent when administrated carefully and with preliminary aspiration. The maximum dose of adrenaline recommended along with LA for a healthy adult subject is 0.2 mg, though this can be lowered to 0.04 mg if patient has severe cardiovascular disease (ASA III and IV) [6].

INCISION AND MUCOPERIOSTEAL FLAP

The design of the elevated muco-perisoteal flaps should provide adequate visibility and accessibility to the operative site. The base of the flap should

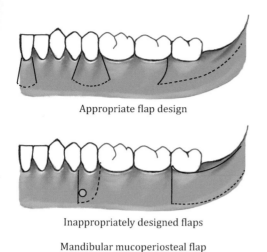

Appropriate flap design

Inappropriately designed flaps

Mandibular mucoperiosteal flap

Figure 10.7 Adequate flap design with a broad base.

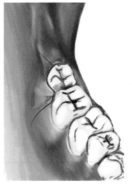 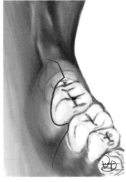

Ward's Incision

Modified Ward's Incision

Common incisions for 3rd molar surgery

Figure 10.8 Standard Ward's incision and modified Ward's incision.

be broader than the free end and should pose an unimpaired blood supply (Figure 10.7). The flap should be planned in such a manner that the healing should be promoted by accurately placing the soft tissue against each other without tension during wound closure. A firm pressure using a pen grasp should be given during incision placement through the mucosal and periosteal layers down to the bone at right angle. The flap should be elevated vertically corresponding to the tooth that needs removal by inserting the sharp end of the periosteal elevator from the mesial end, advancing to the distal end. Bone exposure can be evident if the incision is placed through both the layers of the gingiva down to the bone, else the bone can be seen covered with strands of fibrous periosteum which should be divided with scalpel before continuing to raise the flap.

The preferred surgical blade for the oral mucosal incisions for mandibular third molar surgery is #15 bard parker blade with #3 handle. The most common incision preferred for mandibular third molars is Ward's incision or the modified Ward's incision. Standard Ward's incision starts 6 mm anterior and inferiorly to the junction of anterior two-thirds and distal one-third of mandibular second molar at the attached gingival region with an anterior slant to keep the base of the intended flap broad (without involving the distal papilla of the second molar in the incision, but incorporating it in the flap). The incision is taken upwards to the marginal gingiva of the second molar at the

point of distal one-third of the tooth, and runs cervically involving distal one-third of the second molar and the third molar if completely erupted or at the midpoint of the third molar in partially or unerupted tooth. The incision from this distal point of the tooth is then taken posteriorly and buccally along the external oblique ridge. The mucoperiosteum is then raised from the anterior portion of the incision, using the sharp end of the periosteal elevator, advancing posteriorly exposing the distal bone to the third molar over the ascending ramus (Figure 10.8).

For a modified Ward's incision, which is generally indicated for a larger exposure, the incision starts at the mesial aspect of the distal papilla of the first molar (without involving the papilla in the incision, but incorporating it in the flap). There are various other types of flaps utilized for the third molar surgery which have already been discussed earlier [2,3,7,8] [refer flaps for third molar surgery; Chapter 9] (Figure 10.8).

BONE REMOVAL

The alveolar bone surrounding the tooth or root to be extracted should be adequately exposed once the flap is raised. Once a clean mucoperiosteal flap is raised, the actual depth of impaction can be determined in teeth partially embedded in bone, aiding to decide upon the amount of bone to be removed surrounding the tooth. Bone removal is essential to expose the part of tooth or root, making it free

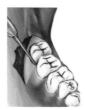

An elevator applied to an adequate mesial point of application should remain in situ without support

Figure 10.9 Elevator in situ without support to offer a purchase point for tooth removal. (Mesial point of application.)

from obstruction providing a point of application for the elevator or forceps and easing the path of removal. The space is created by making buccal and distal gutter, targeting the cervical line of the tooth and to displace the tooth/root into this created space. The buccal cortex provides major strength to the mandible. Hence, bone removal below the cervical line should be judiciously done in order to prevent fracture of the mandible from this weakened point. The bone removal is done in guttering fashion, directing the bur vertically, parallel to the long axis of the tooth. This maintains the integrity of the buccal cortex and prevents complications. Bone removal from the mesial aspect of the impacted tooth should always be precise and needs caution to prevent damage to the root of the adjacent second molar. Sufficient bone removal for creating a purchase point for elevation may be evaluated by engaging the elevator. For instance, for mesial point of elevation, the elevator should remain in situ at 45° without support (Figure 10.9). Once the tooth is extracted, the sharp edges and bony margins should be smoothened and rounded. Rongeur forceps are useful in trimming the sharp bony edges.

Bone removal can be performed either using a dental bur or a chisel and mallet. Though bone removal using sharp chisel is quick and cleaner, a dental bur is usually preferred by most of the clinicians to remove the dense bone under LA as this is more predictable with enhanced operator and patient comfort. Use of postage-stamp method may be employed using a round or flat end fissured bur to remove the bone and also to section the tooth, where required (Figure 10.10). While using a bur with a rotary mechanized instrumentation, it

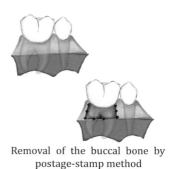

Removal of the buccal bone by postage-stamp method

Figure 10.10 Postage-stamp method.

is essential to prevent the over-heating and damage to the tissues due to the rotary friction by utilizing copious irrigation with sterile normal saline solution (NS) [2,3,7] (Table 10.5).

Bur technique: This is the standard technique followed which is also referred to as "Moore/Gillbe Collar Technique" for the removal of the impacted mandibular third molar using a bur. This technique involves sacrificing the amount of bone using a bur to facilitate the exposure of the "height of contour" of the coronal end or the crown (the most bulbous portion) of the tooth. This procedure involves the use of carbide round and tapered fissure burs with rounded tips (SS White, New Jersey, Lakewood) for bone removal and tooth sectioning. A rose-head or #8 round bur with head diameter (HD) of 2.3 mm can be first used for gross bone removal and defining the area of bone removal around the tooth. A standard fissure bur 702 (HD 1.6 mm) or 703 (HD 2.1 mm) with head length of 7 mm is used to create a "gutter" along the buccal side and the distal surface of the tooth after marking with the round bur and a space is created to displace the tooth (Figure 10.11). A 701 fissured bur with HD 1.2 mm can be used for sectioning the tooth. The lingual soft tissues should be kept protected during the procedure to prevent damage to the lingual nerve [2,3].

ALTERNATIVE TECHNIQUES FOR SPECIAL SCENARIOS

1. *"Lingual split" technique ("Kelsey Fry" or the "split bone" technique):* This is an advocated technique in young patients having elastic bone with prominent grain (trabeculae as seen on radiographs). It involves the use of chisel

Table 10.5 Bone removal

S. No.	Criteria	Chisel and mallet technique	Bur technique (with surgical rotary instrumentation)
1	Technique (based on operator's perception)	Difficult	Easy
2	Patient's acceptance	Not tolerated well when performed	Tolerated well under local anaesthesia
3	Chance of bone fracture	Relatively high	Less possibility
4	Bone healing	Good	Delayed in case of over-heating and inefficient cooling, aggravated by inefficient cutting of bone resulting in thermal necrosis
5	Post-operative oedema	Less	More
6	Dry socket	Less incidence	Relatively high, considering more debris and heat generation. If air-driven instrumentation is used, the chances of emphysema are also more[a]
7	Post-operative infection	Less	High
8	Advantage	Does not cause bone necrosis	Relatively easy to remove deep-seated impactions, impaction in edentulous jaws and geriatric patients
9	Disadvantage	• Difficult to remove deeply buried impactions, impaction in edentulous jaws and geriatric patients • Technique sensitive	Uncontrolled movement of the rotary instrument can cause damage to inferior alveolar nerves, vessels and surrounding soft tissues

[a] Can be avoided, provided proper toilet of the extraction cavity is undertaken utilizing copious saline irrigation and flushing. The intra operative heat generation should be controlled using copious saline irrigation (made cold or kept at room temperature) with the use of rotary instrumentation. In general, air-driven motors should be avoided to prevent chances of air emphysema within the tissue spaces.

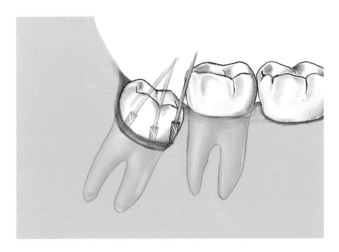

Figure 10.11 A standard fissure bur 702 (HD 1.6 mm) or 703 (HD 2.1 mm) with head length of 7 mm is used to create a "gutter" along the buccal side and the distal surface of the tooth.

and mallet to displace the lingual bone along with a portion of buccal plate to facilitate the removal of mandibular third molar. Lingual split technique was introduced in 1933 by Sir William Kelsey Fry. It was described in detail by James (1936) and Ward (1956). After raising a standard mucoperiosteal flap, a chisel is used to make a vertical stop cut about 5 mm in height and 3 mm width at the buccal cortex distal to the second molar. A second horizontal stop cut of about 4 mm is placed distobuccal

to the third molar by directing the bevel of the chisel downwards, facilitating the removal of the elastic buccal plate encasing the crown. A point of application for the elevator is made with the chisel at the mesial end where the two stop cuts meet, to elevate the tooth. The disto-lingual bone is fractured inwards by directing the chisel from lingual to buccal at 45° angle directing towards the lower second premolar. While making the lingual split care should be taken to direct the edge of the chisel parallel

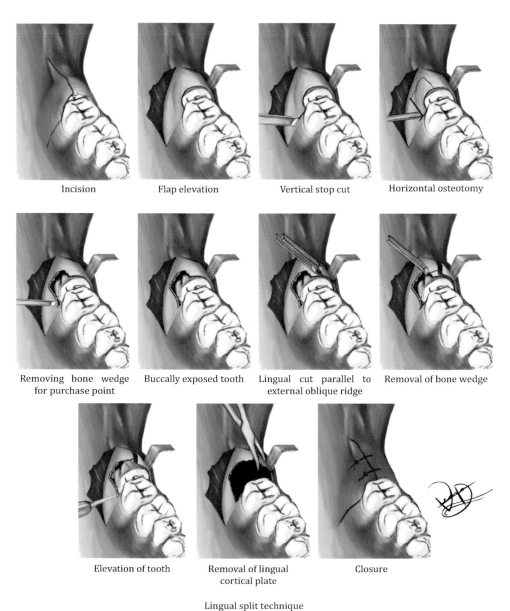

Incision	Flap elevation	Vertical stop cut	Horizontal osteotomy
Removing bone wedge for purchase point	Buccally exposed tooth	Lingual cut parallel to external oblique ridge	Removal of bone wedge
Elevation of tooth	Removal of lingual cortical plate	Closure	

Lingual split technique

Figure 10.12 Lingual split technique. Also referred to as "Kelsey Fry" or the "split bone" technique.

to external oblique line and not to internal oblique line, in order to prevent the splitting of the coronoid process (Figure 10.12).

Several modifications were later proposed for this technique. In 1960, Davis and Lewis proposed a modification wherein they did not elevate the lingual periosteum for the disto-lingual split while sectioning the lingual plate. With the techniques utilizing the lingual bone split, there can be increased risk of injury to the lingual nerve [2,3,7].

2. **Lateral trepanation technique:** It was first described by Bowdler and Henry. This procedure is employed for removing a partially formed unerupted third molar that has not breached the hard and soft tissues overlying it.

In the practice of surgery, the terms "Trepanation" and "Trephination" are used interchangeably. Trephination is the surgical procedure in which a hole is created by the removal of circular piece of bone, while a trepanation is the opening created by this procedure (Stone and Miles, 1990).

A modified S-shaped incision should be placed extending from the retromolar fossa across the external oblique ridge extending up to the mucosa of the mandibular first molar without engaging the marginal gingiva. A 5 mm mucoperiosteal cuff is left distal to the second molar. Raising a clean mucoperiosteal flap and retracting the flap using a Bowdler Henry retractor, the buccal cortical plate is trephined over the mandibular third molar crypt using a round Toller bur followed by placement of vertical cuts in the anterior, running downwards from the anterior most hole. The second cut is made at the posterior end of the crypt at an 45° from the created row of holes. A chisel is used in a vertical direction to out fracture the buccal cortical plate, exposing the third molar lying in the crypt and a Warwick James or Cryer elevator may be applied to ease the tooth out of the crypt.

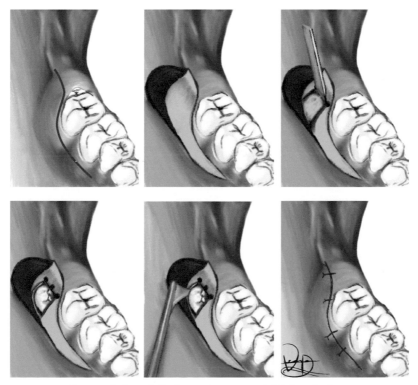

Removal of partially formed unerupted third molar by
Lateral Trepanation Technique

Figure 10.13 Lateral trepanation technique. (Bowdler and Henry.)

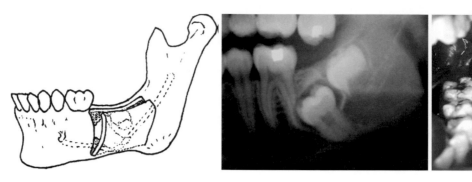

Figure 10.14 Buccal corticotomy for removal of deeply impacted mandibular molars. (Adapted with permission from Tay AB. Buccal corticotomy for removal of deeply impacted mandibular molars. *Br J Oral Maxillofac Surg.* 2007 Jan;45(1):83–4.)

Any follicular remnants in the tooth crypt should be curetted out [2,3,7] (Figure 10.13).

3. ***Buccal corticotomy:*** This technique was advocated by Tay in 2007 as an alternate approach for deeply seated impacted mandibular molars. A trapezoid mucoperiosteal flap is raised followed by elevating and removing a buccal rectangular bony window. The mesial and distal osteotomy cut should extend till the inferior aspect short of the mandibular lower border of the mandible followed by tooth removal and soft tissue closure. Caution should be excised as large buccal shelf osteotomy may make the mandible susceptible to fractures (Figure 10.14).

4. ***Coronectomy (partial odontectomy or intentional root retention):*** Coronectomy is an alternative technique to prevent damage to the inferior alveolar nerve during TAE of lower third molars. Partial odontectomy can be considered most appropriate procedure of choice in older patients with sclerotic non-elastic bone where root(s) of the mandibular molar lie in close relationship with the inferior dental canal. The intention is to prevent permanent nerve injury to the inferior alveolar nerve which may result in dysesthesia. It is rarely advised for young patients until the predictability of nerve injury relates to the high-risk group. Although originally described in 1984 by Ecuyer and Debien in French literature, the concept was introduced by Knutsson et al. (1989) where only the crown of tooth was removed, leaving the root in the socket thereby preventing direct and/or indirect injury to the inferior alveolar nerve

(IAN). Studies have shown that coronectomy reduces the incidence of damage to the IAN and dry socket. Monaco et al. in their clinical study observed that there was no temporary or permanent injury to the inferior alveolar or lingual nerve in patients who underwent coronectomy. It is reported that within the first 12 months, a second surgery would be required in 6% of coronectomy procedures to remove migrated root fragments, especially in younger patients.

Pogrel reviewed three techniques for coronectomy including lingual flap in the first one and sparing the lingual component of the flap in the other two with varied sectioning of the crown. The original technique involves raising a buccal and lingual mucoperiosteal flap, placing a lingual retractor protecting the lingual nerve and the soft tissues. After exposing the crown, it is sectioned using 702-fissured bur from buccal to lingual aspect. The second technique involves raising only the buccal mucoperiosteal flap, sectioning the crown from the occlusal surface using a fissure or round bur, to split and remove in sections. The third technique is similar to the above-mentioned procedure, except the crown is sectioned horizontally from the cervical line as done for complete tooth removal. A fissure bur is taken till two third from the buccal aspect of the crown, further fracturing the crown using a straight elevator. At times, the use of an elevator may result in accidentally mobilizing the roots and failure of the procedure. In any case, coronectomy should include

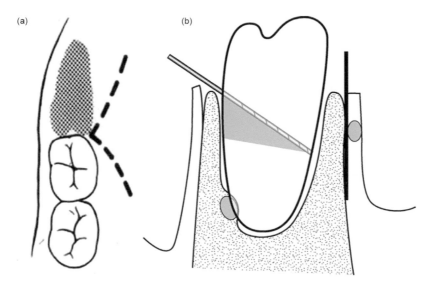

Figure 10.15 (a) The conventional third molar incision extending down the external oblique ridge to the distobuccal line angle of the lower second molar with a buccal releasing incision going no further forward than the midpoint of the first molar to avoid a frequent arteriole located in this area. (b) Diagrammatic representation of coronectomy technique. A lingual retractor has been placed to protect the lingual soft tissues, including the lingual nerve, and a 702 fissure bur is used at approximately a 45° angle to section the crown completely before removal. The grey area represents the portion of the tooth root that is then removed to place them 3–4 mm below the alveolar crest. (Adapted with permission from Pogrel MA. Coronectomy: Partial odontectomy or intentional root retention. *Oral Maxillofac Surg Clin North Am.* 2015 Aug;27(3):373–82.)

portion of the crown 2–3 mm below the alveolar crest, trimming all the sharp edges of the remaining root, and removal of all the enamel, a tension-free and water-tight closure is done for the success of the procedure and to avoid complications [9–12] (Figures 10.15 and 10.16).

TOOTH DIVISION AND REMOVAL OF THE TOOTH (ODONTECTOMY)

Removing the tooth in toto is often difficult in cases with impacted third molars. To overcome the difficulty and to prevent excessive bone removal, the tooth can be removed by splitting the crown and root as separate fragments. The line of withdrawal or the path of exit can be different for each root in a multi-rooted tooth along with the various angulations and position of the third molars in respect to the second molars that determine the lines of sectioning of the tooth and the root for favourable path of removal. Difficulty to retrieve the tooth from socket, the crown and the roots should be sectioned and removed along the individual favourable paths of withdrawal [2,3,7] (Figure 10.17).

In case of a completely erupted (with or without root formation) vertically upright third molar forceps removal or buccal application of elevator can deliver the tooth safely out of the socket provided the alveolar bone is sufficiently elastic and roots are not splayed. While applying the forceps for tooth delivery a "figure-of-eight" motion for luxation of the tooth is more beneficial than a buccal traction, as the presence of the thick external oblique ridge prevents the buccal cortical expansion. A vertical impaction with divergent roots needs sectioning of the crown and root in distal and mesial parts and removal of the former allows easy removal of the mesial segment. A deep vertically impacted molar poses a high surgical difficulty especially if it is below the cervical line of the second molar. Sectioning and removal for vertically impacted mandibular third molars is demonstrated in Figures 10.18–10.22.

In a mesioangular impaction, if the interdental spacing between the third and second molar is sufficient after exposing the crown along with creating

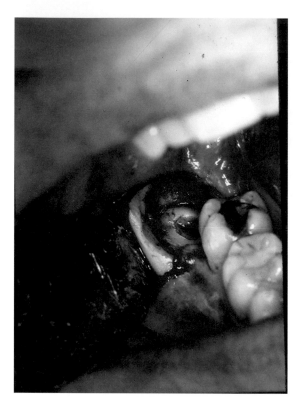

Figure 10.16 Postcoronectomy, note the exposed pulp chamber and the retained root fragments below the rim of the alveolar crest. (Adapted with permission from Pogrel MA. Coronectomy: Partial odontectomy or intentional root retention. *Oral Maxillofac Surg Clin North Am.* 2015 Aug;27(3):373–82.)

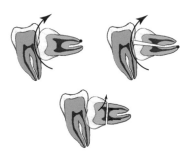

Tooth division to relieve tooth impaction

Figure 10.17 Tooth division (Odontectomy). Note the arch for elevation, if the force is applied on the mesial surface of the impacted tooth as seen in the figure, the tooth will rotate in an arch, the centre of which is at the apex of the distal root. As the cusps of the impacted tooth are below the distal convexity of the second molar tooth, forceful elevation will damage the area distal to second molar, this may also cause the damage to the distal surface of the second molar. Vertical division of the third molar would allow the distal root and the portion of the crown to be delivered, the remaining tooth will rotate along an arch with rotation centred along the mesial root allowing the delivery of the remaining tooth with an elevator. If the surgeon prefers to section the tooth along the cemento-enamel junction, the crown may be delivered by distally pushing it in the space created, the roots may be delivered utilizing the space created by the removal of the crown.

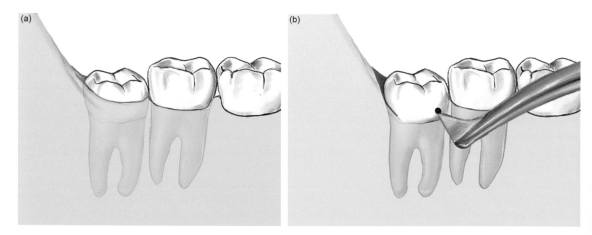

Figure 10.18 Vertical mandibular impacted tooth removal (a); buccal and distal trough created, purchase point placed and elevation using an elevator (b).

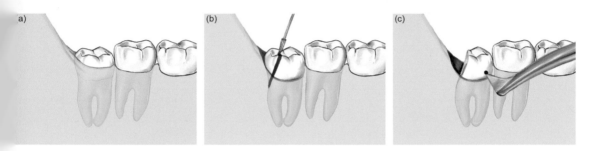

Figure 10.19 Vertical mandibular impacted tooth removal (a); distal crown segment sectioned (b); and removed followed by a purchase point for elevation in the remaining portion of the tooth (c).

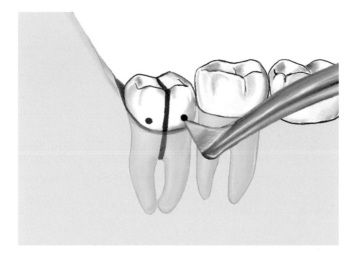

Figure 10.20 Vertical mandibular impacted tooth removal; tooth and root units split vertically and are removed distal followed by mesial with purchase points.

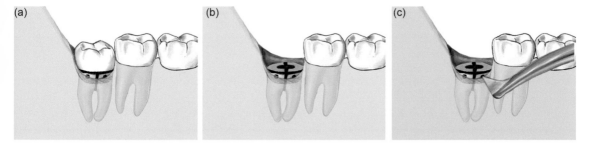

Figure 10.21 Vertical mandibular impacted tooth removal (a); crown removed using a horizontal cut and roots split for removal distal followed by mesial with purchase points (b, c).

a buccal and distal gutter, and the path of removal is not hindered with the distal bone, the tooth can be elevated using a straight elevator at the mesial portion, at the cervical region. Few mesioangular impactions require sectioning of the distal portion of the crown or sectioning of the complete tooth in mesial and distal fragments with roots. Removal of distal segment is done first followed by up righting and elevating the mesial section of the tooth. Sectioning and removal for mesioangular impacted mandibular third molars is demonstrated in Figures 10.23 and 10.24.

Horizontal impactions require adequate bone removal from the buccal and distal aspects so that the area of furcation can be appreciated before

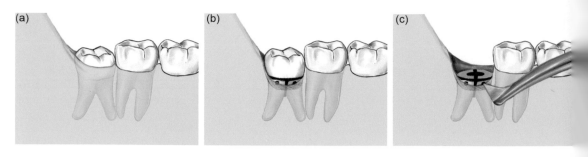

Figure 10.22 Vertical mandibular impacted tooth removal with flared roots (a); crown removed using a horizontal cut (b); and roots split for removal distal followed by mesial with purchase points in case of flared roots (c).

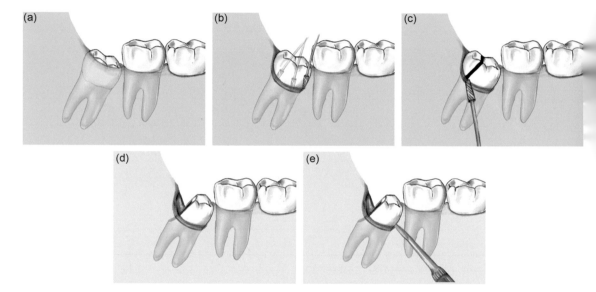

Figure 10.23 Mesioangular mandibular impacted tooth removal; for cases with adequate space for bone removal and point of application between second and third molar (a); buccal and distal trough created and tooth elevated distally (b); with a mesial purchase point. Where needed distal coronal portion may be sectioned and removed separately (c–e).

sectioning the tooth. Sectioning is carried along the long axis of the tooth, followed by vertical sectioning of the crown. This allows the removal of complete crown in two halves followed by the removal of roots separately by making a purchase point between the distal root and the distal bone. Sectioning and removal for horizontally impacted mandibular third molars is demonstrated in Figure 10.25.

Distoangular impactions are considered to be the most difficult ones as the path of removal of the tooth is directed towards the ramus of the mandible. After creating buccal and distal trough at or below the cervical line the crown is section in order to remove the distal portion of the crown after creating a distal space to elevate the crown. If further hindrance or lock on elevation is experienced, sectioning of the remaining crown and its removal is done. The remaining roots are sectioned from the furcation and elevated individually. Sectioning and removal for distoangular impacted mandibular third molar is demonstrated in Figures 10.26–10.28.

Care should be taken to remove all the fragments of root and tooth or the tooth in toto using extraction forceps or a curved haemostat. Judicious bone removal can aid in enhanced healing process as there will be reduction in bone quantity to be resorbed and remodelled thereby retaining the clot which would fill the socket.

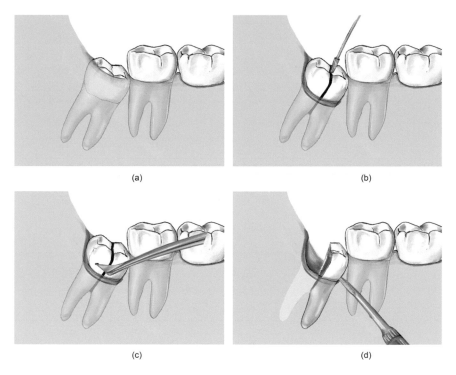

Figure 10.24 Mesioangular mandibular impacted tooth removal; for cases with inadequate space for bone removal and point of application between second and third molar (a). The sectioning of roots with elevation of the distal segment followed by elevation of the mesial segment (b–d).

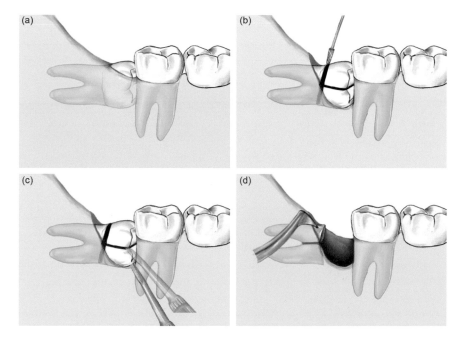

Figure 10.25 Horizontal mandibular impacted tooth removal (a); the crown is sectioned from root and removed as a unit or may need to be sectioned longitudinally for removal. Elevation of roots with a purchase point using an elevator. Roots may need to be sectioned into two pieces and removed separately, with upper followed by lower (b–d).

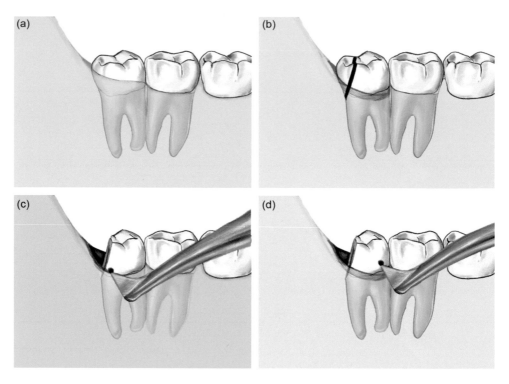

Figure 10.26 Distoangular mandibular impacted tooth removal (a); buccal and distal trough created and distal portion of crown sectioned (b); followed by a purchase point ideally on the distobuccal aspect (c); of the remaining tooth structure by elevation. In case sectioning the crown provides sufficient room for displacing and elevating the tooth, a more buccal and mesial elevation point may be utilized (d).

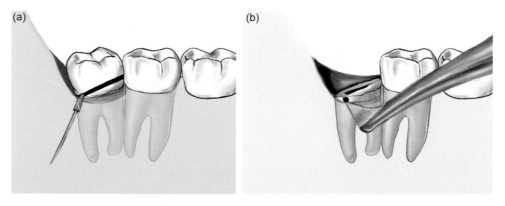

Figure 10.27 Distoangular mandibular impacted tooth removal; crown sectioned horizontally and elevation attempted (a, b).

Any intra operative suspicion of the accidental nerve injury may it be involving IAN or the lingual nerve, should be documented and the patient should to be reviewed at regular intervals to prevent permanent damage. Neuropraxia or partial nerve injury may require a steroid therapy to limit perineural or intra fascicular oedema leading to further ischaemic nerve damage intra operatively and in the post-surgical phase. Some surgeons do prefer supplementation with components of vitamin B-complex to aid in the recovery from neuropraxia or partial nerve injury.

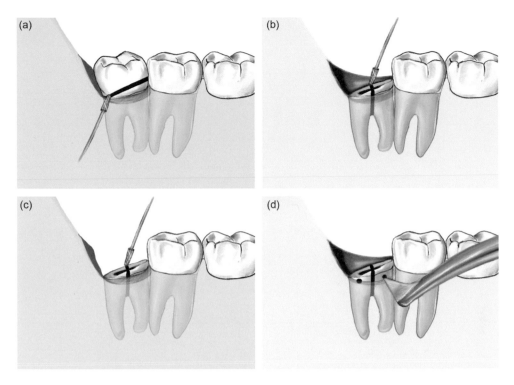

Figure 10.28 Distoangular mandibular impacted tooth removal; in cases where resistance is felt to acceptable moderate elevation force, removal followed by sectioning of the remaining roots and elevation of each root independently is an option (a–d).

Intra operative bleeding either from the inferior dental canal or from the retromolar foramen should be identified. Pressure packing, obliterating the puncture in the canal using bone wax, placement of a haemostatic cellulose mesh or gelatine sponge to stabilize the clot and avoiding further irrigation and suctioning are the measures to be taken before water-tight closure of the wound with sutures.

SOCKET TOILET

Once the removal of the tooth is done, toileting of the wound is essential for an uneventful healing process. The presence of any sharp bony areas should be removed using a rongeur forceps, or a surgical bur and margins are smoothened with a bone file or a bur. Any remnant tooth or root piece should be inspected and removed. The presence of all the follicular substance has to be curetted out of the socket. Once the cavity is debrided of all the particulate matter and has smooth bony margins, the socket should be thoroughly irrigated with normal saline before the closure of the muco-periosteal flap.

SUTURING

In general, a suture should be considered as a foreign body and should be used only if there is a positive indication for its use. The sutures are placed following the third molar surgery to approximate the flap, achieve haemostasis, protect the stabilizing clot, minimize wound contamination by preventing food lodgement and prevent periodontal defects distal to the second molar. Some surgeons do prefer to de-epithelize the margins of the flap both on the buccal and the lingual side before suturing, in cases of partially or completely erupted mandibular third molars. However, this concept is not supported by any available randomized control trial. In general, post-operative sequelae do not alter with or without de-epithelization of the flap margins. A simple interrupted silk suture is preferable in the oral cavity following transalveolar extractions. Forming a soft tissue cuff distal to the second molar is a mandate to avoid the chances of formation of the periodontal defect involving the distal portion of the second molar. This can be achieved by mobilizing the buccal flap, taking the

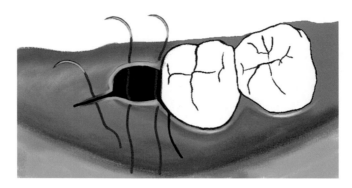

Figure 10.29 Ideal location of sutures after surgical extraction of the mandibular third molar.

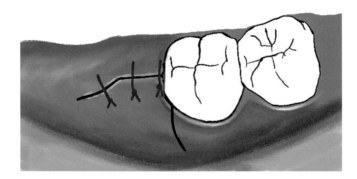

Figure 10.30 Forming a soft tissue cuff distal to the second molar is a mandate to avoid the chances of formation of the periodontal defect involving the distal portion of the second molar. This can be achieved by mobilizing the buccal flap, taking the first needle bite in the free papilla adjacent to the second molar advancing it lingually in an oblique manner (needle to be directed from buccal to mesiolingual direction) to involve sufficient amount of lingual papilla to form a tight cuff along the distal surface of the second molar. Rest of the flap should be closed distal to this cuff using a simple interrupted suture. Anterior releasing incision is usually left unsutured in order to facilitate drainage of the inflammatory exudates.

first bite in the free papilla adjacent to the second molar advancing it lingually in an oblique manner (needle to be directed from buccal to mesiolingual direction) to involve sufficient amount of lingual papilla to form a tight cuff along the distal surface of the second molar. This aids in lesser complications and avoids wound dehiscence as the thinner mucosa attached to the lingual flap can be maximally incorporated along with the buccal papilla for a tight closure. Rest of the flap should be closed distal to this cuff using a simple interrupted suture. Anterior releasing incision is usually left unsutured in order to facilitate drainage of the inflammatory exudates (Figures 10.29 and 10.30). The

flaps on either side should be placed against each other without tension. Once healing is satisfactory, the sutures can be removed, preferably on the 7th post-operative day.

POST-OPERATIVE CARE AND FOLLOW-UP

Post-surgical instructions should be explained verbally/in writing to the patient and a responsible attendant (Table 10.6). The patient should be recalled on 7th day post-operatively for suture removal if the wound healing is satisfactory. If the extraction was traumatic or there is an anticipation

Table 10.6 Post-surgical instructions after transalveolar extraction of the mandibular third molar

1	Pressing or biting a folded gauze (2×2 in.) at the area of extraction for 30–45 minutes after extraction[a].
2	Avoid forceful rinsing and gargling for 24 hours.
3	Avoid spitting for 24 hours.
4	Advise the patient to be on soft or semi-liquid diet consumed at room temperature for 48 hours.
5	Advise cold fomentation externally on the face by wrapping ice in a piece of cloth or a polyethene bag intermittently for 24 hours to reduce oedema.
6	Maintain adequate oral hygiene by rinsing and brushing after 24 hours.
7	Smoking and alcohol consumption should be strictly avoided for 2 weeks after extraction.

[a] There remains no unanimity among the oral and maxillofacial surgeons regarding advocating the ideal time for applying bite pressure over the extraction socket, it is generally agreed upon that the time required for "not only" the **clot formation**, but also the **clot stabilization** and retraction process in an extraction socket should be supplemented with the bite pressure with a gauze piece/pack. After the initial *clot formation* (initial 4–10 minutes), this is followed by fibrin mesh crosslinking and stabilization of the insoluble clot against shear stress. Within a few minutes of clot formation and stabilization, it begins to contract and usually expresses out most of the fluid (serum) from the clot within 20–60 minutes **(clot retraction)** [13].

of any possible complications, then the patient may be followed up on 1st or 3rd post-operative day followed by subsequent visits. In case of anticipated nerve injury, initiation of corticosteroids is essential in the post-operative period, which can be assessed only after the effect of the local anaesthesia wears away. A course of appropriate prophylactic anti biotics and analgesics should be prescribed to prevent possible infection and pain.

CONCLUSION

Each individual step mentioned above should be planned and executed carefully to avoid unwarranted complications. The treatment plan should be tailor-made for each patient depending on the systemic and local factors, type and difficulty of the impaction and proximity to the vital structures. A proper treatment plan and appropriate handling of the soft and hard tissue will result in uneventful surgical outcomes.

Pre-operative assessment of the type of impacted mandibular third molar is an essential criterion to decide on the surgical procedure. It is wise that the details of the procedure and the expected possible surgical risks are informed to the patient prior and documented for medico-legal purpose. Appropriate pre-operative planning and post-operative care can limit uneventful outcomes for both the patient and the operator.

TRANSPLANTATION OF MANDIBULAR THIRD MOLARS

Louis K. Rafetto, DMD, Department of Oral and Maxillofacial Surgery and Hospital Dentistry, Christiana Care Health System, Wilmington, DE, USA
William Synan, DDS Department of Oral and Maxillofacial Surgery, The University of Iowa, College of Dentistry, Iowa City, IA, USA

(*Excerpt adapted with permission from Rafetto LK, Synan W. Surgical management of third molars. Atlas Oral Maxillofac Surg Clin North Am. 2012 Sep;20(2):197–223. doi: 10.1016/j.cxom.2012.07.002.*)

Transplant of a third molar to another site may be an option for replacement of another tooth indicated for removal or already removed. Although a patient's age is not a major risk factor for successful autoplastic transplantation, epidemiologic data indicate better results are achieved when performed at a younger age because the donor tooth (in this case third molar) is still developing and retains its eruptive potential [14] (Figure 10.31).

Advantages

- May provide an alternative to fixed or removable prosthodontics
- Avoids adjacent teeth preparation
- May allow continued development of alveolus in growing patient
- Comparative cost-effectiveness

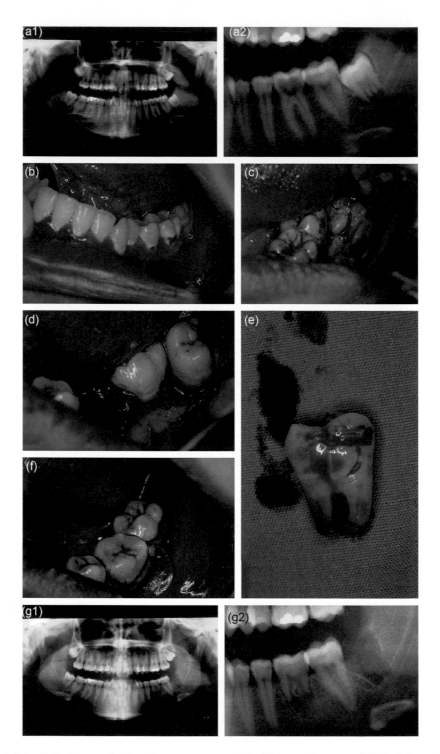

Figure 10.31 (a1,a2) Radiograph of carious, nonrestorable #36, and impacted #38 with partial root formation. (b) Photo of carious, nonrestorable #36. (c) Surgical access to #38. (d) #36 Removed with forceps and #38 elevated and removed from socket. (e) #38 Transplant. (f) #38 Transplanted to site #36. (g1,g2) Radiograph post-transplantation of #38. (Adapted with permission from Rafetto LK, Synan W. Surgical management of third molars. *Atlas Oral Maxillofac Surg Clin North Am.* 2012 Sep;20(2):197–223. doi: 10.1016/j.cxom.2012.07.002.)

Disadvantages

- Technique sensitive
- Has uncertain prognosis
- Risk of transplant loss secondary to complications, such as root resorption and loss of attachment

Factors that Influence Success

- Atraumatic extraction of the transplanted tooth.
- Host site infection and post-operative plaque adversely influence success.
- Minimal handling protects Hertwig root sheath and pulpal tissue.
- Minimize time out of socket to avoid desiccation.
- Appropriate immobilization to allow re-establishment of innervation and vascularity.
- Ideal age for success is 15–19 years.

Contraindications

- Poor oral hygiene.
- Mismatch of alveolar dimension. If recipient site has insufficient space to accommodate donor tooth, resorption of ridge or root may occur.
- Age may present as a relative contraindication.

Impact of Root Development

- Most recommend root development be between one-half to two-thirds of its final length.
- Although higher success rates are achieved with immature roots, they have less root growth after transplantation.
- Although transplantation is feasible for teeth with complete root development, endodontic treatment is usually indicated 7–14 days after transplant.
- Endodontic treatment or apicoectomy during procedure increases the risk of root resorption and failure of the procedure.

Key Points to Success

- Minimal trauma with the extraction of donor third molar and tooth at the recipient site
- Care to preserve periodontium
- Replacement root resorption occurs in teeth with cementum injury
- Donor tooth placed with 1–2 mm of periodontal ligament above osseous crest to achieve an ideal biologic width
- Proper splinting technique
- Rinse with chlorhexidine for several days
- Although some studies show no relation between graft survival and the use of antimicrobials, many surgeons believe they improve clinical outcomes.

Splinting

- Excessive time or rigid splinting adversely affects outcome
- Should not force roots against bony walls of the alveolus (may damage the periodontium)
- Flexible with sutures through the mucosa and over occlusal surface for 7–10 days allows functional movement
- In case graft is used, graft with mature roots should be placed slightly subocclusal to prevent trauma
- Graft with immature roots slightly more depressed to allow for eruption
- Advice soft diet for the first few days

REFERENCES

1. Kim C, Hwang K, Park C. Local anesthesia for mandibular third molar extraction. *J Dent Anesth Pain Med*. 2018;18(5):287–94.
2. Howe GL. *The Extraction of Teeth*, 2nd rev. ed. London: Butterworth-Heinemann Ltd, 1974.
3. Howe GL. *Minor Oral Surgery*. London: Wright, 1985.
4. Bhargava D, Sreekumar K, Deshpande A. Effects of intra-space injection of twin mix versus intraoral-submucosal, intramuscular, intravenous and per-oral administration of dexamethasone on post-operative

sequelae after mandibular impacted third molar surgery: A preliminary clinical comparative study. *Oral Maxillofac Surg.* 2014 Sep;18(3):293–6. doi: 10.1007/s10006-013-0412-7.

5. Bhargava D, Sreekumar K, Rastogi S, Deshpande A, Chakravorty N. A prospective randomized double-blind study to assess the latency and efficacy of twin-mix and 2% lignocaine with 1:200,000 epinephrine in surgical removal of impacted mandibular third molars: A pilot study. *Oral Maxillofac Surg.* 2013 Dec;17(4):275–80. doi: 10.1007/s10006-012-0372-3.

6. Godzieba A, Smektała T, Jędrzejewski M, Sporniak-Tutak K. Clinical assessment of the safe use local anaesthesia with vasoconstrictor agents in cardiovascular compromised patients: A systematic review. *Med Sci Monit.* 2014 Mar;10(20):393–8. doi: 10.12659/MSM.889984.

7. Farish SE, Bouloux GF. General technique of third molar removal. *Oral Maxillofac Surg Clin North Am.* 2007 Feb;19(1):23–43, v–vi. doi: 10.1016/j.coms.2006.11.012.

8. Kale TP, et al. Lingual guttering technique for removal of impacted mandibular third molar. *J Int Oral Health.* 2014;6(4):9–11.

9. Cervera-Espert J, Pérez-Martínez S, Cervera-Ballester J, Peñarrocha-Oltra D, Peñarrocha-Diago M. Coronectomy of impacted mandibular third molars: A meta-analysis and systematic review of the literature. *Med Oral Patol Oral Cir Bucal.* 2016;21(4):e505–13.

10. Monaco G, et al. What are the types and frequencies of complications associated with mandibular third molar coronectomy? A follow up study. *J Oral Maxfac Surg.* 2015;73(7):1246–53.

11. Pogrel MA, Lee JS, Muff DF. Coronectomy: A technique to protect the inferior alveolar nerve. *J Oral Maxillofac Surg.* 2004 Dec;62(12):1447–52. doi: 10.1016/j.joms.2004.08.003.

12. Pogrel MA. Coronectomy: Partial odontectomy or intentional root retention. *Oral Maxillofac Surg Clin North Am.* 2015 Aug;27(3):373–82. doi: 10.1016/j.coms.2015.04.003.

13. Kumar S, Paul A, Chacko R, Deepika S. Time required for haemostasis under pressure from dental extraction socket. *Indian J Dent Res.* 2019 Nov–Dec;30(6):894–8; Hemostasis and blood coagulation. In: Guyton and Hall (eds) *Textbook of Medical Physiology*, 14th ed. Elsevier, 2021, pp. 477–88.

14. Rafetto LK, Synan W. Surgical management of third molars. *Atlas Oral Maxillofac Surg Clin North Am.* 2012 Sep;20(2):197–223. doi: 10.1016/j.cxom.2012.07.002.

11

Periodontal considerations for impacted mandibular third molars

SUMEDHA SRIVASTAVA, JAIDEEP MAHENDRA, AND KHUSHBOO DESAI

INTRODUCTION

Tooth impaction is a condition where a tooth fails to attain its normal functional position. In comparison to other teeth, third molars are most commonly found impacted. The inadequate space between the distal area of the second mandibular molar and the anterior border of the ascending ramus of the mandible leads to mandibular third molar impaction (M3MI). Erratic eruption pathways also contribute to third molar impaction. The reported incidence for impaction is remarkably higher for third molars when compared with other teeth. M3MI has a reported incidence of 66%–77%, being the most common impacted tooth [1]. Its abnormal position and blocked eruption give rise to several problems such as caries, pericoronitis, acute or chronic periapical infections, pain, pathology associated with cystic degeneration and/or neoplastic transformation of the dental follicle. However, in some conditions, the impacted third molar may be asymptomatic with long-lasting localized periodontal defect (pocket) on the distal surface of the adjacent second molar. This may increase the chance of food impaction/lodgement, thus leading to periodontal inflammation and bone loss [2]. It should be noted that M3MI surgical extraction itself may cause periodontal complications on the distal aspect of the root of the adjacent mandibular second molar such as deep pockets, periodontal bone loss, recession, tooth mobility, etc. Hence, management of impacted third molar-associated problems includes treatment of acute symptoms if any, followed by surgical extraction of the impacted tooth. Therefore, preoperative periodontal evaluation both clinically and radiographically including proper diagnosis of periodontal history, type of impaction, reasonable selection of flap design, proper armamentarium and suture type and necessary post-operative interventions, which include various regenerative therapy such as guided tissue regeneration (GTR), bone graft, etc. would aid to reduce the future risk of periodontal defects distal to the second molar after M3MI extraction.

IMPACTION AS A RISK FACTOR FOR PERIODONTAL TISSUES DISTAL TO SECOND MOLAR

Periodontal defect formation before removal and after surgical extraction of the impacted third molar often causes plaque accumulation and further local inflammatory disease. Maintaining proper oral hygiene in posterior areas or the oral cavity is generally difficult, and the unfavourable position of the impacted third molar may attract more plaque accumulation and may pose a risk for the periodontal health of the second molar. Therefore, considerations should be given to minimizing tissue damage around the surgical area. Apart from the vital indications, two of the important reasons for removing impacted third molars are to preserve periodontal health or, in some

DOI: 10.1201/9781003324034-11

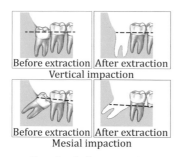

Before extraction | After extraction
Vertical impaction

Before extraction | After extraction
Mesial impaction

Bone level after extraction

Figure 11.1 Bone level after the surgical extraction of the mandibular third molar.

situations, to treat a periodontitis that already exists. Impacted or partially impacted third molars are very frequently associated with loss of the distal attachment and bone distal to the second molar. The kind and magnitude of periodontal damage depend on the situation and type of impaction as reported by Kim et al. They indicated that the incidence of distal alveolar bone loss in the adjacent second molars is closely related to M3MI varies with the impacted type [3]. According to Kugelberg et al. [4], impacted third molars that are most likely to form periodontal pockets and bone defects in the distal part of the second molars is the mesial impaction, followed by the horizontal impaction, and the vertical impaction which has the lowest incidence for such defects [4,5] (Figure 11.1).

EFFECTS ON PERIODONTIUM WITH VARIOUS IMPACTION TYPE

1. In *partially impacted third molars*, due to food particle retention and poor hygiene, is an active source of bacterial entry into the distal area of the second molar. All these lead to poorer gingival and plaque indexes. These indices improve with extraction of the wisdom tooth. If left untreated, deep pockets will develop due to loss of attachment, which augments the anaerobic microbiota causing episodes of acute repeated infections, which, if continued over time, may lead to chronic distal infection of the second molar.
2. *Mesial and horizontal impaction* compromise the distal periodontal attachment of the second molar, which often leads to weakening or eliminating the interdental bone partition

that separates them (Figure 11.1). All this leads to periodontopathogenic bacterial aggression, which ultimately gives rise to periodontal pockets and clinical attachment loss, leading to difficulty in plaque control and often leads to complications such as pericoronitis and even cellulitis or fascial space involvement if the infection progresses.
3. *Non-erupted M3MI* can be divided into completely impacted (completely in bone) and sub-mucosal impacted (completely covered by oral mucosa), which have different effects on post-operative periodontal tissues:
   a. If there is a bone coverage above the M3MI (*bone/hard tissue impaction*), the post-operative periodontal conditions only have a little change [6]. Complete M3MI removal usually results in buccal defects due to bone removal lateral to the third molar.
   b. The sub-mucosal *M3MI* (*sub-mucosal/ soft tissue impaction*) already has a coronal bone wall missing, and the buccal bone wall usually needs to be partially removed intraoperatively. Especially in the coronal plane, the M3MI is in close contact with the second molar, and there is no obvious bone boundary, which causes greater defect in the distal periodontal tissues of the second molar after surgery [7].

TREATMENT

After analysing the existing preoperative periodontal damage caused by the third molar impaction, clinician must decide to undertake measures to avoid any further periodontal damage distal to the second molar during the impaction surgery; for this, various factors should be kept in mind. At the time of the surgical extraction of the impacted third molar, minimally invasive surgical measures should be adopted, and the clinician should limit the injudicious damage or removal of the soft and hard tissues around the second molar tooth. In cases with post-operative damage or deterioration of the periodontal defect distal to the second molar tooth, the treating clinician should use appropriate interceptive therapy to overcome and reduce further periodontal damage.

PERIODONTAL RISK PREDICTORS

Kugelberg has identified a number of "periodontal risk predictors" whose presence is related to an increased likelihood of periodontal damage distal to the second molar or the periodontal sequelae after removal of the adjacent third molar [8]. These factors include:

- Plaque visible on the distal surface of the second molar.
- Probing depth greater than 6 mm on the distal side of the second molar.
- Bone defect greater than 3 mm on the distal side of the second molar.
- Sagittal inclination of the third molar of over 50°.
- Large contact surface area between second and third molars.
- Resorption of the distal root of the second molar.
- Wisdom tooth follicle enlarged mesially over 2.5 mm.
- Smoking.

PREOPERATIVE AND INTRAOPERATIVE CONSIDERATIONS

There are various risk factors that affect the removal of impacted third molars with their effects on the periodontium and have to be considered during the treatment planning phase. These include age, direction of eruption, preoperative bony defects and resorption of second mandibular root surface.

Age: The most common age of third molar eruption is between the ages of 17 and 25. Age is the most pivotal factor as the bone density tends to vary with the age of the individual, thus exerting a significant influence on the extraction of the impacted tooth. Where indicated, early removal of the impacted third molar is reported to be beneficial in preventing periodontal defects distal to the second molar tooth. For instance, tooth extraction is easier when only two-thirds of the roots of the third molar have developed. At this stage, removing the third molars is easier and so is the recovery without adversely affecting the periodontal health. After the roots have fully developed, patients have a greater risk of complications both during and after

the extraction procedure. The difficulty of M3MI extraction increases with age, owing to continuous root development, periodontal ligament thinning, mandibular bone becoming less elastic and the development of hypercementosis [9]. Chiapasco et al. have reported that the periodontal defects of the distal second molar after the third molar surgery over 25 years of age are found to be three times that of those before 25 years old [10].

Armamentarium: Anatomical position, poor accessibility and potential risk of injuries to the surrounding vital structures, nerves, vessels, soft tissues and adjacent teeth during surgeries makes the surgical management of impacted third molar difficult. The factors contributing to the post-operative sequelae are many; out of them, the one with significance is the trauma caused due to the bone removal, which is carried out either by chisel and mallet or by rotary cutting instruments (surgical bur). Previously, chisel and mallet were used as a common tool of choice for extractions, to remove bone and split tooth, which are likely to bring about significant post-operative trauma [11]. The traditional use of chisel for splitting the crown of the mandibular third molar can cause different degrees of periodontal damage, while minimally invasive tooth extraction surgery can effectively promote alveolar bone healing [12]. The concept of minimally "damaging" tooth extraction has emerged with the advent of refined instrumentation, including ultrasonic or piezo-bone knife, 45° contrast-angle surgical handpieces, elongated tooth burs, modified minimally invasive dental elevator or luxators (thinner edge) and buccal retractor, which are widely used now making the surgery more refined. Though there are advantages of minimally "invasive" tooth extraction surgery, this technique may still result in bone loss and periodontal defect formation in the distal aspect of the second molar. Procedures, like ultrasonic osteotome window technique, are advocated to prevent periodontal defects [13].

Flap design: Selection of appropriate flap design for extraction of impacted third molar plays a pivotal role for post-operative periodontal health. Different flap designs affect the probing depth of the post-operative periodontal pocket after the tooth extraction. The few flap designs utilized include standard envelop flap, triangular, Szmyd's and modified flaps (Figure 11.2). On comparing the effects of the envelope flap and the triangular

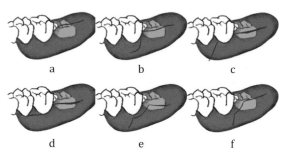

Flap designs used in impacted mandibular third molar extraction

a) Standard envelope flap

b) Standard triangular flap

c) Szmyd flap

d–f) Modification flaps

Figure 11.2 Some of the common flap designs (a–f) used for the impacted mandibular third molar extraction.

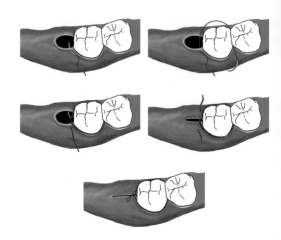

Suturing technique

Figure 11.3 Suturing technique involving the second molar with an intention to prevent periodontal defect distal to the second molar tooth (anchor suture technique).

flap on the periodontal condition of the adjacent second molar, the probing depth of the triangular flap was found significantly less than that of the envelope flap at 3 months after surgery as demonstrated by Korkmaz et al. [14]. Therefore, compared with the envelope flap, the triangular flap design is better for periodontal health [15]. In general, any flap design that allowed advancement of the buccal flap and aids in formation of the distal cuff to the second molar tooth at the time of suturing would have superior periodontal healing.

Suturing technique: Primary and secondary closure are used for wound management after extraction of impacted lower third molars. Studies have shown that different types of suture have different effects on the periodontal tissue. Commonly used sutures are interrupted suture, anchor suture, and the figure-of-eight sutures. The advantage of using anchor suture is that it fixes the distal aspects of the buccal-lingual gingival flaps to the adjacent tooth in an anchor-like manner to avoid the V-shaped gap formation in the distal adjacent tooth (Figure 11.3). However, the figure-of-eight suture is more conducive to the healing of the distal periodontal tissue of the adjacent teeth, which may make the mucosal epithelium closer to the distal root surface of the adjacent tooth to form a barrier to prevent food debris from embedding, thereby protecting the periodontal tissue in this area for regeneration and restoration. Cetinkaya et al. compared the effects of interrupted sutures and anchor

sutures on the periodontal tissue of the adjacent second molar 6 months after M3MI extraction and found that the probing pocket depth (PPD) and clinical attachment level (CAL) distal to second molars in the interrupted suturing group were significantly higher than those in the anchored suturing group, indicating that anchor sutures may be a better choice to maintain the health of periodontal tissues and prevent periodontal problems [16].

POST-OPERATIVE MANAGEMENT OF THE PERIODONTAL DEFECTS

There may be occasions when the removal of third molars can either create or exacerbate periodontal problems on the distal aspect of the lower second molar. After the extraction of impacted mandibular third molars, a significant improvement in the periodontal status on the distal root of second molars can be observed if the surgery is done in accordance with appropriate protocols, endowing a positive effect on the overall periodontal health, else it may aggravate the periodontal problems.

Through multiple regression analysis, Kugelberg et al. demonstrated that the size of the distal bone defect of the second molar after surgery is related to the preoperative periodontal status in addition to the type of impaction [17]. Hence, a thorough preoperative periodontal and radiographic examination is mandatory before M3MI extraction, which should include pre-probing depth, clinical attachment loss, prior history of periodontitis or pericoronitis, pericoronal abscess, radiographic bone loss, and the oral hygiene status. Patients with existing periodontal diseases often progress to develop periodontal pockets after the third molar extraction. Complications of deep M3MI extraction involve formation of intrabony defects at the distal site adjacent to the second molar. To avoid deep intrabony defects and improve bone healing after tooth extraction, the use of regenerative materials like grafts and/or membranes is found effective in controlling pocket depth progression and bone loss.

Periodontal examination records before the third molar extraction

The periodontal pocket, one of the definitive signs of periodontal disease, is the most common parameter that requires assessment before the surgery. Periodontal parameters should be measured at least at three sites in the distal part of the second molar to provide a more accurate and comprehendible periodontal condition. Researchers have also selected five probing sites around the distal region to the second molars, that is, buccal, dis-buccal, mid-distal, dis-lingual, lingual as the multisite measurements which permit the detailed assessment of the distal periodontal status of the second molar [18–21]. Where required, various imaging methods such as intra-oral periapical radiographs, panoramic radiography and cone-beam CT (CBCT) may be utilized to aid in assessing the distal bone level of the second molar in a much better and accurate manner [20].

Post-operative treatment modalities for management of periodontal defects

Proposed interventions to promote periodontal tissue regeneration, including non-surgical periodontal treatment, GTR, use of bone grafts, use of collagen sponge and transplantation of cell active ingredients. The rationale is to create space, stabilization of the wound and cell induction as the key factors, which can be achieved using these treatment modalities.

NON-SURGICAL THERAPY

The main aim of non-surgical periodontal therapy is to control microbial periodontal infection by removing bacterial biofilm, calculus, and toxins from periodontally involved root surfaces. Scaling and root planing, are the widely utilized basic methods for periodontal treatment. Where indicated, manual scaling and root planing on the distal region of the second molar after extraction can completely remove the plaque and calculus in these areas. The simultaneous non-surgical periodontal treatment along with the extraction of the impacted third molar will reduce the risk for the distal pocket formation [22].

LOCAL DRUG DELIVERY

Any residual infective/inflammatory element still harbouring in the periodontal apparatus that is not eradicated by mechanical removal by hand or mechanized instruments is generally treated by local drug delivery system. Local drug delivery systems may involve introducing chlorhexidine gluconate, doxycycline hyclate, metronidazole gel, minocycline ointment, tetracycline fibres, etc. at the site. Local administration of drugs can deliver higher concentrations directly into diseased sites reducing the microbial load. Irrigating systems, fibres, gels, strips, films, microparticles, nanoparticles and low-dose antimicrobial agents are some of the local drug delivery systems available, which aim to deliver antimicrobial agents to sub-gingival diseased sites with minimal or no side effects. However, scientific evidence supporting this treatment after third molar extraction is less [23–26].

PERIODONTAL SURGICAL MANAGEMENT

Some of the surgical procedures only help in repair or reduction in pocket depth; however, some periodontal surgical procedures help in pocket elimination and regeneration of new tissues and alveolar bone distal to the second molar. The various treatment modalities for the management of distal pocket are regenerative osseous surgery, which includes bone grafts and GTR. Platelet-rich plasma (PRP), platelet-rich fibrin (PRF), and growth factors such as bone morphogenetic proteins (BMP) and concentrated growth factor (CGF) may also be used as an adjunct.

Guided tissue regeneration

Periodontal regeneration is defined as a process by which the architecture and function of the periodontium is completely restored [27]. With the advent of GTR restoration of periodontium is being achieved more predictably. GTR is based on the biologic behaviour of different periodontal tissues. It is now known that the periodontal ligament is the most important source of periodontal progenitor regenerative cells. The GTR procedure involves the placement of an occlusive barrier membrane which prevents the epithelium and granulation tissue from the gingiva contacting the treated root surface during the healing, and at the same time, this membrane maintains a space which allows granulation tissue from the periodontal ligament to proliferate in the coronal direction, thereby securing selective population of the root surface with periodontal ligament cells (Figure 11.4). A number of resorbable (reconstituted collagen and polylactic acid membranes) and non-resorbable materials (Goretex or Teflon membranes) have been used successfully in the procedure of GTR. Non-resorbable membrane has the disadvantage that they have to be removed via a second surgical procedure. To overcome this disadvantage biodegradable collagen membranes were developed and are used for GTR. Grafting of osseous defects distal to mandibular second molars with a xenograft plus a membrane predictably resulted in a significant reduction in the PPD, CAL gain, and bone fill, which suggests that grafting the extraction sites with a xenograft along with a membrane has the potential to prevent the formation or restore existing distal periodontal defects [28].

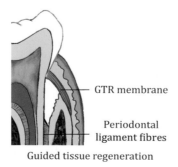

GTR membrane

Periodontal
ligament fibres

Guided tissue regeneration

Figure 11.4 Guided tissue regeneration (GTR).

Bone grafts

The various bone grafts available are autografts, allografts, xenografts and alloplastic material. These materials act either as osteo-genic, osteo-inductive, or osteo-conductive in nature [29]. The objectives of periodontal bone grafts are probing depth reduction, clinical attachment gain, bone fill of the osseous defect and regeneration of the new bone, cementum and periodontal ligament. Due to immunogenic reaction, disease transmission, ethical problems and infection risks allograft bone is currently rarely used in the repair of distal bone defects in the second molar after extraction of the M3MI [30]. In the synthetic bone substitute material, hydroxyapatite (HA) and bioactive glass are chiefly used for the bone defect repair [31].

Platelet-rich plasma and platelet-rich fibrin

Cell active component transplantation stimulates cell proliferation, repair of the bone defects and promotes bone regeneration by releasing various growth factors [32]. PRP is a biological product that is defined as the portion of plasma fraction of autologous blood with a platelet concentration above that of the original whole blood. A supermixture of key cytokines and growth factors is present in platelet granules. Thus, the application of PRP has gained unprecedented attention in regenerative medicine. It is a proven source of growth factors such as platelet-derived growth factors (PDGFs) and transforming growth factor-beta 1 and 2; vascular endothelial growth factors that positively influence repair and regeneration of tissues. PRF has a dense fibrin network with leukocytes, cytokines, structural glycoproteins and also growth factors. PRF is considered as the second-generation platelet concentrate having several advantages over PRP; such as ease of preparation and lack of difficulties with biochemical handling of blood, which makes this preparation strictly autologous. Combining PRP or PRF with autogenous bone in mandibular continuity defects results in significantly faster radiographic maturation and histomorphometrically denser bone regeneration and may be utilized for bone defects distal to the mandibular second molars after the extraction of M3MI [33,34].

Absorbable collagen sponge

The use of absorbable collagen sponge has been investigated for the prevention or repair of bone defects distal to the mandibular second molars after the extraction of M3MI. Collagen sponge is a biocompatible material that fills the extraction socket or the bone defect and acts as a scaffold to prevent the collapse of soft tissue after extraction. It can help reduce the patient's post-operative complications at an early stage and enhance the initial healing of soft tissue and minimize periodontal defects. The collagen sponge acts as an extra cellular matrix, favouring the immigration of osteoblasts, stabilizing blood clot, help soft tissue healing, aid in wound protection and bone reconstruction [35]. It may be utilized for patients with a high risk of developing periodontal defects [36].

CONCLUSION

Surgical procedure itself or the colonization of the subgingival microbiota, due to the difficulties associated with hygiene leads to the development of a periodontal defect in the distal region to the second molars. Adequate presurgical and post-operative measures following an appropriate protocol can reduce the risk of the distal periodontal defect and improve the periodontal health of the second molar from further deterioration after the third molar extraction.

REFERENCES

1. Xiao Y, Huang J, Xiao L. Effects of bone grafting after impacted mandibular third molar extraction for treatment of distal periodontal defects of second molar: A meta-analysis. J Clin Stomatol. 2019;35(2):65–67. doi: 10.1016/j.joms.2018.07.025.
2. Haug RH, Abdul-Majid J, Blakey GH, White RP. Evidenced-based decision making: The third molar. Dent Clin North Am. 2009;53(1):77–96. doi: 10.1016/j.cden.2008.09.004.
3. Kim E, Eo MY, Nguyen TTH, Yang HJ, Myoung H, Kim SM. Spontaneous bone regeneration after surgical extraction of a horizontally impacted mandibular third molar: A retrospective panoramic radiograph analysis. Maxillofac Plast Reconstr Surg. 2019;41(1):4–6. doi: 10.1186/s40902-018-0187-8.
4. Zhang Y, Chen X, Zhou Z, et al. Effects of impacted lower third molar extraction on periodontal tissue of the adjacent second molar. Ther Clin Risk Manag. 2021;17:235–247. doi: 10.2147/TCRM.S298147.
5. Kugelberg CF, Ahlström U, Ericson S, Hugoson A. Periodontal healing after impacted lower third molar surgery: A retrospective study. Int J Oral Surg. 1985;14(1):29–40. doi: 10.1016/s0300-9785(85)80007-7.
6. Yan ZY, Tan Y, Xie XY, He W, Guo CB, Cui NH. Computer-aided three-dimensional assessment of periodontal healing distal to the mandibular second molar after coronectomy of the mandibular third molar: A prospective study. BMC Oral Health. 2020;20(1):264. doi: 10.1186/s12903-020-01250-z.
7. Petsos H, Korte J, Eickholz P, Hoffmann T, Borchard R. Surgical removal of third molars and periodontal tissues of adjacent second molars. J Clin Periodontol. 2016;43(5):453–460. doi: 10.1111/jcpe.12527.
9. Rossi D, Rossi D, Rossi D, et al. Dental supplement: Complication in third molar extractions. J Biol Regul Homeost Agents. 2019;33(3 Suppl. 1):169–172.
10. Chiapasco M, Crescentini M, Romanoni G. Germectomy or delayed removal of mandibular impacted third molars: The relationship between age and incidence of complications. J Oral Maxillofac Surg. 1995;53:418. doi: 10.1016/0278-2391(95)90715-7.
11. Mistry FK, Hegde ND, Hegde MN. Postsurgical consequences in lower third molar surgical extraction using micromotor and piezosurgery. Ann Maxillofac Surg. 2016;6(2):251–259. doi: 10.4103/2231-0746.200334.
12. Coomes AM, Mealey BL, Huynh-Ba G, et al. Buccal bone formation after flapless extraction: A randomized, controlled clinical trial comparing recombinant human bone morphogenetic protein 2/absorba-blecollagen carrier and collagen sponge alone. J Periodontol. 2014;85(4):525–535. doi: 10.1902/jop.2013.130207.
13. Zhang XM, Hou GY, Wang WW, Liao JX, Kang FW. Application of the buccal bone osteotomy with piezosurgery in extracting deeply impacted mandibular third molars. J Oral Maxillofac Surg. 2019;29(1):30–33. doi: 10.2147/TCRM.S298147.

14. Korkmaz YT, Mollaoglu N, Ozmeriç N. Does laterally rotated flap design influence the short-term periodontal status of second molars and postoperative discomfort after partially impacted third molar surgery? *J Oral Maxillofac Surg.* 2015;73(6):1031–1041. doi: 10.1016/j.joms.2015.01.005.

15. Rosa AL, Carneiro MG, Lavrador MA, Novaes AB. Influence of flap design on periodontal healing of second molars after extraction of impacted mandibular third molars. *Oral Surg Oral Med Oral Pathol Oral Radiol Endod.* 2002;93(4):404–407. doi: 10.1067/moe.2002.122823.

16. Cetinkaya BO, Sumer M, Tutkun F, Sandikci EO, Misir F. Influence of different suturing techniques on periodontal health of the adjacent second molars after extraction of impacted mandibular third molars. *Oral Surg Oral Med Oral Pathol Oral Radiol Endod.* 2009;108(2):156–161. doi: 10.1016/j.tripleo.2009.03.024.

17. Kugelberg CF, Ahlström U, Ericson S, Hugoson A, Thilander H. The influence of anatomical, pathophysiological and other factors on periodontal healing after impacted lower third molar surgery: A multiple regression analysis. *J Clin Periodontol.* 1991;18(1):37–43. doi: 10.1111/j.1600-051x.1991.tb01117.x.

18. Orban B, Wentz FM, Everett FG, et al. *Periodontics – A Concept: Theory and Practice.* St Louis, MO: C.V. Mosby Co, 1958, pp. 10–20.

19. Faria AI, Gallas-Torreira M, López-Ratón M. Mandibular second molar periodontal healing after impacted third molar extraction in young adults. *J Oral Maxillofac Surg.* 2012;70(12):2732–2741. doi: 10.1016/j.joms.2012.07.044.

20. Jaroń A, Trybek G. The pattern of mandibular third molar impaction and assessment of surgery difficulty: A retrospective study of radiographs in east Baltic population. *Int J Environ Res Public Health.* 2021;18:6–16. doi: 10.3390/ijerph18116016.

21. Aniko-Włodarczyk M, Jaroń A, Preuss O, Grzywacz A, Trybek G. Evaluation of the effect of surgical extraction of an impacted mandibular third molar on the periodontal status of the second molar – Prospective study. *J Clin Med.* 2021;10(12):26–55. doi: 10.3390/jcm10122655.

22. Xie C, Guo FY, Li XS, Cheng B. Effect of third molar extraction combined with simultaneous periodontal repair on periodontal tissue. *Chin J Aesthet Med.* 2018;27(1):50–55. doi: 10.17219/dmp/948921.

23. Szulc M, Zakrzewska A, Zborowski J. Local drug delivery in periodontitis treatment: A review of contemporary literature. *Dent Med Probl.* 2018;55(3):333–342. doi: 10.17219/dp/94890.

24. Sender-Janeczek, A, Zborowski, J, Szulc, M, Konopka T. New local drug delivery with antibiotic in the nonsurgical treatment of periodontitis – Pilot study. *Appl Sci.* 2019;9(2):50–77. doi: 10.3390/app9235077.

25. Joshi D, Garg T, Goyal AK, Rath G. Advanced drug delivery approaches against periodontitis. *Drug Deliv.* 2016;23(2):363–377. doi: 10.3109/10717544.2014.935531.

26. Brunsvold MA, Melloing JT. Bonegrafts and periodontal regeneration. *Periodontol.* 2000;1993(1):80–91.

27. Cortell-Ballester I, Figueiredo R, Valmaseda-Castellón E, Gay-Escoda C. Effects of collagen resorbable membrane placement after the surgical extraction of impacted lower third molars. *J Oral Maxillofac Surg.* 2015;73(8):1457–1464. doi: 10.1016/j.joms.2015.02.015.

28. Karapataki S, Hugoson A, Kugelberg CF. Healing following GTR treatment of bone defects distal to mandibular 2nd molars after surgical removal of impacted 3rd molars. *J Clin Periodontol.* 2000;27(5):325–32. doi: 10.1034/j.1600-051x.2000.027005325.

29. Nasr HF, Aichelmann Reidy ME, Yukna RA. Bone and bone substitutes. *Periodontol.* 2000;1999(1):74–86.

30. Liang Y, Kang FW. Repair of distal bone defect of the second molar after extraction of fully impacted mandibular third molars. *Stomatol.* 2020;40(1):22–25.

31. Sammartino G, Tia M, Bucci T, Wang HL. Prevention of mandibular third molar extraction-associated periodontal defects: A comparative study. *J Periodontol.* 2009;80(3):389–396. doi: 10.1902/jop.2009.080503.

32. Yelamali T, Saikrishna D. Role of platelet rich fibrin and platelet rich plasma in wound healing of extracted third molar sockets: A comparative study. *J Maxillofac Oral Surg.* 2015;14:410. doi: 10.1007/s12663-014-0638-4.

33. Marx RE, Carlson ER, Eichstaedt RM, Schimmele SR, Strauss JE, Georgeff KR. Platelet-rich plasma: Growth factor enhancement for bone grafts. *Oral Surg Oral Med Oral Pathol Oral Radiol Endod.* 1998;85:638–646.

34. Gandevivala A, Sangle A, Shah D, et al. Autologous platelet-rich plasma after third molar surgery. *Ann Maxillofac Surg.* 2017;7(2):245–249. doi: 10.4103/ams.ams_108_16.

35. Koshinuma S, Murakami S, Noi M, et al. Comparison of the wound healing efficacy of polyglycolic acid sheets with fibrin glue and gelatin sponge dressings in a rat cranial periosteal defect model. *Exp Anim.* 2016;65(4):473–483. doi: 10.1538/expanim.16-0031.

36. Kim JW, Seong TW, Cho S, Kim SJ. Randomized controlled trial on the effectiveness of absorbable collagen sponge after extraction of impacted mandibular third molar: Split-mouth design. *BMC Oral Health.* 2020;20:77. doi: 10.4102/ams108_16.

Complications with impacted mandibular third molar surgery

KISHORE MOTURI, ANIL BUDUMURU, AND R. S. G. SATYASAI

Complications are any adverse, unplanned events that tend to increase the morbidity above what would be expected from a particular operative procedure under normal circumstances. (Dimitroulis, 1997)

It is a well-known fact that any kind of surgery, whether elective or emergency is not devoid of complications and third molar surgery, is not an exception to this. The surgical extraction of impacted third molars is a common oral surgical procedure. It can be preventive or therapeutic and many at times maybe the last resort when all other treatment options have been ruled out. Spectrum of complications includes post-operative pain, swelling, and trismus, nerve damage, hard and soft tissue injury to unanticipated life-threatening injuries. The complications associated with the third molar surgery may or may not be foreseen and may develop from an existing illness, making the treatment difficult and can worsen the prognosis

further sometimes carrying the risk of even death. This topic will highlight all the potential areas of complications after surgical removal of mandibular third molars.

For ease of convenience to understand, all the complications associated with surgical removal of the third molar are categorized as summarized in Figure 12.1 and Table 12.1.

PREOPERATIVE COMPLICATIONS

Complications not only happen during the intra-operative and post-operative periods; lack of proper preoperative assessment can be the starting point of any complication, so the first step in anticipating complications should start from preoperative assessment.

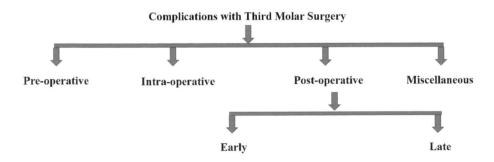

Figure 12.1 Complications with mandibular third molar surgery.

Table 12.1 Complications with mandibular third molar surgery

Preoperative	Intraoperative	Post-operative
Operator related	**Improper surgical site preparation**	**Early**
Inappropriate diagnosis	• Lack of strict asepsis	Pain
Improper medical history	**Inadequate anaesthesia**	Oedema
Improper patient education	• Inadequate volume of anaesthesia	Haemorrhage
Improper armamentarium	• Improper technique	Dry socket
Lack of anatomical knowledge	**During nerve block administration**	Surgical emphysema
Lack of skill and experience	• Needle breakage	Haematoma
Compromising radiographs and	• Intravascular administration of local	Pyrexia
blood investigation	anaesthetic	TMD
Handling by non-surgical	• Accidental administration of	Infection
specialist	formalin/H_2O_2	Osteomyelitis
Lack of good assistance	• Haematoma	Osteonecrosis-BRONJ
Underestimating the difficulty of	**During incision design**	Bad splits during BSSO
surgery	• Wrong selection of incision	**Late**
Patient related	• Bleeding from facial vessels and	Periodontal pocket distal
Unrealistic expectations	retromolar vessels	to adjacent tooth
Patient's social, economic, and	• Lingual nerve damage	TMJ complications or
educational background	**Complication during bone removal**	TMD
	• Laceration of soft tissues	Infection
	• Lip burn	
	• Injury to adjacent tooth	
	• Surgical emphysema	
	• Bur breakage	
	Complication during tooth sectioning	
	• Improper splitting of tooth	
	• Mandibular canal perforation	
	• Bur breakage	
	Complication during elevation of tooth	
	• Fracture of mandible	
	• Displacement of tooth into adjacent	
	spaces	
	• Slipping of elevator	
	• Aspiration of tooth	
	Medical emergencies	
	• Syncope	
	• Hyperventilation	
	• Anaphylaxis	
	• Hypoglycaemia	
	• Respiratory and Cardiac arrest	
	• CVA	
	Miscellaneous	
	• Gauze entrapment	
	• Incomplete removal of dental follicle	
	• Improper surgical area	
	• Complications to surgeon	

Inappropriate diagnosis

Not all cases are the same, and not all pains are the same. Most of the cases can be about abnormalities associated with third molars. However, few cases are challenging due to the nature of referred pain/neuralgia-like conditions where a well-defined diagnosis cannot be predicted at times. This dilemma is called medical uncertainty, and learning to deal with uncertainty by exclusion in the best possible way should be a core competency for any surgeon. The patient should be appropriately counselled when such a situation arises.

Improper patient education

Patient education is an essential component of a planned surgery. The treatment outcome lies mainly on patient's perception of the information provided by the surgeon and the patient's expected outcomes, morbidities, and comorbidities associated with the surgery. Proper patient education ensures that patient understands the need to opt for advanced diagnostics like computed tomography (CT)/cone-beam computed tomography (CBCT) before concluding the treatment plan and explaining the pros and cons of the surgery planned for an existing condition. Proper patient education is a core component to avoid medicolegal problems.

For example, if a patient presents with the proximity of the inferior alveolar nerve to the roots of the mandibular third molar, opting for CBCT will give a detailed picture of their association and help the operator predict the difficulty of the surgery. It will also help educate the patient about the existing condition. The operator can sensitize the patient about possible paraesthesia associated with nerve injury and their prognosis.

Lack of anatomical knowledge

Lack of adequate knowledge on anatomical barriers and vital structures near the vicinity of mandibular molars like facial artery, retromolar vessels, inferior alveolar artery, inferior alveolar nerve, lingual nerve can result in devastating potential complications and can turn an easy surgical extraction into a most difficult one. One should have sound knowledge on the location of these nerves and vessels, adjacent spaces and topographic location of tooth-related to these structures. The best possible way to be familiar with these areas is to master them before attempting a surgical case to minimize the extent of difficulty and complications during the surgery.

Improper armamentarium

A wide array of instruments are available for minor oral surgery, each with its specific uses, advantages, and disadvantages. A surgeon must be familiar with them and their applications – where, when, what, how, and the specific technique involved with each instrument. Standard operating protocols (SOP) have to be maintained and followed regularly for practical instrument usage. Using sterilized instruments, which is a mandate for any surgery, reduces complications by reducing cross-contamination.

Proper armamentarium may not always reduce the surgical difficulty but will reduce the chances of difficulty, thereby decreasing complications.

Lack of skill and knowledge

To be an excellent oral and maxillofacial surgeon takes a lot of commitment, patience, discipline, persistence and hard work which is not possible overnight.

The foundation of skills is essential for delivering optimal care which will take time, and it is a learning curve. One should acquire skill and knowledge; without these, one will eventually land into unanticipated complications that further worsen the prognosis. It is always better to go for a multidisciplinary team approach and perform entirely new surgeries or difficult surgeries under the guidance of a trained and experienced surgical specialist. Where required there should be no reservation to take the help of medical professional assistance (Anaesthetist, General Surgical Specialist, etc.)

Compromising radiographs and blood investigations

The patient characteristics, clinical history, and examination remain essential to guide the investigative choices and are an integral part of the clinical examination. Clinical information is important to correlate with the imaging findings, especially to avoid false-positive imaging diagnosis. A good surgeon listens well to the patient complaints and performs clinical examination before deciding the choice of conventional radiographical investigation or the need for advanced imaging like CBCT. If a pre-existing condition warrants it, then advanced three-dimensional imaging will help majorly in treatment planning. However, this process might not always be possible due to confounding factors like the patient's economic and educational background. It is the responsibility of the surgeon to educate the patient and initiate the treatment only after diagnostic confirmation and the patient's consent. The worst scenario would be to attempt a third molar removal even without an appropriate intra-oral periapical radiograph, making surgery more difficult. Even poor quality radiographs or radiographic artefacts should be critically evaluated and repeat order should be issued for new ones if necessary.

Every patient should be considered as a potential carrier of infection(s). Haemogram should be done on all patients undergoing surgical extraction of the mandibular third molars to rule out bleeding tendencies, anaemia, leukaemia, or viral infections, which can complicate or delay healing and, if not detected preoperatively, can account for intraoperative or post-operative complications. Correlating radiological, blood and histopathological (where required, the third molar involved with cysts or tumour) investigation can take us to the accurate diagnosis and an appropriate management plan.

Immunocompromised patients and missing COVID-19 history

COVID-19 is a SARS-COV2 viral, highly infectious, life-threatening pandemic that affected the globe irrespective of race, religion, country, gender in 2019. It is associated with opportunistic fungal infections like mucormycosis, aspergillosis, and candidiasis (the former are pathological entities, whereas the latter is a regular oral commensal). One should add COVID-19 History as an integral element of patient's case history. Furthermore, special care should be taken in immunocompromised patients, patients on immunosuppressants, organ transplant patients, and diabetic patients with chances of opportunistic infections.

To date, no standard guidelines list the best timing to perform surgery in patients affected by COVID-19 disease, nor is there any note on precautionary measures to be taken or specific investigations (radiological or blood) to be conducted on them before the oral surgical procedure. One should be very careful in recording the following details in COVID-19-affected patients: history severity, medications prescribed, hospitalization stays, loss of smell and taste, and the history of vaccination. After recording the above details, one should examine the patient clinically for any asymptomatic swelling of jaws/face, fullness in the sinus, and any sinus or pus discharge. Discolourations should be noted, and if suspicious, one should go for Paranasal Sinus (PNS) X-ray or CT. One should be cautious as operating intra-orally requires a long duration of mouth opening through the procedure, resulting in breathing difficulty and acute respiratory distress due to damaged lung parenchyma by COVID-19 [1].

Until further guidelines from statutory bodies are issued, a strict and careful examination should be done irrespective of age, keeping in mind the possible complications.

Lack of good assistance

Without saying, it goes, a good surgeon was a good assistant once who escalated through the learning curve. However, we cannot get such skilled people as assistants always. It is necessary to train paramedical or auxiliary staff to the level where they know the kind of procedure being operated on and the type of instrument(s) needed at each stage of the surgery. They should have a good energy level and a good understanding of emergency equipment's location to cope with all kinds of intraoperative complications. A good assistant will help increase the operator's hand-eye coordination, which reduces the incidence of complications.

Handling by non-surgical specialists/ lack of training

Oral and maxillofacial surgery is a specialty of dentistry, but has evolved multiple folds in the last decades; the quantity and quality of time spent to master the skill and knowledge in surgery make a refined oral and maxillofacial surgeon, who is trained to perform intra-oral procedures. In surgery, interventions are irreversible, and a small mistake can put the patient's life at risk. Keeping n mind that the patient should be at ultimate benefit, "it's always better to say *NO* when we *DON'T KNOW*". It is always wise to refer complicated cases to a more trained and skilful specialist or a centre with available facilities.

Underestimating the difficulty of surgery

In this competitive world, speed and accuracy are two essential skills needed for any surgeon to excel. Without appropriate precautions and aptness of the procedure, either of them will be a nightmare for the patient, especially in minor oral surgery. Whether the procedure is very easy or difficult, all the basic principles of minor oral surgery should be followed in every case. Never underestimate the underlying difficulty and respect the available literature.

Unrealistic expectations

There can always be a gap between patients' expectations and the reality of care provided. Within limitations, the best possible care based on the needs and expectations of the patient should be provided. Unrealistic expectations of patients will always lead to complications.

Patient social, economic, and educational background

The expression of pain from the third molar may be of the same nature or presentation for most patients. However, each patient is different in race, religion, community, culture, ethnicity, habits and perceptions. One should understand the patient first before acknowledging the disease of the patient. One should be empathetic towards the patient irrespective of their economic, social, and educational background.

INTRAOPERATIVE COMPLICATIONS

Lack of strict asepsis

Maintenance of strict aseptic conditions is an essential step in any surgical procedure. Several pathogens exist in and around the surgical site and need to be disinfected before the commencement of the surgical procedure. All the surgical instruments that are to be used must be sterilized congruously. The incidence of infection in the postoperative period after third molar surgery is very low even in the absence of an antibiotic regimen if strict asepsis protocol is followed. The frequency of surgical site infection after third molar surgery is reported between 1% and 30% [2].

Prevention: Surgeons should ensure strict sterilization protocol in the operating room. Scrub nurse, circulating nurse, and other assistants should be well trained in following the sterilization protocols. Regular training programmes should be organized for surgeons, nurses, and other assistants in the operating room to sensitize for disinfection and sterilization.

Inadequate anaesthesia

The inadequate volume of anaesthetic agents and improper technique of local anaesthesia are some common causes of insufficient anaesthesia and pain control. The surgery can be dreadful in the absence of proper pain control. Failure of nerve block is frequently seen with inferior alveolar nerve anaesthesia techniques (10%–15%) due to anatomical variation [3]

A proper evaluation of subjective symptoms and objective signs for mandibular anaesthesia should be evaluated before initiating the surgery.

During nerve block administration

NEEDLE BREAKAGE

Needle breakage is a rare complication in current clinical practice. Single-use disposable needles made of reinforced stainless–steel alloys make needle breakage a sporadic incident. Needle breakage can happen during inferior alveolar nerve block (IANB) as the needle has to be redirected within the tissues [3].

Aetiology: In current dental practice, the cause could be due to sudden movement of the patient, usage of short needles for blocks like IANB, complete insertion of the needle up to the hub, bending of needle before/on insertion, and re-use of needles.

Management: Many surgeons advise removing the needle as early as possible to prevent complications from needle migration. However, some surgeons advocate delayed removal after the foreign body fibrosis occurs around the needle, which aids in easy removal. There have been reports of delayed removal (6 months post breakage) of the needle from pterygomandibular space without complications [4].

If one end of a needle is found outside the tissues, it can be retrieved by a haemostat easily. In cases, where it is entirely into the tissue, the needle has to be localized using imaging and explored using an open surgical method.

INTRAVASCULAR ADMINISTRATION OF LOCAL ANAESTHETIC

Intravascular administration of local anaesthetic can be avoided if a proper aspirating technique is followed. Accidental administration into the artery or vein can happen when aspiration is missed before depositing the solution. If administered accidentally, the signs and symptoms depend on the type of the vessel (artery/vein) where the solution gets deposited. It can result in an overdose reaction if large volumes are administered. Management includes patient assurance, monitoring of vitals and symptomatic treatment if needed.

Prevention: One can prevent this safely by two-plane aspiration. After Initial aspiration, rotate the syringe about 45° to reorient the needle bevel relative to the blood vessel wall and aspirate before local anaesthesia deposition [3].

ACCIDENTAL ADMINISTRATION OF FORMALIN, H_2O_2 OR SUCH OTHER CHEMICAL COMPOUNDS AVAILABLE IN OPERATORY

Local anesthetics, H_2O_2, formalin, etc. are clear transparent solutions indistinguishable clinically by their visibility. It is a possibility that operatory staff tends to collect or store formalin or H_2O_2 in empty local anaesthesia bottles [5]. If the solution is withdrawn accidentally and injected, it can cause tissue necrosis at the administration site with a severe pain, burning, and discomfort.

Management: Stop further administration of the solution, once recognized and inject a large volume of saline to dilute the area to prevent tissue damage, explore the area and clear the formalin, H_2O_2 solution if needed.

Prevention: Local anaesthetic bottles should not be used to store any solutions in clinical settings; Health-care workers should be educated about this and should be trained to prevent this kind of untoward incident.

ALLERGIES AND ANAPHYLAXIS TO THE CONTENTS OF THE LOCAL ANAESTHETIC SOLUTION

Theoretically, any individual may develop hypersensitivity to the components of local anaesthetic solution. True allergic reactions to local anaesthetics are rare and represent less than 1% of all adverse local anaesthetic reactions, but when they occur, they may be life-threatening. Management of anaphylaxis is summarized in Table 12.2 and Figure 12.2.

Pain

Many authors have defined and described pain in a detailed manner in literature. However, the attempt to understand pain from patient perception represents one of the oldest and most significant challenges for the health-care delivery. Majority of the patients report with the chief complaint of pain. A component of post-operative discomfort is also expressed as pain. Intraoperatively, the surgery should be performed with minimal discomfort to the patient. To make intra-oral injections more comfortable, "Atraumatic Injection Techniques" should be followed [3]. It is a known fact that more tissue manipulation leads to more damage and ultimately more

Table 12.2 Recommendations for adrenaline use in anaphylaxis

Adrenaline administration

Inject epinephrine/adrenaline intramuscularly in the mid-anterolateral aspect of the thigh

0.01 mg/kg 1:1,000 (1 mg/mL) solution to a maximum of 0.5 mg for adults and 0.3 mg for children (consider child: <35–40 kg body weight)

Record the time of the dose and if required, repeat it in 5–15 minutes

Source: Adapted with permission from Bhargava D. Anaphylaxis: An update. J Maxillofac Oral Surg. 2013 Mar;12(1):48–50. doi: 10.1007/s12663-012-0380-8.

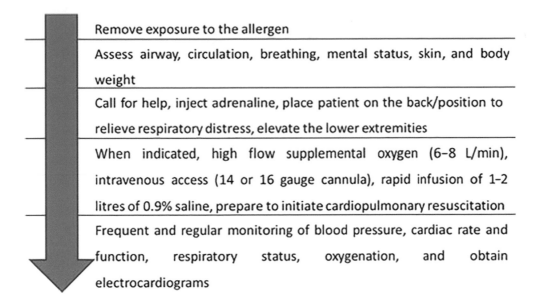

Figure 12.2 Protocol for anaphylaxis management. (Adapted with permission from Bhargava D. Anaphylaxis: An update. *J Maxillofac Oral Surg.* 2013 Mar;12(1):48–50. doi: 10.1007/s12663-012-0380-8.)

pain. Post-operative pain control can be achieved with the use of analgesics at most times. The best time to start analgesia is always before anaesthesia wears off, and an appropriate analgesic based on the kidney and liver status should be selected. However, delayed post-operative pain 3–5 days after the surgery is almost always due to infection or dry socket. In cases where amplified post-operative discomfort is anticipated, the use of parenteral analgesics may be employed (intramuscular injection of diclofenac). Transdermal Ketoprofen and Diclofenac patch have been investigated for post-extraction pain, and are found to be effective [6].

Haematoma

An extravasated blood clot is called haematoma. Haematoma can occur due to intra or extra-oral injections and collection at the site of surgery. It is significantly related to the density of surrounding structures, limiting its extent. For example, haematoma after posterior superior nerve block resulting from injury to pterygoid plexus of veins or maxillary artery can be noted due to the lack of density of surrounding tissue and due to the involvement of infratemporal space. Whereas for IANB, the surrounding

tissue density can limit its extent, which becomes clinically insignificant. Haematoma after mandibular third molar surgery can be due to bone bleed or soft tissue bleed [7]. Haematoma itself can be a potential reservoir for microorganisms. One should control all kinds of bleeding before the closure of the surgical site to prevent further complications.

Importance of surgical area

The surgical area in this context refers to the area where the surgical instruments are aligned properly to make surgery easy. When the surgical area is soiled by cotton or gauge soaked with blood, blood or saliva on the instruments or tray, and poorly arranged armamentarium will increase time to select and collect the instruments, which increases the operating time. Apart from this, there is always a chance of transporting broken burs and tooth fragments accidentally attached to gauge or cotton, which acts as a foreign body embedded in tissues. Good working area builds confidence, reduces working time and decreases more time-bound complications making the patient more comfortable.

Trigeminocardiac reflex

Trigemino cardiac reflex (TCR) is commonly associated with surgical procedures involving orbit. However, cases of TCR are documented for surgical procedures of the maxilla, mandible, and even mandibular third molar removal [8]. TCR can be recognized by the following signs:bradycardia, bradypnoea, hypotension, increased gastric motility.

Aetiology: Bradycardia developed during mandibular third molar surgery is attributed to pressure on the inferior alveolar nerve.

Management: It is usually self-limiting on the removal of stimulus. Atropine and glycopyrrolate can be used. Rarely TCR progresses to cardiac complications, requiring the availability of a defibrillator [9].

Prevention: This can be prevented by giving adequate local anaesthesia, even when the procedure is done under sedation or general anaesthesia. Emergency kit should include atropine and glycopyrrolate, for the management of non-responsive or prolonged bradycardia after removing the neural stimulus.

Aspiration/swallowing of tooth

Accidental swallowing or aspiration of tooth or tooth piece can occur during surgical extraction of the third molar. Blood-coated tooth and slippery surface of the tooth due to saliva can lead to slippage of the tooth from operators' control. It can be swallowed or aspirated. If it is suspected that the tooth is lodged in the upper airway and the patient is choking, perform the Heimlich manoeuvre. A chest X-ray is essential to rule out the accidental aspiration of a tooth into the lungs. An immediate referral to a pulmonologist for bronchoscope-aided retrieval of a foreign body is advised. If the tooth is aspirated, it can probably be into the right lung as the right bronchus is short, broad, and straight [10].

Soft tissue injuries/lacerations

Soft tissue injury in the oral cavity may occur during surgical removal of third molars due to the vulnerability of the soft tissue. Improper handling by the operator or misuse of sharp instruments like blade, bur, elevators, and faulty surgical handpieces that are heated quickly can cause physical injury or thermal burns on coming into contact with soft tissues. Instrument slippage from the point of application (tooth and/or alveolar bone) towards the tongue/floor of the mouth/palate/throat may cause unwarranted injury to the surrounding soft tissues. The reported incidence of soft tissue injuries is around 1.1% [11].

These iatrogenic injuries add to the pain and discomfort in addition to the surgical injury. These can be prevented by using an appropriate armamentarium, proper instrument grip, and adhering to minor oral surgery principles. While using elevators, the surgeon's index finger should extend along the elevator's shank and blade, and the non-dominant hand's fingers are padded with gauze should be placed on the lingual side to prevent damage to soft tissues in case of instrument slippage.

Complication during tooth sectioning

Though time taking, sectioning the tooth prevents complications that can occur with third molar surgery. However, the arc of rotation guides the surgeon regarding the sectioning of the tooth. Arc is drawn such that its diameter extends from the distal root tip to the mesiolingual cusp. An arc that indicates interference with the adjacent tooth designates a requirement for tooth sectioning before elevating it (Figure 12.3).

After sectioning, the distal fragment of the tooth is delivered first so that the mesial fragment can be pushed into the distal space created, thereby avoiding forces on the adjacent tooth. One should always remember while executing the third molar removal surgery that:

"TOOTH BELONGS TO YOU (SURGEON); BONE BELONGS TO THE PATIENT"

The chances of mandibular canal perforation must also be evaluated before mandibular third molar surgery. Rood's criteria/Howe and Poyton's criteria give an idea of the involvement of the mandibular canal. Based on the interpretation of Rood's criteria, CBCT may be advised if needed. The patient should be counselled and informed about the possible complication beforehand regarding post-operative paraesthesia.

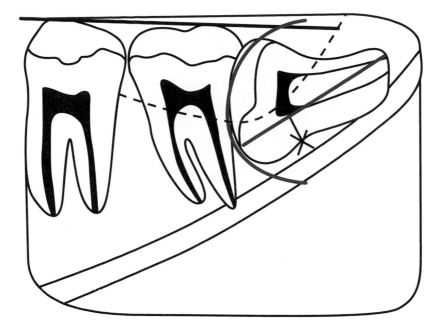

Figure 12.3 Arc of rotation.

Bleeding

Prolonged bleeding in a healthy individual is an unusual complication and warrants further investigations. However, unusual bleeding can occur during third molar surgery when the impacted tooth is close to the inferior alveolar canal. Bleeding from the facial artery may occur when the incision extends along with the mandibular second molar. Bleeding can also be from retromolar vessels. Moghadham has reported life-threatening haemorrhage after mandibular third molar surgery due to the formation of haematoma in sub-mandibular and lateral parapharyngeal spaces [12]. Krauss has reported a case of extensive facial haematoma in a 90 years old woman after mandibular third molar extraction [13].

Preventive measures:
- Proper knowledge of the anatomy of vasculature while placing an incision.
- Thorough medical history of the patient is essential to rule out bleeding disorders.

Management:
- Mechanical methods-application of pressure at the area of bleeding. Bone wax and gelatine sponge or cellulose matrix are useful haemostats for inferior dental canal haemorrhage.
- Ligating the bleeder where necessary. (Facial/ Inferior alveolar vessels, although in extreme cases this has to be planned after taking the patient to the operating room.)
- Pharmacological agents like tranexamic acid, ethamsylate and haemocoagulase may be used with mechanical packs.
- Blood pressure should be monitored.
- Use of electrocautery to achieve haemostasis may be employed. (For soft tissue bleeders/bony canal bleeds need additional interventions.)

Fracture of mandible

Fracture of the mandible after mandibular third molar surgery, though rare is a major complication. Due to its anatomic location at the angle region, the mandibular third molar predisposes the angle-ramus to fracture primarily at the time of surgery or secondarily associated with surgical trauma to the operating site. Factors responsible include deeply positioned impacted tooth, elderly age, endocrine disorders, reduced elasticity of bone, and heavy forces on elevation of the tooth. Sometimes crackling noise may be heard at the time of elevation of tooth indicating fracture. Panoramic radiography and CT will be of great value in ruling out or evaluating iatrogenic fractures and to avoid medicolegal

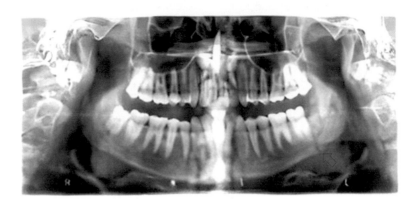

Figure 12.4 Post-operative panoramic radiograph after mandibular third molar surgery. Note the left angle fracture.

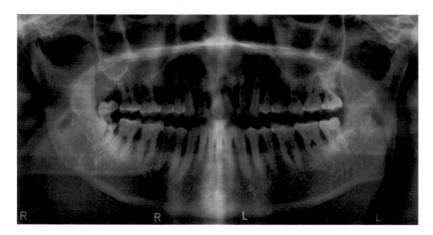

Figure 12.5 A case of attempted mandibular third molar extraction with right mandibular angle fracture.

problems. Women with osteoporosis have a high risk of iatrogenic fracture due to the low resistance to forces while transalveolar extractions [14] (Figures 12.4 and 12.5).

Management: Depending on the fracture site, degree of displacement of fracture segments, patient compliance, open or closed method of reduction, and fixation should be planned.

Complications during bone removal

Bone removal is usually done using a bur or using a chisel and mallet. The use of the bur allows controlled and precise bone cutting. However, a large amount of heat is generated during this procedure and should be countered using a proper irrigating solution (like normal saline). Failure to do so

results in damage to the bone and osteonecrosis. Although clinically it is not practical to monitor the temperature, in theory, the accepted threshold level that is required for the thermal injury on the bone is 47°C for a period of 1 minute [15].

Motorized surgical handpieces tend to get heated on prolong usage or the ones with faulty mechanics. There is every chance that the handpiece could contact surrounding soft tissues and result in thermal injury. It is generally advised to keep a check on the motorized devices regularly during the procedure. If a proper grasp and finger rest are not used, the bur rotation at high speeds could lacerate adjacent soft tissues and damage the adjacent tooth/teeth.

A laceration may also occur due to accidental slipping of the blade, surgical bur, or other sharp nstruments. These iatrogenic injuries add to the pain of surgery. These can be prevented by proper instrument handling. While placing an incision, scalpel has to move with complete conscious control. While using elevators, the surgeon's index finger should extend along the shank and blade of the elevator. This prevents accidental slipping of the elevator. A finger guard (of the hand other than holding the elevator) is always needed at the anticipated area of slippage opposite to the direction of force or the tip of the elevator.

Bur breakage/broken instrument

Some of the instruments used during third molar surgery are vulnerable to fracture intraoperatively (Figure 12.6). It is essential to identify any broken instrument after completing the procedure. The surgical wound toilet is a critical step to ensure that the site is clean and free from any foreign objects.

Preventive measures

- Use only high-quality medical-grade stainless instruments
- Instruments that are too old with worn-out working ends should be discarded
- The instruments must not be used under unreasonably high force.
- Once the surgical procedure is complete, ensure all instruments used in the intraoperative period are intact and not broken. Inspect the surgical site before closure.

Management of broken bur/instruments:

- Explore the surgical site and retrieve the broken instrument.
- Achieve haemostasis to visualize the surgical site properly.
- In case of difficulty, various additional techniques can be used to localize the broken instrument. (Advanced imaging/devices.)

Balaji SM has reported a case of a broken instrument tip in an asymptomatic patient during a routine dental radiograph [16]. Moore UJ has demonstrated the use of a metal detector device to localize a broken instrument [17].

Subcutaneous emphysema

Subcutaneous emphysema is a relatively rare but potentially severe complication with third molar surgical extractions.

Aetiology Occurs when the air from the high-speed dental handpiece is forced into the soft tissue through the reflected flap and invades the adjacent tissue planes, leading to swelling, crepitus (on palpation). Trismus and dysphagia can also result from the emphysema spreading through the fascial planes that can even lead to extensive cervicofacial emphysema, or pneumothorax and pneumomediastinum [18].

At times such a swelling might extend to the supraclavicular area about 24 hours after the surgery; potential reason for this can be attributed to functions like chewing, swallowing and speaking,

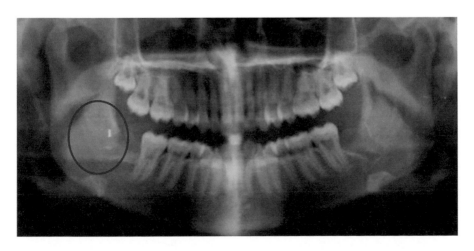

Figure 12.6 Panoramic radiograph demonstrating broken bur head at the surgical site.

which drive the air from primary spaces to loose deeper spaces [19].

Early recognition and prompt diagnosis reduce the risk of further complications. CT will be of great aid in visualizing air accumulation in involved spaces [20].

Management: Usually symptomatic. Antibiotic therapy may be instituted, careful observation of the airway, and monitoring the progression of the extension of the gas is recommended [21]. Most cases of subcutaneous emphysema start resolving after 3–5 days. Patients are advised to avoid increasing the intra-oral pressure, like blowing the nose vigorously or playing musical instruments, as the activities could cause the introduction of more air. If it seems to progress further, incision and drainage (evacuation) will help reduce the spread.

Prevention: Minimal mucoperiosteal flap elevation and gentle reflection. The elevation should not extend to the lingual alveolus of the mandibular third molar area. One should restrict the use of air-driven turbine high-speed handpieces. Prophylactic antibiotic therapy is recommended since the introduction of air and non-sterile water could cause serious infections [22].

Medical emergencies

Medical emergencies may include syncope, hyperventilation, anaphylaxis, seizures, or hypoglycaemia to extreme situations like angina, myocardial infarction and cerebrovascular accidents. These can happen to patients preoperatively (during transport/waiting area/before the start of the treatment due to anxiety), intraoperatively or postoperatively (due to pain/anxiety or because of pharmacological agents used).

The most common medical emergency is Syncope followed by Hyperventilation. Proper case history, stress reduction protocol, atraumatic injection techniques, and sedation in anxious patients can reduce the incidence of emergencies. Every clinical area should be equipped with emergency rescue equipment and an emergency drugs kit. All the staff members should be trained in identifying and using equipment and drugs along with efficiently performing basic life support (BLS). One should not delay mobilizing the patient to a nearby higher medical care facility in cases where it is difficult to manage the emergency at the dental clinical operatory.

Gauze and cotton entrapment to handpiece bur

Most operators have experienced at least once the accidental entrapment of cotton or gauze into rotating bur of handpiece. This maybe perceived by the patient as an accident in their oral cavity during the surgery. Furthermore, he/she would become more anxious during the procedure. All measures should be taken to prevent such an incidents.

POST-OPERATIVE COMPLICATIONS

Trismus

Trismus results from prolonged spasm of the masticatory muscles of the jaw. The transient jaw stiffness usually reaches its peak on the 2nd postoperative day and resolves by the end of the 1st week. It is diagnosed using clinical examination and recording the preoperative maximal interincisal distance (Figure 12.7).

AETIOLOGY

This can result from needle injury to medial pterygoid during local anaesthetic injection, oedema, haematoma or injury to the temporalis tendon or anterior coronoid fibres of the temporalis. More tissue destruction also accounts for oedema which further restricts mouth opening.

PREVENTION

Trismus may not be preventable at all times, minimizing damage to tissues, perioperative steroids therapy, and cold fomentation in the immediate post-operative period, physiotherapy or mouth opening exercises will benefit the patient.

MANAGEMENT

Mouth Opening Exercises: Patients may be advised physiotherapy right from the third post-operative day. The use of stacked ice cream wooden sticks or use of a jaw openers is helpful [23].

NSAIDs and Steroids: Non-opioid analgesics like ibuprofen, ketoprofen, aceclofenac or diclofenac may be employed in the post-operative period. Steroid are not advised in routine post-operative therapy due to the risk of wound infection. In cases with anticipated nerve injury, utilization of steroids in the post-operative phase will also benefit in prevention of surgical oedema. Intraoperative ıse of "twin-mix mandibular anaesthesia technique" has been investigated for prevention of ɾrismus and oedema, and is found beneficial [24]. ℤhang reported a case of persistent trismus up to 30 days after third molar surgery [25]. However, ıt gradually decreased over time after surgical ɗebridement.

MRONJ (Medicines-Related Osteonecrosis of the Jaw)

Medications implicated in the pathogenesis of ꞎosteonecrosis of the jaw include bisphosphonates and monoclonal antibodies. Bisphosphonates are a class of drugs that inhibit farnesyl biphosphate synthase and are used in the treatment of osteoporosis, Paget's disease and metastatic bone disease.

AETIOLOGY

These medications are associated with a disturbed bone healing process and decrease in local bone blood supply.

Patients on intravenous bisphosphonates are at risk of developing MRONJ. It is reported that patients on oral bisphosphonates are at high risk of MRONJ upto at least after 3 years of usage.

PREVENTION

In any case considering the risk, if not contra indicated, discontinue oral bisphosphonates at least 3 months before the oral surgery in consultation with the treating physician.

Evaluate not only the intake of bisphosphonate drugs (current or past) but also other pharmacological therapies (e.g., other antiresorptive agents or drugs with anti-angiogenic activity) and perform a thorough physical examination and medical examination, together with targeted radiologic examinations. "Pain" may not always be present in cases with MRONJ, especially in the early stages.

MANAGEMENT

Treatment of MRONJ is a challenge for clinicians, and an effective and appropriate MRONJ therapy is still to be devised. A multidisciplinary team approach is suggested to evaluate and decide the best therapy for the patient. In most cases, surgical debridement is the first step, followed by prophylactic antibacterial oral rinse and antibiotic therapy. The use of hyperbaric oxygen therapy

is reported in the literature. Local dressing with "iodoform" compound has shown benefit.

Haematoma/organized haematoma

Haematoma gradually expands and organises in a fibrotic capsule. Yoshida has reported a case of organized haematoma developing after extraction of the mandibular third molar [26].

PREVENTIVE MEASURES

The use of aspiration syringes and aspirating before injecting the local anaesthetic will prevent the formation of haematoma. Achieving haemostasis before wound closure is a good surgical practice.

MANAGEMENT

Antibiotic cover to prevent secondary infection. Large post-operative haematomas may be aspirated or drained. Surgical excision is indicated in case of organized non-resolving haematoma with a fibrous capsule.

Incomplete removal of dental follicle

The dental follicle is an ectomesenchymal tissue associated with the development of all the teeth and the third molar is not an exception to this. During third molar surgery, it is imperative to remove the dental follicle completely after delivery of the tooth. The surgical site should be debrided appropriately and irrigated to identify any remnants of the dental follicle. Remnants of the dental follicle may be associated with cystic changes in a considerable number of patients [27,28].

Osteomyelitis

Osteomyelitis is an infection occurring in the medullary cavities of the bone, thereby spreading through Haversian systems of the cortex to extend till the periosteum of the bone. It is relatively common in the mandible owing to its limited blood supply (inferior alveolar vessels and periosteal). Conditions that may predispose include immunocompromised situations like diabetes mellitus, organ transplant patients, AIDS, autoimmune disorders, and patients on long-term immunosuppressant drugs or steroids. There are reported cases of post-operative osteomyelitis after mandibular third molar surgery and this can occur even

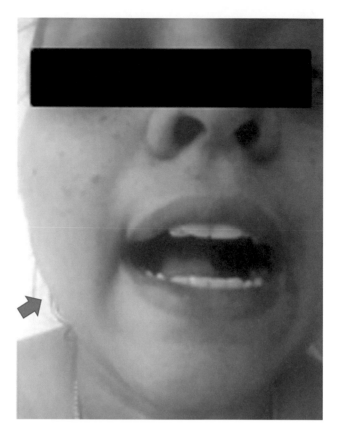

Figure 12.7 Post-operative trismus. Note the extra-oral swelling on the right side of the face, on first post-operative day following transalveolar extraction of #48.

after uncomplicated extraction of the third molar [29,30].

MANAGEMENT

Surgical debridement: Debridement, sequestrectomy, saucerization and decortication should be employed and fresh bleeding should be induced.

HBO therapy (hyperbaric oxygen): Though not available readily at all centres, it has reports of benefit in cases with osteomyelitis involving the facial bones. The procedure involves exposure to 100% oxygen in a large chamber at 2.4–3 atm pressure for 90 minutes sessions or "dives" for as many as 5 days a week, totalling 30 or more sessions. It is expected to promote hypercellularity and hypervascularity.

Pyrexia

Pyrexia is a constant, elevated body temperature above 98.5°F. It can occur in the early post-operative period due to various factors like inadequate

fluid intake, bacteraemia, or rarely due to drug reaction (Drug Fever). The patient should be advised to take plenty of fluids in the post-operative period. The patient should be properly evaluated and if pyrexia continues to exist even after proper fluid intake, antipyretic medications like paracetamol should be prescribed. Intravenous paracetamol and cold sponging may be considered only when the temperature is above 101°F. The patient should be put on antibiotics to control bacteraemia.

Pyrexia may be present even in a preoperative period when there is active pericoronitis, periapical infection, cellulitis, or spreading fascial space infections. A preoperative antibiotic and hydration regimen are helpful in such conditions. Proper sterilization protocol and adequate fluids help prevent post-operative pyrexia. In cases with poor oral hygiene, the patient should be advised to undergo thorough oral prophylaxis before the third molar surgery. This reduces bacteraemia significantly.

Infection

Infection after third molar surgery is common, especially when proper asepsis protocol is not followed during the operative procedure [31]. It can also be seen due to non-compliance of patients to post-operative instructions. Most surgeons prescribe antibiotics in the post-operative period to decrease post-operative infections. However, there is no indication of post-operative antibiotics in healthy individuals [32].

The incidence of infection at the surgical site is more frequent in the early post-operative period than in the late post-operative period. Delayed onset infections, which occur after a month are also reported. Delayed onset infections are usually associated with mesioangular impacted teeth and are caused due to food entrapment in the periodontal defect distal to the second molar tooth.

MANAGEMENT

Empirical antibiotic therapy should be started. Culture and sensitivity test is indicated if there is pus discharge. Furthermore, definitive therapy may be started once the report is obtained.

Surgical debridement, incision and drainage may be required. Delayed periodontal defects may require periodontal therapy.

Delayed paraesthesia

Paraesthesia, if it occurs, is usually seen in the early post-operative period. Delayed paraesthesia in the distribution of the inferior alveolar nerve is rare after third molar surgery. However, Doh RM has reported neurosensory dysfunction that developed 2 weeks after the third molar surgery [33].

AETIOLOGY

Inflammatory exudate, fibrous reorganization of the clot and nerve trauma could be the probable cause for delayed paresthesia.

MANAGEMENT

Non-steroidal anti-inflammatory medication and corticosteroid therapy may be helpful. Although such rare instances require detailed evaluation.

Necrotizing fasciitis

Infection from the third molar can spread to various fascial spaces and result in necrotizing fasciitis. There are a few reports of post-operative necrotizing fasciitis following routine third molar extraction procedures [34].

PREVENTION

Necrotizing fasciitis can rapidly spread along the superficial and deep fascia of the head and neck. If thorough debridement is not done in time, it can spread to deep spaces and even lead to necrotizing mediastinitis.

MANAGEMENT

- Antibiotic therapy,
- Necrosed fascia has to be identified and debrided.
- Regular surgical dressings.

Oedema

Oedema after surgical removal of third molars is very common and is unavoidable, and generally commensurates with the degree of surgical trauma [35]. The patient should be made aware of this fact prior to surgery. Post-operative surgical oedema is usually transudate in nature. Peak swelling will usually occur 48–72 hours after surgery and would gradually decrease [36].

MEASURES TO REDUCE OEDEMA

Careful and gentle manipulation of tissues during the procedure.

Immediate application of ice packs for the first 24 hours with 20 minutes increments is advised to reduce the post-operative oedema. Intramuscular or intravenous administration of glucocorticoids, and oral steroids if needed may be considered. Preventing post-operative trauma to the surgical site is advised.

Temporomandibular joint disorders and dislocations

The removal of third molars has been cited as a factor that may cause temporomandibular joint (TMJ) damage. Furthermore, the surgical trauma caused by third molar surgery has been a risk factor for the progression of TMJ disorder (TMD)-related symptoms [37]. This may be attributed to sustained period of mouth opening and the application of significant forces to the mandible required for the surgical extraction of the mandibular third molars.

The most common problems observed following third molar extraction are joint pain, muscle pain, decreased jaw opening and joint noise (click). This may result from muscular and articular pain as a consequence from muscle and ligament stretching, condyle subluxation, or disc derangement. Studies indicate that TMJ symptoms worsen among patients who already have TMDs. Prior to the third molar surgery, it is critical to identify individuals who have pre-existing joint pain or evidence of dysfunction in their temporomandibular joints and masticatory tissues [38]. Acute TMJ dislocation at the time of the surgery requires reduction of the joint using the prescribed manoeuvre [39].

Periodontal defects

Surgical extraction of the third molar can often result in the formation of a periodontal pocket distal to the second molar, delaying healing and allowing bacteria to colonize the socket, resulting in secondary abscess, or causing mobility, hypersensitivity, or the formation of a periodontal defect. Three critical factors influence periodontal complications at the distal aspect of the second molar: patient's age, third molar impaction type and depth, and presurgical periodontal defect [40].

Other factors that can cause dehiscence include

1. The surgical technique used (procedure and suture),
2. The post-operative care of the wound, and
3. The occurrence of complications during and after the procedure (iatrogenic errors, infection, retraction, resorption or collapse of the flap, and foreign body reaction).

The flap distal to the second molar is first sutured with an appropriate 3–0 absorbable or silk stay-suture with additional suturing as deemed necessary. Tight cervical closure of the distal soft tissues to prevent a distal pocket is advocated [41].

Nerve injuries

Neurosensory impairment is a common complication with extraction of impacted third molars. The inferior alveolar nerve (IAN) injury incidence ranges from 0.35% to 8.4%. The incidence of IAN neurosensory deficit is found highest with horizontal impactions (4.7%) and lowest when the tooth is vertically impacted (0.9%). In most cases, IAN paraesthesia is temporary and recovers within 6–8 months in the post-operative period. Permanent sensory loss is reported to be about 0.7% [42].

The risk factors of post-operative IAN damage include the surgeon's experience, the age and sex of the patient, the degree of operative tissue damage, surgical instrumentation, and post-operative oedema. However, the most critical factor is the anatomical relationship between the impacted third molar and the mandibular canal.

Lingual nerve injury is an uncommon but significant complication in the removal of the mandibular third molar. Juodzbalys et al. have reported the incidence of lingual nerve injury as highest for the distally impacted mandibular teeth (4.0%), followed by horizontal impaction (2.8%), mesial impaction (2.4%), and minimum with vertical impaction (1.9%).

Bad splits during sagittal split osteotomy

Attempting with an unerupted at the time of sagittal split osteotomy increases the operating time and surgical difficulty. That is why many surgeons recommend prior removal of the third molars at least by 6–9 months. Nevertheless, due to the complexity of removal, more bone has to be sacrificed, leading to a bad split during the osteotomy. The overall incidence of the negative splits is reported to be 0.21%–22.72% [43]. An impacted third molar below the external oblique ridge, distoangular or vertical oriented tooth with divergent/supernumerary roots would cause more unfavourable splits when the spreader is not used appropriately during the osteotoly [44].

Dry socket (alveolar osteitis)

Dry socket is a condition presenting as a post-operative sequela after the mandibular third molar extraction. It is characterized by excruciating pain in and around the extraction site area, with or without halitosis, and with partially or completely disintegrated intra-socket blood clot.

Concept of fibrinolytic alveolitis proposed by Brin (1973) stands valid to understand the aetiology of the dry socket. **Birn's hypothesis** explains that the trauma and inflammation cause the release of stable tissue activator from the bony socket and adjacent soft tissues. Tissue activator converts plasminogen (present in the blood clot) to the plasmin. This plasmin causes lysis of the blood clot. The bone devoid of the clot with the nerve endings exposed to the inflammatory mediators causes excruciating pain.

Factors that increase the incidence of dry socket formation include forceful spitting or rinsing leading to loss of clot, smoking, oral contraceptive pills or oestrogen/progesterone pills, Paget's disease, haematological disorders associated with the impaired formation of a blood clot, poor oral hygiene, retained root stump, infection, excessive irrigation/curettage of the socket, and poor tissue handling.

PREVENTION

Gentle intra-operative tissue handling. The patient should be properly educated about the post-operative instructions. Adequate suturing prevents dislodgement of blood clot. Proper medical history should be recorded to rule out the use of contraceptive pills, hormonal therapy or other systemic problems. The patient should be advised to restrain from smoking.

MANAGEMENT

Wound debridement using irrigation to clear the inflammatory mediators that are irritant to the nerves along with obtundent dressings with zinc oxide eugenol or an Iodoform dressing is all that would be required to manage a case with alveolar osteitis. Analgesics may be prescribed for pain management. Treatment should include gently irrigating the area with (warm) saline, and the inserting an obtundent medicated dressing. Ideally, the socket should not be curetted as this will increase the amount of exposed bone and the pain, and remove parts of the blood clot that have not been lysed. The socket should be carefully suctioned of the excess saline followed by the placement of the medication-impregnated dressing. This may need to be repeated every 2–3 days depending on the severity of the pain.

Complications to surgeon

So far, all the possibilities of complications for patients are discussed. Practice of surgery or profession suffers from medicolegal problems or assault from patient or attendants due to unexpected inevitable complications. The clinician is also, always at risk of needlestick injury, injury from scalpel and other sharps, cross-contamination, biting injury on fingers, thermal or chemical injuries. As appropriate ergonomics is an integral part of the exodontia practice, when ignored, spine and posture ailments commonly affect the clinicians practising this medical science.

REFERENCES

1. Aoyama H, Uchida K. Respiratory characteristics and related intraoperative ventilatory management for patients with COVID-19 pneumonia. *J Anesth.* 2021 Jun;35(3):356–360. doi: 10.1007/s00540-020-02845-0.

2. Susarla SM, Sharaf B, Dodson TB. Do antibiotics reduce the frequency of surgical site infections after impacted mandibular third molar surgery? *Oral Maxillofac Surg Clin North Am.* 2011 Nov;23(4):541–546. doi: 10.1016/j.coms.2011.07.007.

3. Malamed SF. *Handbook of Local Anesthesia*, 7th ed. St. Louis, MO: Elsevier, 2020.

4. Ethunandan M, Tran A, Anand R, et al. Needle breakage following inferior alveolar nerve block: Implications and management. *Br Dent J.* 2007;202;395–397.

5. Swami PC, Raval R, Kaur M, Kaur J. Accidental intraoral injection of formalin during extraction: Case report. *Br J Oral Maxillofac Surg.* 2016 Apr;54(3):351–352. doi: 10.1016/j.bjoms.2015.09.016.

6. Bhargava D, Thomas S, Beena S. Comparison between efficacy of transdermal ketoprofen and diclofenac patch in patients undergoing therapeutic extraction – A randomized prospective split mouth study. *J Oral Maxillofac Surg.* 2019 Oct;77(10):1998–2003. doi: 10.1016/j.joms.2019.04.007.

7. Kraus CK, Katz KD. Extensive facial hematoma following third molar removal. *Am J Emerg Med.* 2014 Sep;32(9):1153.e5–6. doi: 10.1016/j.ajem.2014.02.031.

8. Ichiyama T, Watanabe, M, Nariai Y, Sekine J. A case of sinus arrest caused by trigeminocardiac reflex during extraction of an impacted lower third molar. *Japanese J Oral Maxillofac Surg.* 2015;61:182–186. doi: 10.5794/jjoms.61.182.

9. Wang W, Cai H, Ding H, et al. Case report: 2 cases of cardiac arrest caused by rhino-cardiac reflex while disinfecting nasal cavity before endonasal transsphenoidal endoscopic pituitary surgery. *BMC Anesthesiol.* 2021:21;18.

10. Elgazzar RF, Abdelhady AI, Sadakah AA. Aspiration of an impacted lower third molar during its surgical removal under local anaesthesia. *Int J Oral Maxillofac Surg.* 2007 Apr;36(4):362–364.

11. Sayed N, Bakathir A, Pasha M, Al-Sudairy S. Complications of third molar extraction: A retrospective study from a tertiary healthcare center in Oman. *Sultan Qaboos Univ Med J [SQUMJ].* 2019;19(3):e230–e235.

12. Moghadam HG, Caminiti MF. Life-threatening hemorrhage after extraction of third molars: Case report and management protocol. *J Can Dent Assoc.* 2002 Dec;68(11):670–674.

13. Kraus CK, Katz KD. Extensive facial hematoma following third molar removal. *Am J Emerg Med.* 2014;32(9):1153.e5–1153.

14. Chrcanovic BR, Custodio ALN. Considerations of mandibular angle fractures during and after surgery for removal of third molars: A review of the literature. *Oral Maxillofac Surg.* 2010;14:71–80.

15. Isler SC, Cansiz E, Tanyel C, Soluk M, Selvi F, Cebi Z. The effect of irrigation temperature on bone healing. *Int J Med Sci.* 2011;8(8):704–708. doi: 10.7150/ijms.8.704.

16. Balaji SM. Burried broken extraction instrument fragment. *Ann Maxillofac Surg.* 2013;3(1):93–94.

17. Moore UJ, Fanibunda K, Gross MJ. The use of a metal detector for localisation of a metallic foreign body in the floor of the mouth. *Br J Oral Maxillofac Surg.* 1993 Jun;31(3):191–192. doi: 10.1016/0266-4356(93)90125-g.

18. Shackelford D, Casani JAP. Diffuse subcutaneous emphysema, pneumomediastinum, and pneumothorax after dental extraction. *Ann Emerg Med.* 1993;22:248–250.

19. Sekine J, Irie A, Dotsu H, Inokuchi T. Bilateral pneumothorax with extensive subcutaneous emphysema manifested during third molar surgery. A case report. *Int J Oral Maxillofac Surg.* 2000;29:355–357.

20. Matsumoto S, Koyanagi N, Matsuo M, Kurata S, Shiraishi N, Ayuse T, Oi K. A case of wide-spread emphysema following the extraction of mandibular third molar under intravenous sedation. *Masui.* 2001 Mar;50(3):278–280.

21. Kung JC, Chuang FH, Hsu KJ, Shih YL, Chen CM, Huang IY. Extensive subcutaneous emphysema after extraction of a mandibular third molar: A case report. *Kaohsiung J Med Sci.* 2009 Oct;25(10):562–566. doi: 10.1016/S1607-551X(09)70550-9.

22. Gamboa Vidal CA, Vega Pizarro CA, Almeida Arriagada A. Subcutaneous emphysema secondary to dental treatment: A case report. *Med Oral Patol Oral Cir Bucal.* 2007;12:76–78.

23. Shulman DH, Shipman B, Willis FB. Treating trismus with dynamic splinting: A case report. *J Oral Sci.* 2009;51:141–144.

24. Bhargava D, Sreekumar K, Rastogi S, Deshpande A, Chakravorty N. A prospective randomized double-blind study to assess the latency and efficacy of twin-mix and 2% lignocaine with 1:200,000 epinephrine in surgical removal of impacted mandibular third molars: A pilot study. *Oral Maxillofac Surg.* 2013 Dec;17(4):275–280. doi: 10.1007/s10006-012-0372-3.

25. Zhang Y, Zhuang P, Jia B, Xu J, Cui Q, Nie L, Wang Z, Zhang Z. Persistent trismus following mandibular third molar extraction and its management: A case report and literature review. *World Acad Sci J.* 2021;3(1):2.

26. Yoshida S, Matsuzaki Y, Kogou T, Kato H, Ohno K, Watanabe A, Akashi Y, Takano M. A rare case of organized hematoma in the cheek. *J Oral Maxillofac Surg Med Pathol.* 2021;33(4):443–447.

27. Saravana GH, Subhashraj K. Cystic changes in dental follicle associated with radiographically normal impacted mandibular third molar. *Br J Oral Maxillofac Surg.* 2008 Oct;46(7):552–553. doi: 10.1016/j.bjoms.2008.02.008.

28. Dongol A, Sagtani A, Jaisani MR, Singh A, Shrestha A, Pradhan A, Acharya P, Yadav AK, Yadav RP, Mahat AK, Maharjan IK, Pradhan L. Dentigerous cystic changes in the follicles associated with radiographically normal impacted mandibular third molars. *Int J Dent.* 2018 Mar;20:2645878. doi: 10.1155/2018/2645878.

29. Yamamoto S, Taniike N, Yamashita D, Takenobu T. Osteomyelitis of the mandible caused by late fracture following third molar extraction. *Case Rep Dent.* 2019;5421706.

30. Humber CC, Albilia JB, Rittenberg B. Chronic osteomyelitis following an uncomplicated dental extraction. *J Can Dent Assoc.* 2011;77:b98.

31. Al-Asfour A. Postoperative infection after surgical removal of impacted mandibular third molars: An analysis of 110 consecutive procedures. *Med Princ Pract.* 2009;18(1):48–52.

32. Susarla SM, Sharaf B, Dodson TB. Do antibiotics reduce the frequency of surgical site infections after impacted mandibular third molar surgery? *Oral Maxillofac Surg Clin North Am.* 2011 Nov;23(4):541–546. doi: 10.1016/j.coms.2011.07.007.

33. Doh RM, Shin S, You TM. Delayed paresthesia of inferior alveolar nerve after dental surgery: Case report and related pathophysiology. *J Dent Anesth Pain Med.* 2018;18(3):177–182.

34. Hechler BL, Blakey GH. Necrotizing soft tissue infection following routine third molar extraction: Report of two cases and review of the literature. *Int J Oral Maxillofac Surg.* 2019 Dec;48(12):1525–1529.

35. Laskin DM. *Oral and Maxillofacial Surgery*, Vol. 1. St. Louis, MO: Elsevier, 2009.

36. Dym H, Ogle OE, Wettan HL. *Atlas of Minor Oral Surgery*. Philadelphia: Saunders, 2001.

37. Damasceno, YSS, Espinosa, DG, Normando, D. Is the extraction of third molars a risk factor for the temporomandibular disorders? A systematic review. *Clin Oral Invest.* 2020;24(10):3325–3334.

38. Trishala A. Evaluation of an association between impacted teeth and temporomandibular joint disorders. *Eur J Mol Clin Med.* 2020;7(1).

39. Bhargava D, Sivakumar B. Temporomandibular joint hypermobility disorders. In: Bhargava D. (ed) *Temporomandibular Joint Disorders*. Singapore: Springer, 2021. doi: 10.1007/978-981-16-2754-5_18.

40. De Biase A, Mazzucchi G, Di Nardo D, Lollobrigida M, Serafini G, Testarelli L. Prevention of periodontal pocket formation after mandibular third molar extraction using dentin autologous graft: A split mouth case report. *Case Rep Dent.* 2020;2020:1762862.

41. Motamedi MHK. A technique to manage gingival complications of third molar surgery. *Oral Surg Oral Med Oral Pathol Oral Radiol Endod.* 2000;90(2):143–143.

42. Sarikov R, Juodzbalys G. Inferior alveolar nerve injury after mandibular third molar extraction: A literature review. *J Oral Maxillofac Res.* 2014 Dec;5(4):e1. doi: 10.5037/jomr.2014.5401.

43. Balaji SM. Impacted third molars in sagittal split osteotomies in mandibular prognathism and micrognathia. *Ann Maxillofac Surg.* 2014 Jan–Jun;4(1):39–44.

44. Schubert W, Kobienia BJ, Pollock RA. Cross-sectional area of the mandible. *J Oral Maxillofac Surg.* 1997;55:689–692.

Healing after mandibular third molar extraction

EINSTEIN A, SHUBHANGI DURGAKUMAR MISHRA, AND
DARPAN BHARGAVA

INTRODUCTION

Healing of a tooth socket is an observable expression of a highly coordinated series of responses, including biochemical, physiological, cellular and molecular, along with the involvement of several types of cells, hormones, cytokines, growth factors and proteins, all intending to restore the integrity and function of the tissues post extraction of a tooth.

A thorough understanding of the sequence and the intricacies of these responses following a surgical wound will enable the surgeon to target an optimal healing response both by deciding on the most appropriate surgical procedure and by employing advanced biological approaches that enhance the wound healing process.

HEALING OF AN EXTRACTION SOCKET

The process of socket healing in humans can be divided into three distinct yet overlapping phases, namely the inflammatory phase, the proliferative phase and the bone modelling or remodelling phase [1].

The inflammatory phase

The inflammatory phase commences immediately after tooth extraction with the event of haemorrhage and usually lasts for 3–5 days. Trauma to the

tissue and local haemorrhage following the tooth extraction, activate the Hageman factor (factor XII), which initiates the healing cascade via the complement, plasminogen, kinin, and clotting systems.

Formation of a primary platelet plug by the aggregation of platelets within a fibrin matrix results in the physiological phenomenon of haemostasis, plugging the severed vessels and stopping the bleeding in the socket. This clot formation also assists as a reservoir of cytokines and growth factors such as interleukins, TGF-β, PDGF, and VEGF, released during degranulation of the activated platelets.

With the arrest of bleeding, the subsequent event will be marked by persistent vasodilation mediated by histamine, prostaglandins, kinins and leukotrienes and the influx of cellular mediators of inflammation.

With an intent of "cleaning up" the site of the socket for the formation of new tissue, a large number of inflammatory cells start migrating to the wound area within 2–3 days of tooth extraction. Cytokine-mediated chemotaxis helps recruit neutrophils and monocytes. Neutrophils serve to cleanse the wound of contaminating bacteria, dead tissue and degraded tissue components. Activated monocytes (macrophages) proceed with the microdebridement of the wound, through phagocytosis of bacteria and cell debris and further serve as major sources of the mediators of wound healing. Thus, macrophages play a major role in all phases of early wound healing.

DOI: 10.1201/9781003324034-13

The proliferative phase

The proliferative phase is characterized by the formation of granulation tissue, which is composed of inflammatory cells, proliferating new blood vessels and immature fibroblasts that fill up the extraction socket.

Considering the regenerative nature of this phase, the essential primary step is the establishment of a local microcirculation through angiogenesis via the action of growth factors. The fibroblasts migrate into the wound and secrete new matrix and immature type III collagen. Thus, the granulation tissue is gradually replaced by a provisional connective tissue matrix after the socket is sterilized. The appearance of a tissue matrix rich in fibrous and cellular components marks the commencement of the proliferative phase.

The proliferative phase is characterized by rapid and intense fibroplasia and subsequent penetration of blood vessels and osteoblasts into the provisional matrix. Trabeculae of osteoid extend from the alveolus into the clot and osteoclastic activity can be observed along the cortical margins of the socket. Woven bone, a provisional type of bone, can be identified in the healing sockets from 2 weeks to several weeks post extraction, which then gets replaced with lamellar bone and bone marrow.

The surface of the socket is completely reepithelialized with minimal or no scar formation.

The bone modelling/ remodelling phase

The woven bone is replaced with lamellar bone or bone marrow (bone remodelling) and the bone on the socket walls starts resorbing, altering the dimensions of the alveolar ridge (bone modelling). The process of remodelling varies among individuals and a complete replacement of the woven bone with the lamellar bone or bone marrow takes several months to years.

The process of bone modelling occurs earlier than the remodelling, with two-thirds of the process occurring in the first 3 months post extraction. Although bone modelling is equal on the buccal and lingual socket walls, there appears to be a greater vertical bone loss associated with the thinner cortical plate.

Cumulatively, both the processes in this phase result in qualitative and quantitative changes at the site of extraction socket with a resultant dimensional reduction of the ridge.

The histological aspects of the spontaneous wound healing process of extraction socket are depicted in Figure 13.1a–d.

HEALING FOLLOWING MANDIBULAR THIRD MOLAR EXTRACTION

Mandibular third molars are one of the most commonly impacted teeth associated with several clinical concerns such as dental caries, pericoronitis, damage to the adjacent teeth, odontogenic cysts and tumours and temporomandibular joint disorders, thus often demanding an extraction [2]. The healing of the extraction sockets of mandibular third molars that had erupted in a physiologically appropriate position and orientation follows similar phases as those of the healing of sockets of other teeth in the oral cavity.

However, surgical extraction of impacted mandibular third molars, one of the commonest oral surgical procedures and the most complicated when related to greater depth of impaction, associated with notable post-extraction morbidity. The greater surgical insult to the hard and soft tissues due to the reflection of the mucoperiosteal flap, removal of the overlying bone, sectioning of the tooth, removal of the tooth and the socket closure with suturing of the soft tissue flap results in exaggerated inflammatory response exhibiting as pain, swelling, acute trismus, sometimes fever and the like. Furthermore, the less frequent but extremely morbid complications that may occur include infection and nerve damage [3].

ASSESSMENT OF WOUND HEALING AFTER MANDIBULAR THIRD MOLAR EXTRACTION

Clinical assessment

The soft tissue healing is assessed and is supposed to be satisfactory with the tissue colour being pink and similar to the adjacent gingiva; epithelialization at the incision margins with no exposed

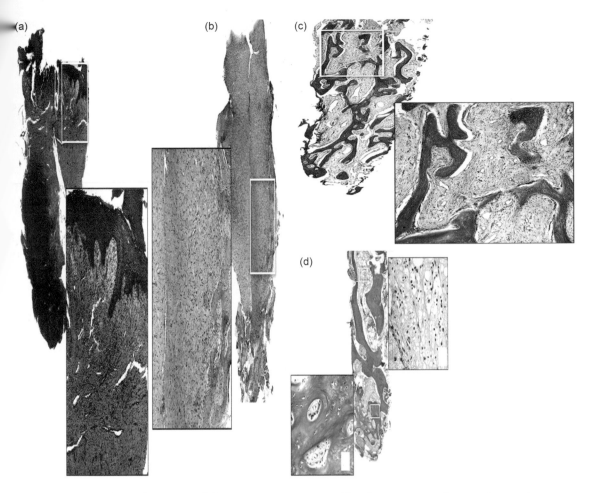

Figure 13.1 Histological aspects of the spontaneous wound healing process of extraction sockets. (a) A biopsy was obtained after 3 weeks of healing. The tissue is rich in vessels, fibroblasts, and inflammatory cells and is characterized as granulation tissue. Original magnification ×2.5. (b) A biopsy was obtained after 4 weeks of healing. The provisional matrix comprises mesenchymal cells densely packed fibres and vessels. Only a few inflammatory cells can be observed. Original magnification ×2.5. (c) Decalcified section obtained from a biopsy sampled after 6 weeks of healing. Note the presence of trabeculae of immature woven bone that occur in a cell and fibre-rich provisional matrix. Original magnification ×2.5. (d) Biopsy was obtained from an extraction wound representing 12 weeks of healing. The tissue comprises of more mature bone; woven bone and lamellar bone that reside in a non-mineralized matrix. Original magnification ×2.5. (Reprinted with permission from: Farina, R. and Trombelli, L. Wound healing of extraction sockets. *Endod Topics*, 2011;25:16–43. doi: 10.1111/etp.12016.)

connective tissue; and the absence of bleeding on palpation, granulation tissue, or suppuration.

Clinical indicators of socket healing also include the absence of pain, measured on various available pain scales; absence of cheek swelling and oedema, assessed by measuring the distances from the tragus to the soft tissue pogonion and from the tragus to the angle of mouth; good periodontal health of the adjacent second molar in terms of the pocket depth on the distobuccal aspect of the second molar; absence of disintegrated blood clots with or without halitosis or necrotic debris; and absence of a denuded socket [4,5].

Radiographic assessment

Although various scoring systems and criteria have been proposed in the literature to assess the bone healing radiographically, a few common parameters to summate are the thickness of the lamina dura distal to the second molar tooth and the density and the trabecular pattern of the newly formed bone [4,5]. Further, radiographic evidence of bone formation may not become apparent until 6–8 weeks post extraction. The bone remodelling process might take 4–6 months to be appreciated on radiographs as a measure for complete healing.

Histological assessment

A histological assessment of wound healing after mandibular third molar extractions is rarely advocated due to the invasiveness of the procedure. However, when performed, the parameters that are assessed histologically include evidence of new bone formation, fibrovascular stroma with angiogenesis, absence of inflammatory infiltrate, regular dispersion of osteocytes, osteoblastic proliferation and differentiation [6].

COMPLICATIONS IN HEALING OF EXTRACTION SOCKET

Knowledge of the myriad of local and systemic factors that can impede the physiologic wound healing process can help the surgeon to predict, prevent and manage such factors and ensure normal wound healing following a surgical procedure such as extraction.

Excessive and prolonged trauma

Excessive and longer duration of traumatic insult to the tissues result in longer healing periods and probable post-surgical morbidity. Thus, minimizing trauma at every stage of the surgical procedure including incision placement, bone removal, handling tissues and suturing should always be on the surgeon's mind, to promote faster healing.

Infectious complications

Prolonged trauma during the surgical procedure, inadvertent or extended exposure of denuded bone, inadequate irrigation during surgery and poor infection control might all lead to failure of formation or disintegration of the blood clot resulting from bacterial colonization of the clot or an adverse inflammatory reaction. Birn suggested that prolonged traumatic insult or the presence of a bacterial infection could induce the release of plasminogen tissue activators in the post-extraction socket, resulting in the plasmin induction of fibrinolysis leading to disintegration of the clot [7,8].

These infectious complications might include dry alveolar osteitis, suppurative osteitis, necrotic osteitis and/or fibrous healing. The localized alveolar osteitis, commonly referred to as dry socket, is characterized by considerable delay in healing owing to the absence of a healthy granulation tissue. Further, bone modelling might proceed at a much slower pace. Patients usually present with foul smelling, dry and bare socket that are open or partially covered with hyperplastic epithelium. Suppurative osteitis presents with a purulent yellow-greenish appearance and intense persistent pain.

Infectious complications are observed more among women, probably associated with the increased intake of oral contraceptives; more with increasing age; and more common among smokers. The complications are also related to the surgical technique and skills employed, cooling systems employed during bone cutting, and improper antibiotic coverage.

Use of medications

Usage of drugs that interfere with the physiologic process of healing might result in post-extraction healing. A classic example is the systemic use of corticosteroids, which impair wound healing owing to their anti-inflammatory action and their inhibiting action on fibroplasia and epithelialization [9].

Pathological states

Patients with type 2 diabetes mellitus have impaired and unpredictable healing following extraction owing to modifications in the expression of mediators such as TGF-β. Uncontrolled hyperglycaemia results in alteration of the leucocyte function, impairment of phagocytosis and chemotaxis, and increased risk of infections [10].

Immunodeficiency states including HIV/AIDS manifest with a decreased resistance to infections resulting in defective healing.

Tissue perfusion is a major factor in ensuring adequate and timely healing. Lack of oxygenation (hypoxia) results in slower and interrupted deposition of the collagen matrix, delaying the normal healing process. Patients with previous oral radiation therapy or anti-angiogenic treatments are at risk for such hypoxia-related complications because of the narrowing of the blood vessels, which then decrease the flow of blood to the tissues.

ADVANCED BIOLOGIC APPROACHES TO ENHANCE WOUND HEALING AFTER MANDIBULAR THIRD MOLAR EXTRACTION

The cognizance of the clinical complications or morbidity associated with the healing of wounds after extraction of mandibular third molars has made researchers attempt the exploitation of the four elementary events of wound healing, namely angiogenesis, immune defence, trapping of circulating stem cells, and re-epithelialization, to augment wound healing post extraction. Histologically and biochemically, bone regeneration is facilitated by three vital elements, the scaffolds that include collagen, bone minerals, etc.; the formative cells like fibroblasts and osteoblasts; and the signalling molecules in the form of growth factors.

Suturing

Suturing aids in hastening the soft tissue recovery by reducing post-extraction bleeding and narrowing the site of wound created by surgical extraction of mandibular third molars. Further, it prevents infection of the wound by protecting the blood clots and avoiding the entry of food into the socket. In surgical extractions not incorporating post-extraction suturing, a high possibility of formation of a wedge gap in relation to the adjacent second molar has been noticed [11].

Suturing with buccal drainage

A mandibular third molar socket is generally sutured not too firmly, and the wound was conventionally left unsutured at the turning point of incision that is adjacent to the distal side of the second molar to facilitate drainage between the distal side of the second molar and mesial side of the third molar in some of the proposed flap designs. However, it was often found that patients in such cases would avoid chewing from the operated side with the apprehension of food entering the extraction socket. Moreover, it was observed that such kind of drainage delayed wound healing.

Thus, the accepted norm is to allow drainage from the area where the mesiobuccal incision starts from the distobuccal aspect of the second molar region and not the mesiobuccal region of the adjacent tooth, as was done conventionally. While suturing, sutures may be placed at the distal incision and the superior alveolar area. The anterior buccal releasing incision is left unsutured, this establishes successful buccal drainage and has been surveyed to be more acceptable by patients solving the problems of facial swelling or food impaction post-surgical extraction [12].

Platelet-rich fibrin

Platelet-rich fibrin has been rightfully described by researchers as a stimulative agent for the chemotaxis of human mesenchymal stem cells at the site of tissue injury. Platelets act as an autologous source of growth factors including PDGF, IGF and TGF-β, stored in the α-granules. Their isolation from peripheral blood and incorporation at the site of extraction socket along with the fibrin matrix delivers high concentrations of growth factors at the site of bone regeneration [4].

Dentin autologous graft and other graft materials

The development of a periodontal pocket distal to the second molar is a threat to uneventful healing of the wound after mandibular third molar extraction. As an innovative approach, there are reports of the extraction socket being grafted with ground dentin from the extracted third molar and this has shown to reduce the pocket depth, although such newer grafting techniques require controlled trials with larger patient sample before applying in the regular practice [13]. Conventionally autogenous or xenografts have been employed to restore bone defects. Alloplastic substitutes are also preferred where indicated. Utilization of such grafts may require a combination approach with guided

Table 13.1 Combination of different reconstructive technologies on the healing of extraction sockets: histological aspects. Only results of controlled (pre-clinical and clinical) studies evaluating the effect of the combined approach versus either the spontaneous healing or each reconstructive technology when used alone have been included

Authors	Year	Animal/ human	Materials		Observation intervals (time elapsed from socket grafting)	Comparison between test treatment and spontaneous healing	Comparison between test treatment and single reconstructive technology
			Test treatment	Control treatment/s			
GRAFT+MEMBRANE							
(112) Becker	1996	Human	DFDBA+ePTFE membrane	DFDBA	4–13 months	—	No adjunctive effect of ePTFE membrane over DFDBA
(100) Dies	1996	Human	DFDBA or DBBM+ePTFE membrane	DFDBA, DBBM	6–9 months	—	Graft residual particles retard/impair bone regeneration compared to ePTFE membrane alone
(113) Smukler	1999	Human	DFDBA+ePTFE membrane	Spontaneous healing	8–23 months	No adjunctive effect of ePTFE membrane over spontaneous healing	—
(114) Iasella	2003	Human	FDBA+collagen membrane	Spontaneous healing	4–6 months	More bone in experimental sites, but including also non vital bone	—
(115) Molly	2008	Human	DBBM, PLA/PGA or CC+ePTFE membrane	ePTFE membrane	6 months	—	Sites treated with DBMM+ePTFE membrane had lower % of viable bone compared to membrane alone, while PLA/PGA+ePTFE membrane or CC+ePTFE membrane did not
GRAFT+BIOACTIVE AGENTS							
(116) Brandao	2002	Animal (rat)	HA+BMPs	Spontaneous healing, HA	7–42 days	No differences in the amount of bone between HA+BMPs and spontaneous healing at 7 days. HA+BMPs resulted in a delayed healing in terms % of new bone at 21 days, but not at 42 days when compared to spontaneous healing	No differences in the amount of bone between HA+BMPs and HA at 7 days. HA+BMPs resulted in a delayed healing in terms % of new bone at 21 days, but not at 42 days compared to HA

Table 13.1 (Continued) Combination of different reconstructive technologies on the healing of extraction sockets. histological appraisal... only... controlled (pre-clinical and clinical) studies evaluating the effect of the combined approach versus either the spontaneous healing or each reconstructive technology when used alone have been included

| Authors | Year | Animal/ human | Materials | | Observation intervals (time elapsed from socket grafting) | Comparison between test treatment and spontaneous healing | Comparison between test treatment and single treatment and single reconstructive technology |
			Test treatment	Control treatment/s			
(117) Shi	2007	Animal (dog)	CS+PRP	Spontaneous healing, CS	8 weeks	CS+PRP promoted bone formation compared to spontaneous healing	The addition of PRP to CS resulted in the enhancement of bone regeneration in the early phase of healing
(118) Neiva	2008	Human	xenograft/ P15+collagen dressing material	Collagen dressing material	16 weeks	—	No differences in vital bone, marrow, and fibrous tissue between xenograft/ P15+collagen dressing and collagen dressing alone
GRAFT + SOFT TISSUE GRAFT							
(119) Luczyszyn	2005	Human	HA+ADM	ADM	6 months	—	Frequent presence of HA particles enclosed in fibrous connective tissue in sites treated with HA+ADM, not in ADM group
STEM CELLS							
(120) De Kok	2005	Animal (dog)	HA/ TCP+BMMSCs	Spontaneous healing, TCP	49 days	No difference in new bone formation area between HA/ TCP+BMMSCs and spontaneous healing	Significantly greater new bone formation area in HA/ TCP+BMMSCs compared to HA/TCP
(121) Marei	2005	Animal (rabbit)	PLA/ PGA+BMMSCs	Spontaneous healing, PLA/PGA	2 weeks, 4 weeks	Evidence of active bone deposition in PLA/ PGA+BMMSCs at 4 weeks, not in spontaneous healing	Evidence of active bone deposition in PLA/ PGA+BMMSCs at 4 weeks, not in PLA/PGA

DFDBA: demineralized freeze dried bone allograft; ePTFE: expanded polytetrafluoroethylene; DBBM: deproteinized bovine bone mineral; FDBA: freeze dried bone allograft; PLA/PGA: polylactic/polyglycolic acid; CC: calcium carbonate ceramic; HA: hydroxyapatite; BMP: bone morphogenetic protein; CS: calcium sulphate; PRP: platelet-rich plasma; P15: peptide 15; ADM: acellular dermal matrix; TCP: tricalcium phosphate; BMMSCs: bone marrow mesenchymal stem cells.
This table was adapted with permission from Farina, R. and Trombelli, L. Wound healing of extraction sockets. Endod Topics, 2011;25:16–43. doi: https://doi.org/10.1111/ etp.12016; The references cited at the author's column in the table can be followed for further reading at: https://doi.org/10.1111/etp.12016

Table 13.2 Combination of different reconstructive technologies on the healing of extraction sockets: clinical aspects. Only results of controlled (pre-clinical and clinical) studies evaluating the effects of the combined approach versus either the spontaneous healing or each reconstructive technology when used alone have been included

Authors	Year	Animal/ human	Materials		Observation intervals (time elapsed from socket grafting)	Comparison between test treatment and spontaneous healing	Comparison between test treatment and single reconstructive technology
			Test treatment	Control treatment/s			
GRAFT+MEMBRANE							
(114) Iasella	2003	Human	FDBA+collagen membrane	Spontaneous healing	4–6 months	1.6 mm less horizontal contraction for FDBA+collagen membrane compared to spontaneous healing; vertical gain in experimental sockets, vertical loss in control sockets (inter-group difference: 2.2 mm)	—
(102) Pinho	2006	Human	Autologous bone+titanium membrane	Titanium membrane	6 months	—	No difference in vertical and horizontal changes between treatments
(122) Kim	2008	Animal (dog)	DBBM+collagen membrane	Spontaneous healing, DBBM	4 months	Greater bone augmentation in DBBM+collagen membrane compared to spontaneous healing	Greater bone augmentation in DBBM+collagen membrane compared to DBBM
GRAFT+BIOACTIVE AGENTS							
(117) Shi	2007	Animal (dog)	CS+PRP	Spontaneous healing, CS	2 months	Significantly less reduction in ridge height in CS+PRP compared to spontaneous healing at anterior sites	No significant difference in the reduction of ridge height between CS+PRP and CS

(Continued)

Table 13.2 (*Continued*) Combination of different reconstructive technologies on the healing of extraction sockets: clinical aspects. Only results of controlled (pre-clinical and clinical) studies evaluating the effects of the combined approach versus either the spontaneous healing or each reconstructive technology when used alone have been included

Authors	Year	Animal/ human	Materials		Observation intervals (time elapsed from socket grafting)	Comparison between test treatment and spontaneous healing	Comparison between test treatment and single reconstructive technology
			Test treatment	Control treatment/s			
GRAFT + SOFT TISSUE GRAFT							
(119) Luczyszyn	2005	Human	HA+ADM	ADM	6 months	—	Less horizontal ridge resorption in HA+ADM compared to ADM
(30) Fickl	2008a	Animal (dog)	DBBM+free soft tissue graft	Spontaneous healing	2–4 months	Lower resorption rate of buccal and lingual crest compared to spontaneous healing	—
(93) Fickl	2008b	Animal (dog)	DBBM+free soft tissue graft	Spontaneous healing, DBBM	4 months	No difference in vertical changes and lower horizontal (at 1 mm from the crest) resorption compared to spontaneous healing	Greater vertical changes and lower horizontal resorption (at 1 mm from the crest) compared to DBBM
(94) Fickl	2008c	Animal (dog)	DBBM+free soft tissue graft	Spontaneous healing, DBBM	2–4 months	Lower resorption of buccal crest compared to spontaneous healing	No difference in buccal and lingual crest resorption compared to DBBM

FDBA: freeze dried bone allograft; DBBM: deproteinized bovine bone mineral; CS: calcium sulphate; PRP: platelet-rich plasma; HA: hydroxyapatite; ADM: acellular dermal matrix. This table was adapted with permission from Farina, R. and Trombelli, L. Wound healing of extraction sockets. *Endod Topics*, 2011;25:16–43. doi: https://doi.org/10.1111/etp.12016; The references cited at the author's column in the table can be followed for further reading at: https://doi.org/10.1111/etp.12016

tissue regeneration therapy and/or substitution of growth factors (Tables 13.1 and 13.2).

Absorbable collagen sponge

Enhanced post-surgical healing of the soft tissues and a reduction in the periodontal defects has been observed with the placement of an absorbable collagen sponge in the mandibular third molar extraction sockets. The sponge imitates an extracellular matrix, favouring osteoblast recruitment, blood clot stabilization, wound protection, soft tissue and bone regeneration [14]. The fear with collagen matrix is that it may act as a nidus for infection in cases where the bacterial colonization takes place.

Various regenerative measures utilized to limit the defect distal to mandibular second molars and promote healing at the extraction defect sites are summarized in Tables 13.1 and 13.2.

REFERENCES

1. Araújo MG, Silva CO, Misawa M, Sukekava F. Alveolar socket healing: What can we learn? *Periodontol.* 2015;68(1):122–134. doi: 10.1111/prd.12082.

2. Jerjes W, Upile T, Nhembe F, et al. Experience in third molar surgery: An update. *Br Dent J.* 2010;209(1):E1. doi: 10.1038/sj.bdj.2010.581.

3. Clauser B, Barone R, Briccoli L, Baleani A. Complications in surgical removal of mandibular third molars. *Minerva Stomatol.* 2009;58(7–8):359–366.

4. Dutta SR, Singh P, Passi D, Patter P. Mandibular third molar extraction wound healing with and without platelet rich plasma: A comparative prospective study. *J Maxillofac Oral Surg.* 2015;14(3):808–815. doi: 10.1007/s12663-014-0738-1.

5. Jeyaraj PE, Chakranarayan A. Soft tissue healing and bony regeneration of impacted mandibular third molar extraction sockets, following postoperative incorporation of platelet-rich fibrin. *Ann Maxillofac Surg.* 2018;8(1):10–18. doi: 10.4103/ams.ams_185_17.

6. Hauser F, Gaydarov N, Badoud I, Vazquez L, Bernard JP, Ammann P. Clinical and histological evaluation of post extraction platelet-rich fibrin socket filling: A prospective randomized controlled study. *Implant Dent.* 2013;22(3):295–303. doi: 10.1097/ID.0b013e3182906eb3.

7. Gowda GG, Viswanath D, Kumar M, Umashankar DN. Dry socket (alveolar osteitis): Incidence, pathogenesis, prevention and management. *J Indian Acad Oral Med Radiol.* 2013;25(3):196–199.

8. Mamoun J. Dry socket etiology, diagnosis, and clinical treatment techniques. *J Korean Assoc Oral Maxillofac Surg.* 2018;44(2):52–58. doi: 10.5125/jkaoms.2018.44.2.52.

9. Kylmaniemi M, Oikarinen A, Oikarinen K, Salo T. Effects of dexamethasone and cell proliferation on the expression of matrix metalloproteinases in human mucosal normal and malignant cells. *J Dent Res.* 1996;75:919–926.

10. Yamano S, Kuo WP, Sukotjo C. Downregulated gene expression of TGF-beta in diabetic oral wound healing. *J Craniomaxillofac Surg.* 2013;41: e42–e48.

11. Osunde OD, Adebola RA, Saheeb BD. A comparative study of the effect of suture-less and multiple suture techniques on inflammatory complications following third molar surgery. *Int J Oral Maxillofac Surg.* 2012;41(10):1275–1279. doi: 10.1016/j.ijom.2012.04.009.

12. Hu T, Zhang J, Ma JZ, et al. A novel method in the removal of impacted mandibular third molar: Buccal drainage. *Sci Rep.* 2017;7(1):12602. doi: 10.1038/s41598-017-12722-8.

13. Sánchez-Labrador L, Martín-Ares M, Ortega-Aranegui R, López-Quiles J, Martínez-González JM. Autogenous dentin graft in bone defects after lower third molar extraction: A split-mouth clinical trial. *Materials (Basel).* 2020;13(14):3090. doi: 10.3390/ma13143090.

14. Kim JW, Seong TW, Cho S, Kim SJ. Randomized controlled trial on the effectiveness of absorbable collagen sponge after extraction of impacted mandibular third molar: Split-mouth design. *BMC Oral Health.* 2020;20(1): 77. doi: 10.1186/s12903-020-1063-3.

Advances in surgical extraction of the mandibular third molars

SUNDAR RAMALINGAM AND DARPAN BHARGAVA

According to Darwin's Origin of Species, it is not the most intellectual of the species that survives; it is not the strongest that survives; but the species that survives is the one that is able best to adapt and adjust to the changing environment in which it finds itself.

– Leon C. Megginson

Historical evidence of tooth extraction as a treatment for dental ailments dates back to the Neolithic age (10,000–4,500 BCE), and have been documented by historians during every major civilization. Even the instruments used for removing teeth have evolved from early drills made out of bones and shells to mechanical levers and rudimentary forceps. However, in the early 17th century, extractions were relegated as the last resort treatment and something done only by barbers, who were considered persons with pretentious medical skills and not real clinicians, leading to a diminution in advancement. Nevertheless, most of the currently used elevators and forceps were designed and developed during the renaissance ages not only by surgeons, but also by barbers [1]. It was not until the 18th century that techniques of third molar extraction gained prominence. Although not documented, knowledge about the surgical approaches and use of chisels, osteotomes and mallets for third molar removal were passed on from surgeon to surgeon, until the first manual was published in 1906 by the National Dental Association of America [1]. This was followed by published literature on surgical techniques for third molar removal by eminent dentists and oral surgeons throughout the earlier part of the 20th century. Which included Charles Edmund Kells (1918), George Winter (1926), Kurt Thoma (1932), William Kelsey Fry (1933), Wilfred Fish (1934), Warwick James (1937), Ward (1956), and Gustav Kruger (1959) [1]. While majority of these techniques are still being used or are referred to, the last few decades have witnessed a voluminous growth in evidenced-based research data with respect to surgical removal of impacted and non-impacted mandibular third molars. Some of these advances pertain to flaps and surgical approaches, bone and tooth cutting techniques, wound healing, preventing lingual and inferior alveolar nerve injury, and alternative strategies for mandibular third molar removal [2].

SURGICAL FLAPS FOR MANDIBULAR THIRD MOLAR REMOVAL

Several flap techniques with innovative modifications have been proposed and utilized for mandibular third molar removal over the last century.

DOI: 10.1201/9781003324034-14

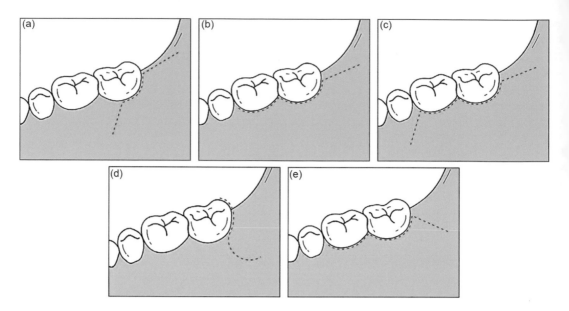

Figure 14.1 Conventional and newer flap designs for mandibular third molar surgery: (a) Triangular flap described by Ward, 1956. (b) and (c) Envelope flap without and with anterior/mesial releasing incision described by Kruger, 1959. (d) Comma flap described by Nageshwar, 2002 and (e) Distal-triangular flap (also reported as reverse triangular flap or modified envelope flap). (Modified from: Sifuentes-Cervantes JS, Carrillo-Morales F, et al. Third molar surgery: Past, present, and the future. *Oral Surg Oral Med Oral Pathol Oral Radiol.* 2021;132(5):523–531; Liu JY, Liu C, et al. Distal-triangular flap design for impacted mandibular third molars: A randomized controlled trial. *Hua Xi Kou Qiang Yi Xue Za Zhi.* 2021;39(5):598–604; Mudjono H, Rahajoe PS, et al. The effect of triangular and reversed triangular flap designs to post third molar odontectomy complications (a pilot study). *J Clin Exp Dent.* 2020;12(4): e327–334; Xie Q, Wei S, et al. Modified envelope flap, a novel incision design, can relieve complications after extraction of fully horizontal impacted mandibular third molar. *J Dent Sci.* 2021;16(2):718–722.)

Nevertheless, they all fall under one of the two main flap designs, namely triangular and envelope flaps (Figure 14.1) [1,2]. The most recent Cochrane Collaboration Systematic Review, originally published in 2014 and updated in the year 2020, found scarce evidence to classify one flap design better over the other in terms of post-extraction bleeding, socket healing, incidence of dry socket and permanent nerve injuries [3]. While a weak evidence favouring non-envelope flaps was reported with respect to reduced pain and swelling during the early postoperative period (24 hours), envelope flaps were associated with a similar weak evidence of reducing incidence of trismus post extraction. Interestingly, no particular flap design is seen to have a clear advantage over other flap designs with regard to postoperative sequelae experienced by patients [4]. Evidence suggests that, under common clinical circumstances, the choice of a given flap design is primarily based on the position of the impacted mandibular third molar, and only

secondarily by the surgeon's clinical experience, duration of surgical procedure anticipated and potential comorbidities [4]. Nevertheless, the last two decades within 21st century, has not witnessed a dearth of newer flap designs and modifications to existing ones. The distolingually based comma flap (Figure 14.1) proposed by Nageshwar (2002), envisages a smooth curvilinear incision beginning from the distal surface of the second molar and extending distobuccally to a point below it [5]. In comparison to conventional flap designs, it was claimed that the comma flap resulted in reduced postoperative pain and swelling, better periodontal healing and no evidence of lingual nerve injury. A modified envelope flap with a distobuccally placed releasing incision (Figure 14.1) has been reported with differing terminologies such as distal-triangular flap [6], reverse triangular flap [7], and modified envelope flap [8]. Although there were no significant differences in any of the postoperative outcomes in comparison with conventional flap designs, authors have claimed that the above flap designs provided better surgical exposure with minimal mouth opening, enhanced wound healing and reduced risk of reactionary haemorrhage due to ease of flap re-approximation. Inspite of all the above modifications and innovations in terms of flap design, invasive soft tissue elevation and manipulation are considered as the main factors associated with better surgical access at the cost of increased patient discomfort and poor postoperative quality of life outcomes [4,9]. Finally, as an alternative to any form of soft tissue manipulation a flapless approach utilizing contra-angled handpiece to section the crown and roots, and remove the tooth in a piecemeal fashion has also been proposed [10,11]. Nonetheless, the flapless technique is feasible only for removal of impacted mandibular third molars with partially or completely exposed clinical crowns.

LINGUAL NERVE PROTECTION DURING THIRD MOLAR REMOVAL SURGERY

The anatomic course of the lingual nerve in the medial aspect of the mandibular third molar, makes it susceptible to injury during the surgical removal of the tooth. Lingual nerve damage resulting in permanent or temporary sensorineural loss is not only a severe complication, but also is a matter of medicolegal significance [12]. Earlier studies had reportedly identified the lingual nerve farther away from the lingual wall of the mandibular third molar socket. Based on a cadaveric study, Mendes et al. (2013) reported the horizontal distance between the lingual cortical plate and the lingual nerve to be in the range of 2 mm to 11 mm, with a mean distance of 4.4 ± 2.4 mm, and the vertical distance ranged from 12 to 29 mm, with a mean of 16.8 ± 5.7 mm [13]. With the advances in radiographic techniques this anatomical relationship has been investigated further and based on magnetic resonance imaging (MRI) study, the lingual nerve has been identified even close to the third molar. Accordingly, the mean horizontal distance was 1.05 ± 1.0 mm, the mean vertical distance was 4.65 ± 1.2 mm, and the diameter of the lingual nerve in the vicinity of the third molar was 1.06 ± 0.2 mm [14]. These findings indicate an even greater responsibility for oral surgeons to be aware of the close proximity of the lingual nerve during

mandibular third molar surgery and therefore avoid iatrogenic injuries to it.

The argument that lingual flap elevation and retraction using specific instruments, especially in cases requiring distal bone removal or lingual splitting, has found takers on both sides of the spectrum. Based on a qualitative review, Steel et al. (2021) reported a greater incidence of lingual nerve injuries with lingual retractors in general, and more specifically with repurposed instruments (periosteal elevators used as standby lingual flap retractors) than with specific instruments like Hovell's or Walter's lingual retractors [2]. On the other hand, Petroni et al. (2021) based on a meta-analysis of 11 studies comparing lingual flap retraction against no lingual flap retraction, reported similar outcomes in terms of lingual nerve injury and further claimed that retraction of lingual flap provided better access and lingual soft tissue protection [12]. Out of 5,938 cases of third molar surgery without a lingual flap, temporary lingual nerve paresthesia was reported in $1.92\% \pm 0.02\%$ and permanent loss of sensation was seen in $0.49\% \pm 0.006\%$. Similarly, out of 3,866 cases of third molar removal with lingual flap retraction, $2.98\% \pm 0.03\%$ of temporary loss and $0.1\% \pm 0.003\%$ of permanent loss in lingual nerve function were reported [12]. Based on the most recent Cochrane Collaboration Systematic Review (2020), the placement of sub-periosteal lingual retractor neither aided nor abetted the incidence of lingual nerve injury [3]. In summary, the risk of lingual nerve injury exists inspite of the advances in our knowledge and understanding of the anatomy and better surgical techniques, with temporary injuries that take up to 2–6 months to recover being reported more frequently than permanent loss of sensation [2,3]. While the position of the mandibular third molar in terms of distolingual angulation and lower eruption levels are unfavourable, the surgeon's level of experience and the use of specific purpose-built lingual retractors where required, are important factors which can help eliminate lingual nerve morbidity.

INFERIOR ALVEOLAR NERVE PRESERVATION DURING THIRD MOLAR REMOVAL SURGERY

Injury to the inferior alveolar nerve (IAN) has been reported as a complication of mandibular third molar removal since long, and could result in up

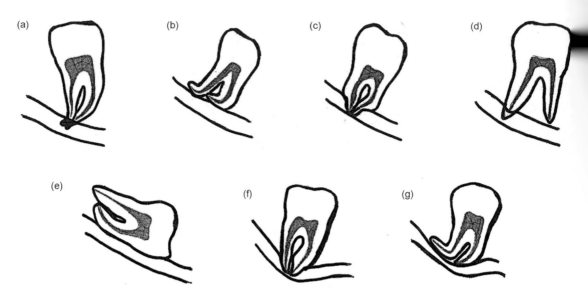

Figure 14.2 Radiographic classification of the relationship between mandibular third molar roots and inferior alveolar nerve (IAN) canal, Rood and Shehab (1990): (a) Root darkening. (b) Root deflection. (c) Root narrowing. (d) Dark and bifid root apex. (e) Interruption of IAN canal white line. (f) IAN canal diversion and (g) IAN canal narrowing. (Modified from: Rood JP, Shehab BA. The radiological prediction of inferior alveolar nerve injury during third molar surgery. *Br J Oral Maxillofac Surg.* 1990;28(1):20–25.)

to 3.6% permanent neurosensory loss and up to 8% temporary sensory disturbances [15]. While age and difficulty of surgery are considered as contributing factors, the key predisposing factor for IAN injury is its close anatomic proximity to the roots of the mandibular third molar [15,16]. Based on periapical radiograph and orthopantomogram (OPG), Rood and Shehab (1990) (Figure 14.2) system to analyse proximity and relationship of the IAN to mandibular third molar roots [17]. Accordingly, they were root darkening, deflection or narrowing, bifid and dark apex, interruption of white line of IAN canal, and IAN canal diversion or narrowing. While it was considered that an evidence of either canal diversion, root darkening or disturbance of the lamina dura, based on periapical radiograph or OPG, as a clear pointer of risk for IAN injury, the advent of dental cone-beam computed tomography (CBCT) in the last decade has radicalized preoperative decision making, in this regard [15,18,19]. Based on a study of 135 patients, Elkhateeb and Awad (2018), reported statistically significant CBCT evidence of direct contact between the root and IAN canal for the most commonly cited predictors of IAN injury in OPG, namely IAN canal interruption and narrowing, and root darkening [20]. Using CBCT Maglione et al. (2015) described

a comprehensive classification scheme which can help understand the three-dimensional orientation of the IAN canal with respect to the mandibular third molar roots (Table 14.1) [19]. Applying the above classification to a subset of 69 patients who underwent mandibular third molar removal, it was observed that the classification scheme functioned as a reliable preoperative radiographic predictor and helped reduce the risk of intra operative IAN injury and postoperative neurosensory morbidity [18].

The practice of leaving in place fractured root fragments, was the traditional method of minimizing IAN injury during mandibular third molar removal [15]. Originally described in 1984 by Ecuyer and Debien, coronectomy is a procedure which involved deliberate sectioning of only the coronal portion of the tooth (coronectomy) and leaving behind the root fragment close to the IAN [2,15,16]. While coronectomy has gained parlance in the last three decades as a technique to minimize postoperative IAN sensory loss, the success of the technique is plagued by several concerns relating to reoperation rates, complications other than IAN injury and measure of effectiveness [2]. Although, large-scale studies about third molar coronectomy or comparing them with complete

Table 14.1 Classification of the relationship between inferior alveolar nerve canal and mandibular third molar based on cone-beam computed tomography imaging, along with representative image outlining a section passing coronally through the tooth and perpendicular to the long axis of IAN canal

Class/description	Subtype	Representative image (Left–lingual/right–buccal)
Class 0 – IAN canal not seen in the section	–	
Class 1 – IAN canal is apical or buccal to the root apex	**1A** – Distance between IAN canal and root>2 mm	
	1B – Distance between IAN canal and root<2 mm	
Class 2 – IAN canal is lingual to the root apex	**2A** – Distance between IAN canal and root>2 mm	
	2B – Distance between IAN canal and root<2 mm	
Class 3 – IAN canal is apical or buccal to the root apex and in contact with it	**3A** – Diameter of IAN canal preserved at point of contact	
	3B – Diameter of IAN canal narrowed at point of contact or shows cortical loss	
Class 4 – IAN canal is lingual to the root apex and in contact with it	**4A** – Diameter of IAN canal preserved at point of contact	
	4B – Diameter of IAN canal narrowed at point of contact or shows cortical loss	

(Continued)

Table 14.1 (*Continued*) Classification of the relationship between inferior alveolar nerve canal and mandibular third molar based on cone-beam computed tomography imaging, along with representative image outlining a section passing coronally through the tooth and perpendicular to the long axis of IAN canal

Class/description	Subtype	Representative image (*Left–lingual/right–buccal*)
Class 5 – IAN canal is between the two roots, and not in contact with them	**5A** – Distance between IAN canal and root>2mm	
	5B – Distance between IAN canal and root<2mm	
Class 6 – IAN canal is between the two roots, and in contact with one of them	**6A** – Diameter of IAN canal preserved at point of contact	
	6B – Diameter of IAN canal narrowed at point of contact or shows cortical loss	
Class 7 – IAN canal is between fused roots	-	

Source: Modified from Maglione M, Costantinides F, et al. Classification of impacted mandibular third molars on cone-beam CT images. *J Clin Exp Dent.* 2015;7(2): e224–31.

Note: IAN, inferior alveolar nerve.

removal are not available, pooled data from the literature indicate success rates for coronectomy as high as 93% [2,21]. These studies also indicate failure rates ranging up to 9.4%, with the predominant cause for failure being inadvertent root mobilization during coronectomy leading to extraction or conversion of a planned coronectomy to extraction. Incidentally, the risk of extraction of a third molar originally slated for coronectomy was higher among young females and patients with radiographic presentation of conical roots which narrowed closer to the IAN canal [2]. While coronal migration of the roots or root exposure were reported as a major complication during the early postoperative phase, minor complications such as socket dehiscence, wound infection and pulpitis have also been reported. Interestingly, enamel retention has been implicated in most cases reporting with a dry socket like foreign body type reaction, thereby underscoring the need for removing all enamel during coronectomy [2].

Out of the three randomized control trials (RCT) comparing coronectomy and complete removal of third molars, identified by the most recent Cochrane Collaboration Systematic Review by Bailey et al. (2020) [3], two RCTs were excluded due to high risk of bias [15,22]. The remaining RCT by Singh et al. (2018) reported no differences between the two techniques in terms of outcomes such as postoperative pain, swelling, rismus, wound infection and dehiscence, periodontal pocket and sensorineural deficit [23]. However, they reported significant yet asymptomatic coronal migration of the roots up to 3.43 mm in 6 months. Based on pooled data, root migration due to persisting eruptive forces are reported in up to 97% of patients undergoing coronectomy, and ranged from 1 to 4 mm. While most root migration occurs in younger patients in either a mesial direction or a distal rotation within 12 months, it has also been reported as late as 24 months post coronectomy [2]. Root migration and exposure has also been reported as the main reason for reoperation and removal of root fragments after coronectomy. Based on a pooled data of 2,062 coronectomies, Barcellos et al. (2019) reported 105 teeth (5.1%) which required reoperation [24]. Out of which 53.3% were due to root migration and exposure, followed by other minor causes such as infection, pain and enamel retention, with each one of them ranging between 9% and 11%. Nevertheless, eruption of the roots into the oral cavity has only been reported in approximately 2% of the cases and reoperation to remove the exposed or coronally migrated roots was dictated purely based on symptomatology and was not associated with IAN injury or paresthesia [2,24,25].

The most important consideration while making a treatment decision of coronectomy of the mandibular third molar, is avoiding risk of IAN injury. Pooled data from systematic reviews have indicated a clear statistical association between coronectomy and reduction in nerve injury, in addition to no significant differences in terms of generic sequelae such as pain, swelling, trismus, postoperative infection and dry socket [3]. Based on a review of 14 studies reporting 2,087 coronectomies, including 152 cases of failure due to inadvertent root mobilization or extraction, Dalle Carbonare et al. (2017) reported 0.5% incidence of transient IAN injury and 0.05% permanent damage, when coronectomy was performed successfully [21]. On the contrary, failed coronectomies resulted in a greater risk of IAN injury ranging from 2.6% temporary paresthesia to 1.3% permanent neurosensory deficit. Furthermore, the risk of lingual nerve injury as a result of coronectomy is only as low as 0.05%, which was not permanent [21]. Similarly, based on a meta-analysis of four studies, Pitros et al. (2020) reported a pooled odds ratio of 1.6 for IAN injury when third molars in close proximity to the IAN were extracted. This however, decreased by 84% when coronectomy was preferred over extraction [26]. In one of the longest and largest reported series of mandibular third molar coronectomy cases, Leung and Cheung (2016), reported only one case of paresthesia due to IAN injury out of 612 procedures (0.16%), which eventually recovered over a 5-year follow-up period [25]. No evidence of lingual nerve injury was reported in the above mentioned case series. In yet another systematic review of 2,176 coronectomies from 16 studies, Póvoa et al. (2021) reported 0.59% and 0.22% risk of injury to the inferior alveolar and lingual nerves, respectively [27].

Although voluminous clinical and follow-up data regarding mandibular third molar coronectomy is available in the literature, due to the dearth of RCTs comparing coronectomy with extraction, and the risk of bias in those reported thus far, a clear superiority of coronectomy over extraction is not demonstrable [2,3]. Nevertheless, coronectomy is a safe procedure as it is associated with similar, if not better, postoperative symptoms when compared to complete removal and also decreases risk of IAN injury. In the absence of preoperative CBCT and utilizing only conventional radiographs, coronectomy is also seen as an economic alternative to complete removal of impacted mandibular third molars [26]. It is therefore imperative that a decision to perform coronectomy for a mandibular third molar be based on clinical and radiographic evidence of proximity to IAN and shared decision making with the patient [2,26,27]. Moreover, it must be borne in mind that during the procedure, care must be exercised to avoid residual enamel and inadvertent mobilization of root fragments, in addition to adhering to a strict postoperative follow-up protocol for at least 6–12 months (Figure 14.3).

LASERS IN MANDIBULAR THIRD MOLAR SURGERY

Ever since the first demonstration of a prototype usable laser (light amplification by stimulated emission of radiation) in 1960, medical applications for the same have been endeavoured. The earliest evidence of medical laser dates back to 1967, when low-level laser therapy (LLLT) was used by Hungarian physician Endre Mester to stimulate

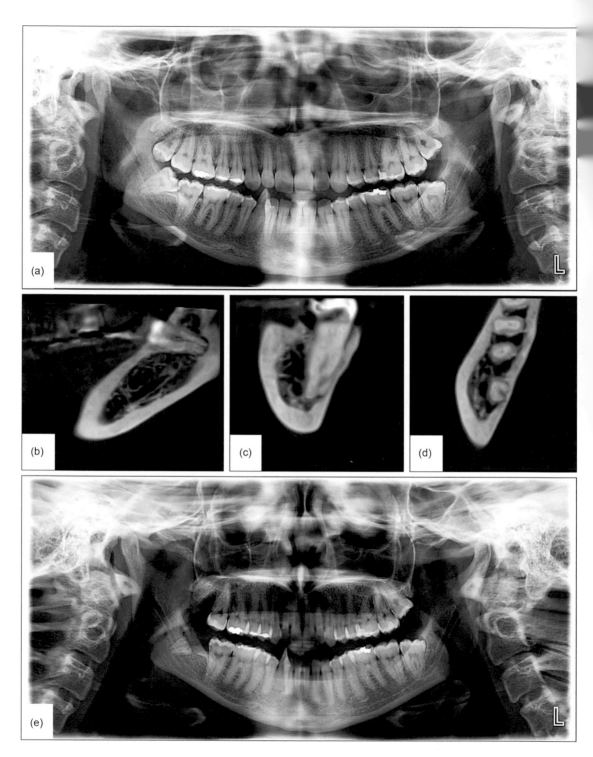

Figure 14.3 Perioperative radiographic assessment of a coronectomy patient: (a) Preoperative ortho-pantomograph (OPG) showing impacted right mandibular third molar (tooth #48) with close proximity to the inferior alveolar nerve (IAN) canal. (b–d) Cone-beam computed tomographic (CBCT) sections showing three-dimensional relationship of the tooth #48 root and IAN canal and (e) postoperative OPG showing coronectomy done in the tooth #48.

Table 14.2 The International Engineering Consortium (IEC) standard 60825 classification for medical laser

Class 3 lasers	Low energy lasers	Utilized for adjunctive treatment of inflammation and accelerating healing
Class 4 lasers	High energy lasers	Used for soft and hard tissue ablation

soft tissue healing in chronic ulcers [28,29]. In dentistry lasers are being used either in the form of *low energy lasers* for adjunctive treatment of inflammation and accelerating healing, and the *high energy lasers* for soft and hard tissue ablation. Accordingly, the International Engineering Consortium (IEC standard 60825) classifies them either as Class 3 or Class 4 lasers, respectively [30] (Table 14.2).

Operating in a near-infrared wavelength range of 660–905 nm and a power output ranging between 10 and 500 mW, LLLT works based on a photochemical process and is usually applied at the site of tissue injury for a period of 30–60 seconds, several times in a week [30]. This form of laser energy is capable of penetrating soft and hard tissues without damaging them, thereby potentially decreasing inflammation, enhancing wound healing and regeneration, and relieving pain. In addition to soft lasers, near-infrared light from LED (light emitting diode) sources have also been shown to elicit similar responses to LLLT. Between 2014 and 2017, consensus statements by the North American Association for Photobiomodulation Therapy and World Association of Laser Therapy, have suggested a blanket term of "Photobiomodulation Therapy" to encompass all forms of LLLT and low energy light treatments [29]. The mechanism of action of photobiomodulation therapy is based on the concept of "light mediated vasodilation", described by RF Furchgott in 1968. According to which low energy light activates cytochrome-C-oxidase (COX) in the mitochondria of mammalian cells leading to reversal of inhibition of cellular respiration, which is the cause for hypoxia in injured tissue [30]. Activated COX is capable of displacing nitric oxide (NO) from the mitochondria, leading to an increased cellular oxidative potential through reactive oxygen species (ROS). In addition, photobiomodulation activates signalling molecules and upregulates transcription factors, leading to proliferation of fibroblasts, epithelial cells, vascular endothelium and lymphocytes. All of this put together results in angiogenesis,

neovascularization and hastened collagen biosynthesis [30]. Moreover, a biphasic dose response curve has been observed with LLLT, wherein low intensity laser radiation is capable of stimulating the aforementioned molecular cascade, and higher intensity radiation is capable of blocking the nociceptive a-delta and c-fibre nerve endings [29,30]. Following mandibular third molar surgery, the biostimulatory properties of LLLT and photobiomodulation have shown beneficial effects on clinical prognosis. In addition to being non-invasive, non-toxic and non-complicating, postoperative low intensity light/laser radiation reportedly reduces pain and inflammation, decreases the incidence of alveolar osteitis, stimulates socket healing and promotes bone regeneration [29].

In the last two decades, advances have been made in the field of high energy, pulsed lasers for both soft and hard tissue surgical applications. Some of them include CO_2, neodymium-doped yttrium aluminium garnet (Nd:YAG) and Erbium-doped yttrium aluminium garnet (Er:YAG) lasers [31]. Amongst these, Er:YAG laser has become one of the most commonly used lasers for bone and soft tissue ablation, including ophthalmic, dermatological, otolaryngology and orthopaedic procedures [28]. Operating at a wavelength of 2,940 nm, and with power outputs ranging from 2,000 to 5,000 mW, Er:YAG laser has a very high absorption coefficient for water (chromophore specific to Er:YAG laser) in all tissue types and works based on a principle of photon induced thermomechanical ablation (Figure 14.4) [32,33]. When a pulsed beam of Er:YAG laser is applied on tissue, it heats up the water molecules in the vicinity of the incident beam up to a depth 5–40 μm per pulse, depending upon the tissue type (soft tissue penetration deeper than in hard tissue), vaporizes water to steam within a confined space, which explodes to cause the desired tissue ablation effect [28,34]. It has further been noted that Er:YAG laser exhibits similar ablative characteristics on hydroxyapatite based mineralized tissues [33]. Furthermore, thermomechanical ablation based on vaporization of biological water molecules, results in minimal carbonization (charring) and extremely small zones of thermal necrosis. Histological studies have shown zones of thermal necrosis not exceeding 30–40 μm when using Er:YAG laser, and this is nearly 5–6 times smaller in comparison to that which is seen with other types of lasers [28].

Based on a micro-computed tomographic study, Zeitouni et al. (2017) reported intact trabecular porosity in bone margins which were cut using Er:YAG laser, in contrast to the collapsed trabecular bone margins on bone cut with rotary burs [35]. They further hypothesized that bone that was cut by laser exposed the marrow spaces to the injury site leading to hastened cellular migration and proliferation, and early wound healing. These favourable characteristics have rendered Er:YAG laser as the preferred choice for all forms of dental treatment including tooth cutting and preparation, gingival and oral mucosal procedures and also for bone removal during the third molar surgery. Several studies have compared the use of Er:YAG laser as against conventional surgical burs, for the removal of mandibular third molars [33,36,37]. Although the time required for surgery using laser is considerably longer than with surgical burs, the postoperative sequelae of pain, swelling and trismus remains either comparable or better with the use of lasers. Nevertheless, the use of lasers for mandibular third molar removal was found better in terms of health-related quality of life outcomes, especially among anxious patients, and resulted in better postoperative wound healing. Recent advancements to the conventionally used fibre-optic laser delivery systems in oral surgery, in the form of robotic delivery systems for osteotomy (CARLO® – Cold Ablation Robot-Guided Er:YAG Laser Osteotomy), have lent further credence to the use of lasers in mandibular third molar surgery [38,39].

PIEZOSURGERY FOR MANDIBULAR THIRD MOLAR REMOVAL

The use of piezoelectric technology for cutting mineralized tissue has also gained prominence during the later part of the 20th century, and in the last two decades has become an interesting component of oral surgical procedures requiring bone cutting without damage to adjoining vital soft tissue structures. Some of the earliest reports indicating alveolar bone cutting using piezoelectric

instrumentation dates back to the 1970s by Horton et al. [40]. Piezoelectric surgery or piezosurgery utilizes the physical concept of ultrasonic vibrations generated in piezoelectric microcrystals and ceramics in response to flow of electric current charge through them. This leads to a linear oscillatory phenomenon in micro-scale with frequencies ranging from 26,000 to 38,000 Hz, which when applied over a cutting tip is translated to precise and efficient cutting of mineralized tissues such as bone and teeth (Figure 14.4) [29]. In order to reduce thermal tissue damage during cutting, piezosurgical handpieces are provided with an in-built coolant irrigation system directed at the surgical site. Nevertheless, visualization of the surgical site is enhanced due to the "cavitation effect" (physically induced air-water bubbles) provided by the cutting tip vibrating at ultrasonic frequencies and the resultant diminished bleeding [29]. The primary advantages of piezosurgery in oral surgery include safe, efficient and precise cutting of bone and teeth without damaging soft tissue and vital structures such as nerves and mucosal lining. Additionally, they provide operator comfort, better visualization and minimal postoperative discomfort to patients [29,40,41].

Several studies have compared piezosurgery and conventional rotary instruments for mandibular third molar removal. Based on systematic reviews and meta-analyses of such studies Liu et al. (2018) and Cicciù et al. (2021) have reported that piezosurgery is less traumatic and is associated with faster socket healing, because of its ability to selectively cut mineralized tissue and spare all soft tissues, including nerves and blood vessels [40,41]. Third molar removals done with piezosurgery resulted in reduced intra operative and postoperative bleeding, decreased thermal tissue damage and less frequent incidence of postoperative alveolar osteitis or delayed healing. Although both systematic reviews were in agreement that piezosurgery was slower for tooth sectioning than conventional rotary instruments and no significant differences in cutting efficiency were reported [40,41]. Nevertheless, postoperative swelling associated with piezosurgery was significantly lower than that of conventional rotary drilling. Based on the above reviews, neurological complications were seldom noticed with both techniques, and postoperative pain and swelling with piezosurgery

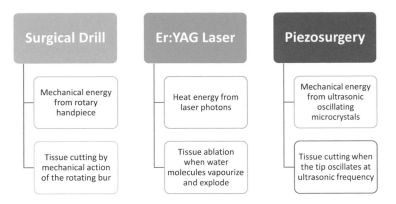

Figure 14.4 Biomechanical principles using various methods utilized for bone and tooth cutting during mandibular third molar surgery.

was either less or similar to that when removal was done using rotary instrumentation.

Clinical studies comparing piezosurgery with Er:YAG laser for mandibular third molar removal have also been reported by Keyhan et al. (2019) and Civak et al. (2021) [31,36]. Interestingly, both studies reported significantly increased surgical time with laser than with piezosurgery. In terms of the postoperative sequelae, although not statistically significant, pain, trismus and swelling were severe among patients treated using laser surgery. Based on yet another study, Silva et al. (2020) suggested piezosurgery not only for bone removal and tooth sectioning during mandibular third molar removal, but also for flap elevation owing to the favourable postoperative outcomes [42]. In spite of the greater operating time required to remove a mandibular third molar with piezosurgery than with rotary drills, whenever available, using a piezosurgery instrument offers safe, efficient and precise hard tissue cutting ability and minimal postoperative morbidity (Figure 14.4).

CURRENT PERSPECTIVES IN DECISION MAKING FOR THE ASYMPTOMATIC MANDIBULAR THIRD MOLAR

It is noteworthy that the last two decades have witnessed several advances in mandibular third molar surgery, pertaining to flap techniques, prevention of injury to the lingual and inferior alveolar nerves, radiographic assessment, and methods of bone and tooth cutting. In spite of these developments, controversies surrounding perioperative decision making are still encountered [2]. The timing of mandibular third molar removal and the choice of prophylactically removing asymptomatic third molars have always been a point of contention. One of the established set of protocols being followed are the National Institute for Health and Care Excellence (NICE) guidelines (2000). According to which, asymptomatic teeth either need not be removed at all or can be delayed until they are symptomatic or are associated with a pathology. However, applying these guidelines over the last two decades, it has been noted that the average age for mandibular third molar removal has increased from 21–25 to 32 years and above, without any decrease in the number of teeth removed. Moreover, the proportion of third molars removed due to dental caries has also increased. Considering the increased postoperative morbidity associated with mandibular third molar removal beyond 24 years of age, the NICE guidelines are being reviewed as on date (January 2022) [2]. Based on systematic protocol reviews conducted by individual institutions, while making a decision to retain or extract the asymptomatic mandibular third molar, it is imperative to consider the morbidity that might be associated with an older age of patient at the time of removal. Moreover, it has been observed that a strategy of prophylactically removing asymptomatic mandibular third molars could cost lesser than a wait and watch policy, in addition to improving quality of life outcomes.

REFERENCES

1. Sifuentes-Cervantes JS, et al. Third molar surgery: Past, present, and the future. *Oral Surg Oral Med Oral Pathol Oral Radiol.* 2021;132(5):523–531.

2. Steel BJ, et al. Current thinking in lower third molar surgery. *Br J Oral Maxillofac Surg.* 2021;60(3):257–265.

3. Bailey E, et al. Surgical techniques for the removal of mandibular wisdom teeth. *Cochrane Database Syst Rev.* 2020;7(7):CD004345.

4. Marco GDE, et al. The influence of flap design on patients' experiencing pain, swelling, and trismus after mandibular third molar surgery: A scoping systematic review. *J Appl Oral Sci.* 2021;29:e20200932.

5. Nageshwar. Comma incision for impacted mandibular third molars. *J Oral Maxillofac Surg.* 2002;60(12):1506–1509.

6. Liu JY, et al. Distal-triangular flap design for impacted mandibular third molars: A randomized controlled trial. *Hua Xi Kou Qiang Yi Xue Za Zhi.* 2021;39(5):598–604.

7. Mudjono H, Rahajoe PS, Astuti ER. The effect of triangular and reversed triangular flap designs to post third molar odontectomy complications (a pilot study). *J Clin Exp Dent.* 2020;12(4):e327–e334.

8. Xie Q, et al. Modified envelope flap: A novel incision design, can relieve complications after extraction of fully horizontal impacted mandibular third molar. *J Dent Sci.* 2021;16(2):718–722.

9. Khiabani K, Amirzade-Iranaq MH, Babadi A. Does minimal-invasive envelope flap reduce side effects compared to conventional envelope flap following impacted third molar surgery? A split-mouth randomized clinical trial. *J Oral Maxillofac Surg.* 2021;79(12):2411–2420.

10. Chu H, et al. Clinical application of flap or flapless buccal surgery on the extractions of mesially/horizontally impacted 3rd molar with high or medium position impact: A comparative study. *J Stomatol Oral Maxillofac Surg.* 2020;121(5):490–495.

11. Materni A, et al. Flapless surgical approach to extract impacted inferior third molars: A retrospective clinical study. *J Clin Med.* 2021;10(4):593.

12. Petroni G, et al. Lingual flap protection during third molar surgery: A literature review. *Eur J Dent.* 2021;15(4):776–781.

13. Mendes MB, de Carvalho Leite Leal Nunes CM, de Almeida Lopes MC. Anatomical relationship of lingual nerve to the region of mandibular third molar. *J Oral Maxillofac Res.* 2013;4(4):e2.

14. Al-Haj Husain A, et al. Preoperative visualization of the lingual nerve by 3D double-echo steady-state MRI in surgical third molar extraction treatment. *Clin Oral Investig.* 2021;26(2):2043–2053.

15. Renton T, et al. A randomised controlled clinical trial to compare the incidence of injury to the inferior alveolar nerve as a result of coronectomy and removal of mandibular third molars. *Br J Oral Maxillofac Surg.* 2005;43(1):7–12.

16. Lamiae H, et al. Coronectomy of mandibular wisdom teeth: A case series. *Int J Surg Case Rep.* 2021;90:106673.

17. Rood JP, Shehab BA. The radiological prediction of inferior alveolar nerve injury during third molar surgery. *Br J Oral Maxillofac Surg.* 1990;28(1):20–25.

18. Awad S, ElKhateeb SM. Prediction of neurosensory disorders after impacted third molar extraction based on cone beam CT Maglione's classification: A pilot study. *Saudi Dent J.* 2021;33(7):601–607.

19. Maglione M, Costantinides F, Bazzocchi G. Classification of impacted mandibular third molars on cone-beam CT images. *J Clin Exp Dent.* 2015;7(2):e224–e231.

20. Elkhateeb SM, Awad SS. Accuracy of panoramic radiographic predictor signs in the assessment of proximity of impacted third molars with the mandibular canal. *J Taibah Univ Med Sci.* 2018;13(3):254–261.

21. Dalle Carbonare M, et al. Injury to the inferior alveolar and lingual nerves in successful and failed coronectomies: Systematic review. *Br J Oral Maxillofac Surg.* 2017;55(9):892–898.

22. Leung YY, Cheung LK. Safety of coronectomy versus excision of wisdom teeth: A randomized controlled trial. *Oral Surg Oral Med Oral Pathol Oral Radiol Endod.* 2009;108(6):821–827.

23. Singh K, et al. Impacted mandibular third molar: Comparison of coronectomy with odontectomy. *Indian J Dent Res.* 2018;29(5):605–610.

24. Barcellos BM, et al. What are the parameters for reoperation in mandibular third molars submitted to coronectomy? A systematic review. *J Oral Maxillofac Surg.* 2019;77(6):1108–1115.

25. Leung YY, Cheung LK. Long-term morbidities of coronectomy on lower third molar. *Oral Surg Oral Med Oral Pathol Oral Radiol.* 2016;121(1):5–11.

26. Pitros P, et al. A systematic review of the complications of high-risk third molar removal and coronectomy: Development of a decision tree model and preliminary health economic analysis to assist in treatment planning. *Br J Oral Maxillofac Surg.* 2020;58(9):e16–e24.

27. Póvoa RCS, et al. Does the coronectomy a feasible and safe procedure to avoid the inferior alveolar nerve injury during third molars extractions? A systematic review. *Healthcare (Basel).* 2021;9(6):750.

28. Bornstein ES, Lomke MA. The safety and effectiveness of dental Er:YAG lasers: A literature review with specific reference to bone. *Dent Today.* 2003;22(10):129–133.

29. Costa DL, et al. Use of lasers and piezoelectric in intraoral surgery. *Oral Maxillofac Surg Clin North Am.* 2021;33(2):275–285.

30. Cotler HB, et al. The use of low level laser therapy (LLLT) for musculoskeletal pain. *MOJ Orthoped Rheumatol.* 2015;2(5):00068.

31. Keyhan SO, et al. Use of piezoelectric surgery and Er:YAG laser: Which one is more effective during impacted third molar surgery? *Maxillofac Plast Reconstr Surg.* 2019;41(1):29.

32. Baek KW, et al. A comparative investigation of bone surface after cutting with mechanical tools and Er:YAG laser. *Lasers Surg Med.* 2015;47(5):426–432.

33. Giovannacci I, et al. Erbium yttrium-aluminum-garnet laser versus traditional bur in the extraction of impacted mandibular third molars: Analysis of intra- and postoperative differences. *J Craniofac Surg.* 2018;29(8):2282–2286.

34. Pantawane MV, et al. Evolution of surface morphology of Er:YAG laser-machined human bone. *Lasers Med Sci.* 2020;35(7):1477–1485.

35. Zeitouni J, et al. The effects of the Er:YAG laser on trabecular bone micro-architecture: Comparison with conventional dental drilling by micro-computed tomographic and histological techniques. *F1000Res.* 2017;6:1133.

36. Civak T, et al. Postoperative evaluation of Er:YAG laser, piezosurgery, and rotary systems used for osteotomy in mandibular third-molar extractions. *J Craniomaxillofac Surg.* 2021;49(1):64–69.

37. Passi D, et al. Laser vs bur for bone cutting in impacted mandibular third molar surgery: A randomized controlled trial. *J Oral Biol Craniofac Res.* 2013;3(2):57–62.

38. Baek KW, et al. Comparing the bone healing after cold ablation robot-guided Er:YAG laser osteotomy and piezoelectric osteotomy – A pilot study in a minipig mandible. *Lasers Surg Med.* 2021;53(3):291–299.

39. Ureel M, et al. Cold ablation robot-guided laser osteotome (CARLO(®)): From bench to bedside. *J Clin Med.* 2021;10(3):450.

40. Liu J, et al. Piezosurgery vs conventional rotary instrument in the third molar surgery: A systematic review and meta-analysis of randomized controlled trials. *J Dent Sci.* 2018;13(4):342–349.

41. Cicciù M, et al. Piezoelectric bone surgery for impacted lower third molar extraction compared with conventional rotary instruments: A systematic review, meta-analysis, and trial sequential analysis. *Int J Oral Maxillofac Surg.* 2021;50(1):121–131.

42. Silva LD, et al. Influence of surgical ultrasound used in the detachment of flaps, osteotomy and odontosection in lower third molar surgeries: A prospective, randomized, and "split-mouth" clinical study. *Med Oral Patol Oral Cir Bucal.* 2020;25(4):e461–e467.

15

Medico-legal considerations and informed consent for mandibular third molar extractions

GEORGE PAUL

INTRODUCTION

Informed consent for surgical treatment is an essential component that has evolved over the last few decades. It derived legal stature based on the four ethical principles of medical or dental practice, namely

1. Autonomy
2. Beneficence
3. Non-malfeasance
4. Justice

By and large, informed consent represents the first ethical principle of autonomy or the rights of patients to decide what can or cannot be done to their bodies with full disclosure of the benefits and risks of a procedure.

The *Merriam-Webster Dictionary* has a simple definition for informed consent which states that "consent to surgery by a patient or to participation in a medical experiment by a subject after achieving an understanding of what is involved" [1]. However, in practice, it entails several other issues that include, but is not limited to the consent being obtained after full disclosure of benefits and risks without coercion and should include a choice of accepted alternate procedures including the option of "no surgery" in a language or communication format that is understood by the person giving consent.

Historically informed consent gained sanctity with the *Schloendorf v. Society of New York Hospitals* (1914) which established willingness by a patient as a necessary aspect of doing a procedure. However, the component of basing such consent on credible information as a legally binding principle was accepted through several cases in the 1960s and 1970s that include *Salgo v. Le Land Stanford and several others* [2].

DOES SURGICAL REMOVAL OF THIRD MOLARS NEED INFORMED CONSENT?

While it is customary to obtain informed consent in writing, it can be an implied or even oral consent for inconsequential procedures. It is strongly recommended that informed consent for even minor surgical procedures like extractions and surgical removal of impacted third molars should be reduced to writing to make it legally unequivocal.

In view of the increased litigation related to surgical dentistry, it is strongly advised that informed consent be obtained for all dento-alveolar surgeries, despite some studies indicating that anxiety levels and indecision in patients increase with disclosures of risks [3,4].

DOI: 10.1201/9781003324034-15

WHAT ARE MATERIAL RISKS THAT NEED TO BE DISCLOSED?

Minor and major surgery are relative terms. Many dental surgical procedures including extractions and impacted molar removals are commonly referred to as minor surgery, although such a classification is not accurate. Every surgical procedure, whether done under local or general anaesthesia, carries some elements of risk or possibility of unwanted sequelae [5].

The question often asked is how one decides on what risks are material or relevant for the sake of an informed consent. This is decided by the "the prudent patient test" which determines what a reasonable patient in the position of a plaintiff (complainant) would attach significance to, in coming to a decision on the treatment advice given. The surgeon must foresee what side effect or complication a patient may consider to be significant. A patient may not place significance on mild pain and swelling after an extraction. It is therefore may not be necessary to obtain informed consent for the same. However, a patient may be upset over a prolonged or permanent paraesthesia after the surgical removal of wisdom teeth. Therefore, when surgical intervention to remove a difficult impacted last molar is contemplated, it may be wise to obtain consent after explaining the possibility of transient or permanent paraesthesia [5].

The ability to discern, that the patient might perceive, as worth knowing about before a procedure is called the *"prudent patient test"* [6]. This would of course mean all relevant details of benefits and risks in a patient-centred milieu.

THE INFORMED CONSENT DOCUMENT SHOULD INCLUDE

1. The purpose of the proposed procedure;
2. A summary of the surgical approach;
3. Expected benefits and limitations;
4. A description of post-operative recovery; possible complications and known side effects, including those that are rare;
5. Risks associated with anaesthesia, analgesics, and antibiotics; appropriate alternatives, including the option of no treatment or surgery at all.

The informed consent document may need to take into consideration the following principles and the surgeon and his team can make appropriate changes to accommodate them. These have been enunciated by Lord Scarman in the case of *Sidaway v. Board of Governors of Bethlehem Royal Hospital*

1. The individual should be an adult of sound mind and should have the legal mental capacity to choose what happens to his body.
2. It should offer a choice that entails an opportunity to evaluate knowledgeably the options available and the risks attendant on each (including no surgery option)
3. The doctor should therefore disclose all material risks. The material risks are determined by the "prudent patient test" which determines what a "reasonable" patient in a position of a plaintiff (complainant) would attach significance to, in coming to a decision on the treatment given.

   In addition to this [5]
4. All informed consent must be in a language understood by the patient.
5. In the case of illiterates, the informed consent must be read to them in the presence of an independent witness who must sign on the space provided.
6. In the case of a child, a parent or guardian can sign on behalf of the child.

SOME COMMON BENEFITS AND RISKS OF MANDIBULAR THIRD MOLARS

Benefits to the patient, in terms of prevention or cure/indications:

1. Repeated pericoronitis
2. Damage/caries to adjacent teeth
3. Interference in prosthetic rehabilitation (crowns on adjacent teeth or construction of prosthesis)
4. Orthodontic indications
5. Existing or high risk for pathology like cysts or tumours
6. Trauma to the adjacent soft tissues
7. Intractable neurologic pain associated with compression from tooth

Routine extraction of non-symptomatic third molars in anticipation of possible pathology or fractures is not an accepted indication on a risk/benefit or cost/benefit ratio [7,8].

Common risks that may be considered relevant for the purpose of informed consent include:

1. Pain and swelling beyond what is expected in a normal extraction
2. Restricted mouth opening and pain while swallowing
3. Soreness of oral mucosa or commissure due to stretching and unavoidable thermal injury
4. Unexpected bleeding
5. Neuro-sensory disturbance (paraesthesia/hypoesthesia/or anaesthesia) of lip and/or tongue which may be transient or permanent
6. Necessity to leave behind root stumps if they pose a greater risk of nerve damage or bleeding
7. Injury to the root or crown of adjacent teeth
8. Fracture of mandible due to unavoidable circumstances
9. Dry socket causing delayed healing
10. Unexpected infection

VALIDITY OF INFORMED CONSENT

Any informed consent can be challenged if it is not

1. Voluntary (no coercion or inducement)
2. If the patient is not competent or has incapacity due to mental status or age of consent
3. Non-disclosure of benefits and risks

NEGLIGENCE RELATED TO NON-DISCLOSURE

Negligence has four components:

1. Duty of care
2. Violation of that duty
3. Injury or disutility
4. Injury should be due to violation

Any injury caused without an informed consent is considered a negligent act. It is considered negligence by virtue of non-disclosure of the risk of injury. An expected injury or sequelae becomes a negligent act if the patient was not warned of the same, prior to the surgery (informed consent).

However, it must be remembered that merely having an informed consent does not necessarily excuse an injury that could have been avoided. So, the duty of care cannot be waived merely on account of an informed consent.

CONCLUSION

The informed consent document is patient-centric permitting the surgeon to perform a procedure with full disclosure. Impacted third molar surgery, when indicated, is a complex procedure that can have a number of unexpected sequelae. It is imperative that the indication for removal and the possible complications are clearly explained to the patient, preferably in a written format. This avoids unnecessary breach in a doctor–patient relationship and provides safeguards for the surgeon against unnecessary medico-legal litigations.

REFERENCES

1. https://www.merriam-webster.com/dictionary/informed%20consent</ds>.
2. Faden RR, Beauchamp TL. *A History and Theory of Informed Consent*. New York: Oxford University Press, 1986, pp. 28 and 123.
3. Ferrús-Torres E, Valmaseda-Castellón E, Berini-Aytés L, Gay-Escoda C. Informed consent in oral surgery: The value of written information. *J Oral Maxillofac Surg*. 2011;69:54–8.
4. Goldberger JJ, Kruse J, Kadish AH, Passman R, Bergner DW. Effect of informed consent format on patient anxiety, knowledge, and satisfaction. *Am Heart J*. 2011;162:780–5.e1.
5. Paul G, Rai M. Medicolegal issues in maxillofacial surgery. In: Bonanthaya K, Panneerselvam E, Manuel S, Kumar VV, Rai A (eds) *Oral and Maxillofacial Surgery for the Clinician*. Singapore: Springer, 2021.
6. Lee A. 'Bolam' to 'montgomery' is result of evolutionary change of medical practice towards 'patient-centred care'. *Postgrad Med J*. 2017 Jan;93(1095):46–50.
7. da Costa MG, Pazzini CA, Pantuzo MCG, Jorge MLR, Marques LS. Is there justification for prophylactic extraction of third molars? Systematic review. *Braz. Oral Res*. 2013 Mar–Apr;27(2):183–8.

8. Prasad TS, Sujatha G, Priya RS, Ramasamy M. Knowledge, attitude, and practice of senior dental students toward management of complications in exodontia. *Indian J Dent Res.* 2019 Sep–Oct;30(5): 794–7.

PROTOTYPE CONSENT FORMAT

Consent Form for Wisdom Tooth Removal/Impacted Third Molar Surgery

PATIENT NAME:
AGE/SEX:
DATE OF PROCEDURE:
DIAGNOSIS:
TREATMENT PLAN:

DECLARATION

My doctor has explained in the language that I understand, that there are certain benefits and risks associated with my proposed treatment and in this specific instance they include, but are not limited to:

1. Prolonged bleeding from the extraction site.
2. Injury/loosening of adjacent teeth or fillings/restorations/prosthesis.
3. Post-operative infection/dry socket at the surgical site.
4. Stretching of the corners of the mouth that may cause injury to tissue/lips.
5. Restricted mouth opening during healing related to swelling and muscle soreness.
6. Restricted mouth opening related to stress on the jaw joints (TMJ), especially when a previous TMJ problem exists.
7. A residual small piece of root in the socket may be left in situ, when/if it carries a risk of other complications related to nerve injury or jaw fracture.
8. Injury to the nerve structure adjacent to the teeth, causing numbness, tingling, or sensory disturbances on the chin, lip, cheek, gums, or tongue and which may persist for several weeks months, or in rare instances permanently.
9. I understand, that during the course of the treatment, unforeseen conditions may result that may require a change in the treatment plan or procedure, I authorize my doctor to use professional judgement to perform such additional procedure(s) that may be necessary to complete my surgery or manage any untoward complication(s) encountered.

I hereby understand that the proposed procedure involves the administration of local anaesthesia/general anaesthesia/sedation for the removal of my wisdom tooth. I understand that the tissue will be opened along with bone removal to remove my wisdom tooth/teeth. I have also been explained that the tooth may not be removed fully at all instances but will be removed in sections and sutures will be placed to close the tissue at the site of tooth removal. I am fully aware of the procedure and the possible risks and complications associated with it and understand that a perfect result is not guaranteed. The doctor also provided ample opportunities to ask any doubts and questions regarding the procedure and the answers were provided to my satisfaction.

I *accept/decline* to undergo the surgical procedure explained to me by the doctor.

S. No.	Name of the person	Designation	Signature with date and place
1		Doctor	
2		Patient	
3		Patient's relative/attendant (relationship to the patient)	

In case the patient is a minor, the consent should be obtained from the parents/guardian.

16

Pharmacology relevant to mandibular third molar surgery

GEORGAKOPOULOU ELENI AND DARPAN BHARGAVA

INTRODUCTION

Administration of appropriate local anaesthesia, or opting to operate difficult third molar surgery under general anaesthesia is an important aspect in reducing intraoperative discomfort, patient's anxiety and stress, thereby making the surgical procedure undisturbed and aids in positive treatment outcome. Also, appropriate antibiotic and analgesic regime prevents secondary infection and controls inflammation along with pain at the surgical site, promoting uneventful healing. Accumulation of food debris at the surgical site may increase the risk of dry socket, infection and delayed healing. To prevent these complications, maintenance of good oral hygiene using antiseptic rinses and gels is usually preferred. The basics of pharmacology of drugs and agents that may find its application in mandibular third molar surgery are discussed.

LOCAL ANAESTHESIA

Topical local anaesthesia

Topical anaesthesia work by blocking impulses from pain receptors on peripheral sensory nerve fibres. They are used to control discomfort during needling for local anaesthesia for third molar extractions. Topical anaesthetics must have high mucosal permeability to reach free nerve terminals. However, they only inhibit pain sensations in the mucosal surface layer.

Vasoconstrictors impair mucosal permeability and are therefore not added to topical local anaesthetics, and these agents are more concentrated than an injectable local anaesthetics to facilitate diffusion through the mucosa [1]. Commonly used topical anaesthetic agents include benzocaine, lidocaine, tetracaine and prilocaine.

Benzocaine is a local anaesthetic which is chemically ethyl ester of p-aminobenzoic acid (PABA). PABA is more likely to cause allergic reaction when compared to amide-based local anaesthetics. Due to its low water solubility, benzocaine residues remain on the applied surface for a long time. It comes in 6%–20% concentration spray, gel, gel patch, ointment or solution. Agents manufactured to 20% concentration normally produce an impact in 30 seconds, but it takes 2–3 minutes to obtain acceptable depth and intensity. Pre-injection benzocaine anaesthesia lasts for 5–15 minutes after onset [1].

Tetracaine is a PABA ester. Solubility and anaesthetic effectiveness of this drug is improved by substituting butyl for one of the p-amino groups. Tetracaine is the most potent dental topical anaesthetic, 5–8 times more effective than cocaine. Concentrations range from 0.2% to 2.0% in spray solutions and ointments. Action begins in 2 minutes and lasts for 20 minutes to an hour. Even in healthy individuals, dosages should be restricted to 20 mg (1 mL for 2% solutions) in every session due to rapid mucous membrane absorption to prevent an overdose [1].

DOI: 10.1201/9781003324034-16

Lidocaine is the only amide-based topical anaesthetic drug that may also be injected. Lidocaine is used in dentistry as a 2% or 5% gel, 4% or 5% solution, 5% ointment, and 10% or 15% aerosol spray. Desired action of this drug is achieved in 1–2 minutes and lasts for 15–20 minutes, with peak efficacy at 5 minutes. While 5% ointments are as potent as 20% benzocaine, their effect is more gradual, taking 3 minutes or longer to establish appropriate analgesia [1].

Prilocaine is a secondary amide which is used with other topical anaesthetics. Prilocaine is reasonably safe for usage in pregnant women (Category B) [1].

Local anaesthesia solution for injection

Commonly used injectable solutions for injection may contain lignocaine, mepivacaine, articaine, bupivacaine, and ropivacaine.

Local anaesthesia for the third molar surgery is achieved using various formulations and is considered the most optimal method for anaesthetizing the area for surgery and makes the surgical procedure comfortable for the patient. Local anaesthesia is achieved by stabilizing the neuronal membrane and inhibiting nerve impulse initiation and transmission raising the threshold for electrical excitation in the nerve, delaying nerve impulse propagation and lowering the action potential rise rate. Anaesthesia progresses according to the diameter, myelination and conduction velocity of the afflicted nerve fibres. Epinephrine is a commonly used vasoconstrictor added to local anaesthetic agent to decrease absorption, hence extending tissue concentration and duration of the local anaesthetics [2]. Lignocaine, mepivacaine, bupivacaine and ropivacaine are amide-linked local anaesthetics. Amide-based local anaesthetics are metabolized in the liver.

Lidocaine is a local amino amide anaesthetic agent. It is the most common and preferred drug of choice for local anaesthesia injection. True allergic reaction to lidocaine is rare [3]. The usual concentration of lidocaine utilized for injection is 2% (20 mg/mL). Maximum recommended dose for lignocaine is 7 mg/kg. Maximum recommended adult dose in 24 hours should be limited to 500 mg [3].

Mepivacaine 3% (30 mg/mL) and mepivacaine 2% (20 mg/mL) with or without levonordefrin

1:20,000 are sterile injectable solutions. The recommended dose for mepivacaine is 6.6 mg/kg. The maximum dosage for adults should be limited to 400 mg [3,4].

Articaine is a hybrid molecule. Although classified as an amide, it possesses both amide and ester characteristics. Articaine with or without epinephrine is a sterile aqueous solution containing 4% articaine HCl (40 mg/mL). The recommended dose for articaine is 7 mg/kg body weight. Dose for adults should not exceed 500 mg [5,6].

Bupivacaine is an aminoacyl local anaesthetic. It is a mepivacaine and lidocaine homologue. Bupivacaine in a sterile isotonic solution available as 0.5% with or without epinephrine for injection. The recommended dose for bupivacaine is 2 mg/kg body weight with a maximum adult dose of 90 mg in 24 hours. Anaesthesia lasts for 2–3 times longer than lidocaine and mepivacaine, in many cases up to 7 hours [7].

Ropivacaine is an amino amide class anaesthetic. Unlike most other local anaesthetics, epinephrine has no effect on the start or duration of ropivacaine action and systemic absorption in humans [8]. Single dosage containers of ropivacaine HCl injection are available in concentrations of 0.2%, 0.5%, 0.75%, and 1% (10 mg/mL). Adults tolerate a cumulative dosage of up to 770 mg taken over 24 hours well [8]. Ropivacaine and bupivacaine have considerably longer soft tissue anaesthesia than lidocaine [9]. Although ropivacaine has limited utility for exodontia, it is a drug of choice for post-surgical analgesia.

INHALATIONAL SEDATION

Nitrous oxide (laughing gas) is a chemical substance having the formula N_2O. Gaseous at room temperature with a nice, somewhat sweet aroma and flavour. It is an anaesthetic and analgesic agent used in surgery and dentistry [10].

For patients unable to undergo regular dental treatments, or to finish therapies pleasantly for both the professional and the patient, nitrous oxide-oxygen combination $(N_2O\text{-}O_2)$ may be employed. Nitrous oxide acts in a tri-folded manner providing analgesia, anxiolysis and anaesthesia. The American Society of Anaesthesiologists (ASA) classifies procedural sedation as mild or moderate. ASA has recognized nitrous oxide administered at a concentration of 50% or less as a mild sedation medication. Concentrations >50% increase the risk of moderate or profound drowsiness and should generally be avoided. As a result of nitrous oxide-oxygen inhalation, the patient displays indications of depressed consciousness (e.g., calm, somnolent patient who appears detached and confident) but retains verbal contact throughout the therapy and all critical functions (e.g., preservation of airway patency and spontaneous ventilation) [11].

ANXIOLYTICS AND SEDATIVES

Benzodiazepines

Benzodiazepines, which are anxiolytic and amnesic, have been used to reduce patient anxiety during oral surgery. Midazolam, a benzodiazepine with a half-life of 1.3–2.2 hours, may be employed for third molar extraction surgery considering its safety profile. Parenteral (for intravenous sedation, the dose is titrated at 0.05–0.15 mg/kg), oral (0.25–0.5 mg/kg) or nasal (0.2 mg/kg) midazolam is available. The most commonly reported adverse effects are drowsiness, loss of coordination, confusion and reduced blood oxygen saturation [12].

Compared to midazolam, diazepam has a better sedative effect. Diazepam is discouraged from use considering its long-lasting effect with a duration of action of more than 12 hours. Diazepam is highly lipophilic which has quick onset of action with quick redistribution. Diazepam is mostly broken down by the microsomal enzymes to several active metabolites, mainly desmethyldiazepam. The average half-live of oral diazepam and desmethyldiazepam is about 46 hours and 100 hours, respectively. Oral diazepam (5–10 mg) is a reliable anti-anxiety drug for minor oral surgical procedures.

While using sedatives, assuring patient safety requires monitoring respiratory function, practitioner expertise and training, as well as equipment and medications used to manage airway and ventilation, in case the need arises [12].

Propofol

Propofol is a sedative-hypnotic used for sedation, to induce and maintain anaesthesia. Intravenous infusion of a therapeutic dosage of propofol induces hypnosis with little stimulation in around 40 seconds (the time for one arm-brain circulation).

The induction is pleasant, but there is no muscular relaxation and reflexes are usually not lowered sufficiently. Administration causes build-up and delays recovery. Propofol lacks analgesic property [13,14]. It may be utilized for sedation during monitored anaesthesia care for patients undergoing procedures, always under a supervision of a competent anaesthetist.

Dexmedetomidine

Dexmedetomidine hydrochloride injection is a sedative and selective alpha 2-adrenergic agonist. It acts on adrenoreceptors which are present in most of the tissues including cardiovascular, nervous, and respiratory systems and is more potent than clonidine. It produces excellent sedation and has a minimal depressive effect on the respiratory system [15]. Dexmedetomidine may find its application for sedation in minor oral surgical procedures.

Although widely available as intravenous preparation, during the extraction of third molars, where available dexmedetomidine may be administered using a more convenient intra-nasal route as a spray with an initial dose of 1.0 µg/kg and an additional dose repeated after 20 minutes of 0.5 µg/kg after administration of local anaesthesia [16].

ANTIBIOTICS

Streptococci, anaerobic gram-positive cocci and anaerobic gram-negative rods have been most frequently associated with infections following the removal of third molars. The antibiotic agent used for optimal prophylaxis should have good bone penetrance, be active against the required microorganisms and be widely distributed in body fluids [17].

For the institution of antibiotics, the following strategies should be followed for any surgical procedure: (1) There must be a substantial evidence and relationship between surgical technique and infection to justify antibiotic use; (2) the best antibiotic, considering the regional microbiota, for the surgical operation must be chosen; (3) at the time of operation, the antibiotic level must be high and (4) the smallest effective antibiotic exposure period must be used [17].

Penicillin

Amoxicillin and amoxicillin in combination with clavulanic acid (beta-lactamase inhibitor) is the most preferred antibiotic both for oral and parenteral administration prescribed prophylactically or in cases of infections related to third molar surgery. Amoxicillin is a penicillin derivative drug that is bactericidal for both Gram-positive and Gram-negative bacteria. It works by inhibiting peptidoglycan layer synthesis by binding to penicillin-binding protein in the cell wall and destroys the structural integrity [18]. Amoxicillin when given in combination with clavulanic acid has an extended spectrum for microbes as it also has a coverage to methicillin-sensitive *Staphylococcus aureus* and other species. Bacteria resistant to beta lactams produce beta-lactamase enzyme and destroy the beta-lactam ring. To overcome this beta-lactamase inhibitor is added to beta lactams that restores the function of these antimicrobials. Some common adverse effects to this medication include nausea, vomiting, diarrhoea, and abdominal discomfort.

The commonly recommended dosage and administration for adults is 500 mg every 8 hours or amoxicillin + clavulanic acid (500 + 125) 625 mg every 12 hours. Parenteral dose for intravenous infusion is 1 g amoxicillin every 8 hours or amoxicillin + clavulanic (augmentin) 1.2 g every 12 hours [18].

For prophylaxis against bacterial endocarditis in individuals with congenital or acquired valvular heart diseases or prosthesis undergoing third molar surgery should be administered, in a dose of 2 g of amoxicillin orally 60 minutes prior to the surgery [19]. In cases with penicillin allergy, erythromycin and clindamycin are the alternatives to be considered.

Cephalosporins

Cephalosporins are classified as beta-lactam antibiotics that kill bacteria by inhibiting cell wall production and cover a wide range of Gram-positive (Gm+) and Gram-negative (Gm−) bacterial infections. They act against aerobic bacteria and when combined with metronidazole also provide coverage for anaerobic infections. First-generation cephalosporins cover most of the Gm+ cocci. The drugs in this category include cefazolin, cefadroxil and cephalexin, which are commonly used for surgical prophylaxis. Second-generation cephalosporins are less effective against Gm+ cocci but show more efficacy towards Gm− bacilli (cefuroxime, cefprozil, and cefoxitin). Third-generation cephalosporins include cefotaxime, cefdinir, ceftazidime, ceftriaxone, cefpodoxime, and cefixime. Cefixime has been the most commonly used oral drug for third molar surgery as this class has extended Gm− coverage. Cefixime in adult oral dose can be taken as 400 mg in two divided doses i.e., 200 mg every 12 hours. Cefixime is also given in combination with clavulanic acid (cefixime 200 mg + clavulanic acid 125 mg), as it extends the spectrum by inhibiting beta-lactamase enzyme. Oral suspension dose in cases of patients of 45 kg or less is 4 mg/kg every 12 hours, available as 50 mg/5 mL or 100 mg/5 mL suspension or powder-distil water preparations. Cefotaxime 1 g every 12 hours, administered intravenously, is commonly used parenteral cephalosporin for minor oral surgical procedures [20].

Clavulanic acid

Clavulanic acid is a beta-lactamase inhibitor that is commonly coupled with penicillins and cephalosporins to combat antibiotic resistance by blocking their breakdown by beta-lactamase enzymes, hence expanding the spectrum of bacteria susceptible to these antibiotics. Clavulanic acid is produced from *Streptomyces clavuligerus* bacterium [21].

Erythromycin

Erythromycin (macrolide antibiotic) is bacteriostatic with usual adult dose of 250–500 mg every 6 hours. However, the drug is rarely recommended due to potential adverse effects such as gastrointestinal problems, hepatotoxicity and bacterial resistance. People on simvastatin or colchicine, or who have porphyria, should not be prescribed with this drug. It is an alternate antibiotic for penicillin allergy sufferers [22].

Clindamycin

Clindamycin is a bacteriostatic antibiotic for aerobic and anaerobic coverage. It is effective against bone, joint and dental infections. The antimicrobial spectra cover over 75% of bacteria found in odontogenic infections. Clindamycin is reportedly more effective than penicillin and metronidazole in treating chronic infections. Clindamycin is also suitable for those allergic to beta-lactam antibiotics. In general, for oral administration, 300 mg every 8 hours is considered optimum therapeutic dosage. It is also recommended for prophylaxis in penicillin-allergic individuals [22].

Metronidazole (for anaerobic coverage)

Metronidazole is a bactericidal drug that inhibits protein synthesis by interacting with DNA and results in loss of helical structure and strand breakage. It is targeted to anaerobes, protozoal and microaerophilic bacteria and does not affect the aerobic microbiota. Amoxicillin and metronidazole together cover most oral bacteria. The usual adult oral dose is tablet 400 mg every 6 hours. The extended release (ER) preparations are available: dose 600 mg once daily (1 hour before or 2 hours after the meal). Intravenous dose, which is advised for space infections, is 5 mg/mL (100 mL) or 500 mg/100 mL (3 times in 24 hours). Infusion solution should be administered over 30–60 minutes. Oral suspension of 200 mg/5 mL is available. Metronidazole can interact with alcohol (disulfiram-like reaction; causing headache, nausea, vomiting and abdominal cramps), disulfiram, warfarin, and hydantoin anticonvulsants [22].

ANALGESICS

Non-steroidal anti-inflammatory drugs

Tissue injury causes arachidonic acid secretion. Cyclooxygenase (COX) is essential to convert arachidonic acid into eicosanoids i.e., prostaglandins, thromboxane and prostacyclin. Thromboxane aids in platelet adhesion, prostaglandins cause vasodilation resulting in increased vascular permeability, fluid and white blood cell extravasation, all leading to inflammation, raise the temperature set-point in the hypothalamus and cause nociception that results in painful stimulus in the body. The mechanism of action of NSAIDs is inhibition of COX enzyme and thus has antipyretic, analgesic and anti-inflammatory action. The two main isoforms of COX are COX-1 and COX-2.

COX-1 is a constitutive enzyme that is required to maintain gastrointestinal mucosal lining, kidney function, and platelet aggregation. While COX-2 is activated by specific events (inducible isoenzyme) during an inflammatory response. Coxib, or selective COX-2 inhibitors (celecoxib, etoricoxib, and lumiracoxib), were created based on the concept that selective COX-2 inhibition would have anti-inflammatory benefits without the unpleasant side effects (especially in the stomach) associated with COX-1 inhibition. They find limited application considering their reported cardiovascular complications [23].

Acetaminophen (paracetamol) is also a non-opioid analgesic having antipyretic and analgesic action with a low incidence of adverse effects. It has proven to be a safe and effective drug for relieving the post-operative pain following the surgical removal of lower wisdom teeth [24,25]. Acetaminophen is also grouped with NSAIDs; however, it is considered to have a relatively weak anti-inflammatory property. It has been assumed that paracetamol is a selective inhibitor of the COX-3 enzyme, a cyclo-oxygenase-1 variant, in the central nervous system and acts as a pro-drug which is deacylated to p-aminophenol and in turn conjugate with arachidonic acid to form N-arachidonoyl-phenol-amine. This product is an endogenous cannabinoid, acting on CB1 receptors and also acts as an agonist at TRPV1 receptors [26]. This central inhibition mechanism explains the antipyretic and analgesic effect of paracetamol. Usual adult dose: 500–1,000 mg 3–4 times daily (maximum not more than 4 g in 24 hours) [27].

Surgical extraction of an impacted third molar causes immediate post-operative discomfort that is mostly due to surgical trauma and inflammation. NSAIDs are thus suitable and effective analgesics and anti-inflammatory drugs [24]. Commonly used NSAIDs and their recommended dose for third molar surgery are summarized in Table 16.1

Opioids

Tramadol hydrochloride is a synthetic opioid analgesic. Oral tablet forms are available in combination with paracetamol containing 37.5 mg of tramadol hydrochloride and 325 mg of acetaminophen. Tramadol is considered for patients where NSAIDs are contraindicated or for relieving post-operative acute phase discomfort after impacted third molar surgery [26].

Table 16.1 Usual adult dose of commonly prescribed NSAIDs in oral surgery [25]

NSAIDs	Usual adult dosage
Ibuprofen	400 mg in every 6 hours
Diclofenac	50 mg in every 8–12 hours
	100 mg extended release once daily
Aceclofenac	100 mg in every 12 hours
Piroxicam	20 mg once daily
Ketorolac	10 mg in every 4–6 hours
Nimesulide	100 mg in every 12 hours
Aspirin/acetyl salicylic acid	325 mg in every 4–6 hours

CORTICOSTEROIDS (TO SUPRESS POST-SURGICAL OEDEMA, PAIN AND FOR NEUROPRAXIC NERVE INJURY)

Corticosteroids have a strong anti-inflammatory property. They inhibit vascular dilatation, reduce liquid transudation and oedema formation, also reduce cell exudates and deposition of fibrin around the inflamed tissues. Corticosteroids function by decreasing the release of phospholipase A2 and stimulating the secretion of lipocortin (phospholipase A2 inhibitory protein) that inhibits leukocytic chemotaxis, fibroblast function and endothelial cells proliferation along with suppression of various other chemical inflammatory mediators to the inflamed tissues [28]. Corticosteroids, when combined with NSAIDs, potentially control post-operative pain and inflammation. They are the inhibitors of leukotriene inflammatory pathway.

It can be administered preoperatively for third molar surgical extractions along with local anaesthesia (twin mix) in the ratio of 1.8 mL of lidocaine 2% with adrenaline and 1 mL of dexamethasone solution (4 mg/mL), total 2.8 mL solution in the pterygomandibular space. This combination has been proven to significantly reduce post-operative oedema, trismus and patient discomfort. Preferred parenteral dose for intravenous injection in the immediate first hour of surgery is 2 mL of 4 mg/mL i.e., 8 mg dexamethasone injection. In case of suspicion of nerve injury, the patient is advised oral methylprednisolone during the post-operative period. The recommended dose of 1 mg/kg body weight may be advised which should be ideally tapered over a week. The usual starting dose is 40–60 mg of oral methylprednisolone to limit

the post-traumatic nerve ischaemia. Nerve injury is usually confirmed once the effect of local anaesthesia wears off and the patient presents with residual paraesthesia.

ENZYME PREPARATIONS

Serratiopeptidase

Serratiopeptidase is a protein (proteolytic) enzyme derived from the silkworm enterobacteria *Serratia* E15. This enzyme is used mainly for its anti-inflammatory, fibrinolytic, caseinolytic, and analgesic properties. It decreases the viscosity of exudate thus facilitating drainage and alleviating pain by inhibiting the secretion of bradykinin. Serratiopeptidase is believed to be effective in treating post-operative trismus and inflammation in third molar surgery. Its use is contraindicated in cases with abscess and active space infections as this facilitates the spread of infection due to its fibrinolytic action [29]. Adults' dose is 10 mg serratiopeptidase every 6–8 hours (range 15–60 mg) and is often prescribed in combination with NSAIDs (aceclofenac and diclofenac) [30]. Patients on blood thinners should be cautious in taking serratiopeptidase combination formulations [29,30]. The evidence and pooled data through randomized controlled trials on the efficacy of serratiopeptidase is limited.

Bromelain, trypsin, and rutoside

Combination of bromelain (90 mg), trypsin (48 mg), and rutoside (100 mg) with diclofenac (50 mg) is prescribed by few surgeons to reduce post-operative inflammation and oedema and enhance better wound healing. Bromelain helps to educe neutrophil migration and pro-inflamma-ory cytokines secretion thus, having anti-inflammatory properties [31]. Rutoside trihydrate inhibits pro-inflammatory genes transcription in macrophages [32,33]. Trypsin offers anti-oxidant effects and affects the protease-activated receptor 2 activation, thereby reducing inflammatory response.

Trypsin and chymotrypsin

The proposed mechanism of action of trypsin-chymotrypsin is that these enzymes combine with α1-antitrypsin (protease inhibitor) and do not leave plasmin free for fibrinolytic activity during an acute tissue injury facilitating reduced oedema and improve the healing process. This combination is prescribed in a non-infected third molar surgery to prevent inflammation and oedema. Stomach ache, diarrhoea, itching, skin rash and shortness of breath are a few adverse effects of this formulation. The dosage is 100,000 Armour unit enzymatic activity every 8–12 hours while keeping the enteric coating intact, swallowing the whole tablet without breakage [34,35].

TOPICAL ORAL AGENTS

Chlorhexidine

Chlorhexidine is a biguanide compound known for its antiseptic and antibacterial properties. It works by reacting with negatively charged microbial surface and destroying the membrane integrity causing leakage of intracellular components and cell death. It is used as a mouth rinse in the form of chlorhexidine gluconate 0.2% w/v concentration to reduce bacterial load at the surgical site to prevent the incidence of infection and alveolar osteitis. It is also available in gel form for local application over the surgical site as 1.0% w/w chlorhexidine gluconate gel or in combination with metronidazole (contains 1% w/w metronidazole and 0.25% w/w chlorhexidine gluconate). After mandibular third molar surgery, a single application of chlorhexidine gel has been reported to reduce the incidence of alveolar osteitis by 30%–40% [36,37,39].

Octenidine

Octenidine dihydrochloride works against Gram-positive and Gram-negative bacteria and has a cationic surfactant derived from pyridine. It is used as an antiseptic rinse in 0.1% w/v concentration.

Povidone iodine

Iodine povidone/betadine 2% w/v is generally used as an antiseptic mouth rinse to prevent surgical site infection in third molar surgery. It can penetrate microbial cell membranes and cause oxidization of nucleotides, proteins and fatty acids resulting in cell death [38,39].

Stabilized chlorine dioxide

Stabilized chlorine dioxide is an antimicrobial and oxidizing agent that destroys the cell wall and cell membrane of the microbes and allows intracellular chemicals to leach out causing cell death. The stabilized chlorine dioxide 0.1% based rinse has shown to be more effective than the phenol-based rinse regimen [40].

TOPICAL WOUND DRESSINGS

Reso-Pac

Reso-Pac dressings are zinc oxide or eugenol free and can be used for cases with eugenol allergy. It contains carboxy methyl cellulose and is biocompatible with human gingival fibroblast cells. It is used over surgical wound for wound protection and also acts as haemostatic agent [41,42]. Reso-pac use after third molar surgery is documented, but lacks evidence backed by randomized controlled trials.

Ozone gel

Ozone gel has been discovered to be an effective topical treatment that significantly improves post-operative patient comfort and can be used to aid post-operative pain medication. It is an antimicrobial and immune-stimulating agent. It is an unoxidized olive oil and medical-grade ozone suspension with 0.25 parts ozone and 99.75 parts oxygen and can be applied over the surgical wound every 12 hours [43]. Ozone gel use after third molar surgery is documented, but lacks evidence backed by randomized controlled trials.

STYPTICS

Styptics are local haemostatics that are used on bleeding surgical site. The commonly used styptics are summarized in Table 16.2.

OBTUNDENTS

These agents are required for dressing in cases of dry socket. After irrigating the wound, of the debris and inflammatory mediators using betadine or warm saline, the dressing is placed to promote wound healing. Curettage of the wound is avoided in order to preserve any residual clot that occupies the socket.

Zinc oxide eugenol

Zinc oxide eugenol (ZOE) dressing is prepared by mixing the zinc oxide powder (zinc oxide 80.0%, polymethyl methacrylate 20.0%, zinc stearate, acetate and thymol in traces) and eugenol oil (eugenol 85% and olive oil 15%) impregnated in cotton pellets. ZOE

has been used to treat dry sockets in the form of intra-alveolar dressings possessing its sedative, antimicrobial, and obtundent characteristics [44].

Iodoform

Iodoform is an amber-yellow powder with a distinctive odour. The active component is triiodomethane (CHI3). It stops capillary bleeding and has mild analgesic properties. It is believed to initiate neovascularization that aids in healing by mild irritant effect. Iodoform is appropriate for dry socket dressing material since it is non-irritating, antimicrobial and stable to oral fluids and blood [45]. For oral dressings, it is usually mixed with glycerine or liquid paraffin. For an obtundent effect, it is usually mixed with ZOE for treating cases with dry socket.

Alvogyl

Alvogyl (contains 15.8 gm of iodoform, 13.7 gm eugenol B.P., and 25.7 gm butamben) is preferable for dry socket treatment since it takes less time

Table 16.2 Styptics

Agent	Method of use	Mechanism
Adrenaline	Soaked on sterile cotton or gauge piece	Vasoconstriction
Thrombin powder	Dusted over the bleeding surface	Augments clotting cascade
Fibrin	Applied over bleeding surface	Augments clotting cascade
Gelatin foam	Can be inserted into the bleeding socket	Tamponade effect by absorbing blood + scaffold for clot formation
Oxidized cellulose	Can be inserted into the bleeding socket	Lowers the local pH and causes denaturation of globulin and albumin + scaffold for clot formation
Bone wax	Can be smeared on bleeding bone	Mechanical obstruction
Tannic acid	Local application with a pressure pack	Astringent
Haemocoagulase (a topical preparation, prepared from *Bothrops jararaca* or atrox snake venom)	Topical application	Enzymatic
Feracrylum (1%)	Topical application	Actives thrombin

o relieve pain completely, requires fewer dressng changes and heals the socket faster clinically. After debriding the socket by normal saline irrigation, alvogyl fibres are placed in the socket to cover the denuded bone. It is reported to reliably decrease pain in cases of alveolar osteitis [46,47].

SURGICAL IRRIGANT

NS (0.9% NaCl solution, sterile normal saline) is used for wound debridement and as a coolant while using surgical rotary instrumentation. It is preferred by most surgeons as an effective agent to clean and irrigate the third molar socket before suturing.

GABA ANALOGUES

Gabapentin (for surgical neurogenic pain)

Gabapentin is a GABA analogue used to treat neuropathic pain. The medication controls GABA release without binding to receptors. Gabapentin binds to N-type calcium channels in the brain, reducing calcium influx into neurons. For traumatic trigeminal neuropathy following third molar surgery, gabapentin is advised as 300 mg daily and increased by 300 mg every 2–3 days as tolerated. The daily dosage cap is 1,800 mg. Gabapentin causes sleepiness, dizziness, ataxia, headaches, and tremors. This GABA analogue has few drug interactions [48].

REFERENCES

1. Lee HS. Recent advances in topical anesthesia. *J Dent Anesth Pain Med.* 2016 Dec;16(4):237–244.
2. St George G, Morgan A, Meechan J, Moles DR, Needleman I, Ng YL, Petrie A. Injectable local anaesthetic agents for dental anaesthesia. *Cochrane Database Syst Rev.* 2018 Jul;7(7):CD006487.
3. Bahar E, Yoon H. Lidocaine: A local anesthetic, its adverse effects and management. *Medicina (Kaunas).* 2021 Jul;57(8):782.
4. Porto GG, Vasconcelos BCE, Gomes ACA, Albert D. Evaluation of lidocaine and mepivacaine for inferior third molar surgery. *Med Oral Patol Oral Cir Bucal.* 2007;12:E60–E64.
5. Shruthi R, Kedarnath N, Mamatha N, Rajaram P, Bhadrashetty D. Articaine for surgical removal of impacted third molar: A comparison with lignocaine. *J Int Oral Health.* 2013;5(1):48–53.
6. Sreekumar K, Bhargava D. Comparison of onset and duration of action of soft tissue and pulpal anesthesia with three volumes of 4% articaine with 1:100,000 epinephrine in maxillary infiltration anesthesia. *Oral Maxillofac Surg.* 2011 Dec;15(4):195–199.
7. Bouloux GF, Punnia-Moorthy A. Bupivacaine versus lidocaine for third molar surgery: A double-blind, randomized, crossover study. *J Oral Maxillofac Surg.* 1999;57(5):510–514; discussion 515.
8. Brković B, Andrić M, Ćalasan D, Milić M, Stepić J, Vučetić M, Brajković D, Todorović L. Efficacy and safety of 1% ropivacaine for postoperative analgesia after lower third molar surgery: A prospective, randomized, double-blinded clinical study. *Clin Oral Investig.* 2017 Apr;21(3):779–785.
9. Amorim KS, Gercina AC, Ramiro FMS, Medeiros LA, de Araújo JSM, Groppo FC, Souza LMA. Can local anesthesia with ropivacaine provide postoperative analgesia in extraction of impacted mandibular third molars? A randomized clinical trial. *Oral Surg Oral Med Oral Pathol Oral Radiol.* 2021 May;131(5):512–518.
10. de Moares MB, Barbier WS, Raldi FV, Nascimento RD, Dos Santos LM, Loureiro Sato FR. Comparison of three anxiety management protocols for extraction of third molars with the use of midazolam, diazepam, and nitrous oxide: A randomized clinical trial. *J Oral Maxillofac Surg.* 2019;77(11):2258.e1–2258.e8.
11. Rossit M, Gil-Manich V, Ribera-Uribe JM. Success rate of nitrous oxide-oxygen procedural sedation in dental patients: Systematic review and meta-analysis. *J Dent Anesth Pain Med.* 2021;21(6):527–545.
12. Chen Q, Wang L, Ge L, Gao Y, Wang H. The anxiolytic effect of midazolam in third molar extraction: A systematic review. *PLoS One.* 2015;10(4):e0121410.
13. Parworth LP, Frost DE, Zuniga JR, Bennett T. Propofol and fentanyl compared with midazolam and fentanyl during third molar surgery. *J Oral Maxillofac Surg.* 1998;56:447.

14. Kramer KJ, Ganzberg S, Prior S, Rashid RG. Comparison of propofol-remifentanil versus propofol-ketamine deep sedation for third molar surgery. *Anesth Prog.* 2012 Fall;59(3):107–117.

15. Ryu DS, Lee DW, Choi SC, Oh IH. Sedation protocol using dexmedetomidine for third molar extraction. *J Oral Maxillofac Surg.* 2016 May;74(5):926.e1–7.

16. Ustun Y, Gunduz M, Erdogan O, Benlidayi ME. Dexmedetomidine versus midazolam in outpatient third molar surgery. *J Oral Maxillofac Surg* 2006;64:1353.

17. Martin MV, Kanatas AN, Hardy P. Antibiotic prophylaxis and third molar surgery. *Br Dent J.* 2005 Mar;198(6):327–330. doi: 10.1038/sj.bdj.4812170.

18. Menon RK, Gopinath D, Li KY, Leung YY, Botelho MG. Does the use of amoxicillin/amoxicillin-clavulanic acid in third molar surgery reduce the risk of postoperative infection? A systematic review with meta-analysis. *Int J Oral Maxillofac Surg.* 2019 Feb;48(2):263–273.

19. Taubert KA, Dajani AS. Preventing bacterial endocarditis: American Heart Association guidelines. *Am Fam Physician.* 1998 Feb;57(3):457–468.

20. Vlcek D, Razavi A, Kuttenberger JJ. Antibiotics in third molar surgery. *Swiss Dent J.* 2014;124(3):294–302.

21. Ren YF, Malmstrom HS. Effectiveness of antibiotic prophylaxis in third molar surgery: A meta-analysis of randomized controlled clinical trials. *J Oral Maxillofac Surg.* 2007 Oct;65(10):1909–1921.

22. Ahmadi H, Ebrahimi A, Ahmadi F. Antibiotic therapy in dentistry. *Int J Dent.* 2021 Jan;2021:6667624.

23. Poveda Roda R, Bagán JV, Jiménez Soriano Y, Gallud Romero L. Use of nonsteroidal antiinflammatory drugs in dental practice: A review. *Med Oral Patol Oral Cir Bucal.* 2007;12(1):E10–E18.

24. Levrini L, Carraro M, Rizzo S, Salgarello S, Bertelli E, Pelliccioni GA, Garau V, Bandettini M, Caputi S, Lörincz A, Szűcs A. Prescriptions of NSAIDs to patients undergoing third molar surgery: An observational, prospective, multicentre survey. *Clin Drug Investig.* 2008;28(10):657–68.

25. Weil K, Hooper L, Afzal Z, Esposito M, Worthington HV, van Wijk A, et al. Paracetamol for pain relief after surgical removal of lower wisdom teeth. *Cochrane Database Syst Revs.* 2007, Issue 3. doi: 10.1002/14651858.CD004487.pub2.

26. Bromley L, Brandner B. *Oxford Pain Management Library: Acute Pain.* Oxford: Oxford University Press, 2010.

27. Graham GG, Scott KF. Mechanism of action of paracetamol. *Am J Ther.* 2005 Jan–Feb;12(1):46–55. doi: 10.1097/00045391-200501000-00008.

28. Araújo RZ, Pinto Júnior AAC, Sigua-Rodriguez EA, Olate S, Fonseca Alves LC, de Castro WH. Pain control in third molar surgery. *Int J Odontostomato* (Print). 2016;385–391.

29. Tiwari M. The role of serratiopeptidase in the resolution of inflammation. *Asian J Pharm Sci.* 2017 May;12(3):209–215. doi: 10.1016/j.ajps.2017.01.003.

30. Tamimi Z, Al Habashneh R, Hamad I, Al-Ghazawi M, Roqa'a AA, Kharashgeh H. Efficacy of serratiopeptidase after impacted third molar surgery: A randomized controlled clinical trial. *BMC Oral Health.* 2021 Mar;21(1):91. doi: 10.1186/s12903-021-01451-0.

31. Mendes ML, Do Nascimento-Júnior EM, Reinheimer DM, Martins-Filho PR. Efficacy of proteolytic enzyme bromelain on health outcomes after third molar surgery: Systematic review and meta-analysis of randomized clinical trials. *Med Oral Patol Oral Cir Bucal.* 2019 Jan;24(1):e61–e69. doi: 10.4317/medoral.22731.

32. Ganeshpurkar A, Saluja AK. The pharmacological potential of rutin. *Saudi Pharm J.* 2017 Feb;25(2):149–164. doi: 10.1016/j.jsps.2016.04.025.

33. Wala LJ, Choudhary A, Reddy BC. Clinical evaluation of anti-inflammatory properties of combination of bromelain, trypsin and rutoside with combination of ibuprofen, trypsin and chymotrypsin following third molar extraction – A comparative study. *J Med Sci Clin Res.* 2020;8(2):464–468.

34. Shah D, Mital K. The role of trypsin: Chymotrypsin in tissue repair. *Adv Ther.* 2018 Jan;35(1):31–42. doi: 10.1007/s12325-017-0648-y.

35. Al-Moraissi EA, Al-Zendani EA, Al-Selwi AM. Efficacy of submucosal injection of chymotrypsin, oral serratiopeptidase or oral dexamethasone in reducing postoperative complications following impacted lower third molar surgery: A prospective, randomized, double-blind, controlled clinical trial. *Front Oral Health.* 2020;1:575176.

36. Teshome A. The efficacy of chlorhexidine gel in the prevention of alveolar osteitis after mandibular third molar extraction: A systematic review and meta-analysis. *BMC Oral Health.* 2017 May;17(1):82. doi: 10.1186/s12903-017-0376-3.

37. Kaur J, Raval R, Bansal A, Kumawat V. Repercussions of intraalveolar placement of combination of 0.2% chlorhexidine & 10 mg metronidazole gel on the occurrence of dry sockets – A randomized control trial. *J Clin Exp Dent.* 2017 Feb;9(2):e284–e288. doi: 10.4317/jced.53262.

38. Mahmoud Hashemi H, Mohammadi F, Hasheminasab M, Mahmoud Hashemi A, Zahraei S, Mahmoud Hashemi T. Effect of low-concentration povidone iodine on postoperative complications after third molar surgery: A pilot split-mouth study. *J Oral Maxillofac Surg.* 2015 Jan;73(1):18–21. doi: 10.1016/j.joms.2014.06.454.

39. Rodríguez Sánchez F, Rodríguez Andrés C, Arteagoitia Calvo I. Does chlorhexidine prevent alveolar osteitis after third molar extractions? Systematic review and meta-analysis. *J Oral Maxillofac Surg.* 2017 May;75(5):901–914. doi: 10.1016/j.joms.2017.01.002.

40. https://drugs.ncats.io/drug/8061YMS4RM.

41. Kadkhodazadeh M, Baghani Z, Torshabi M, Basirat B. In vitro comparison of biological effects of coe-pak and reso-pac periodontal dressings. *J Oral Maxillofac Res.* 2017 Mar;8(1):e3. doi: 10.5037/jomr.2017.8103.

42. Raghavan SL, Panneerselvam E, Mudigonda SK, Raja KKVB. Protection of an intraoral surgical wound with a new dressing: A randomised controlled clinical trial. *Br J Oral Maxillofac Surg.* 2020 Sep;58(7):766–770. doi: 10.1016/j.bjoms.2020.03.017.

43. Sivalingam VP, Panneerselvam E, Raja KV, Gopi G. Does topical ozone therapy improve patient comfort after surgical removal of impacted mandibular third molar? A randomized controlled trial. *J Oral Maxillofac Surg.* 2017 Jan;75(1):51.e1–51.e9. doi: 10.1016/j.joms.2016.09.014.

44. Reeshma S, Dain CP. Comparison of platelet-rich fibrin with zinc oxide eugenol in the relief of pain in alveolar osteitis. *Health Sci Rep.* 2021 Aug;4(3):e354. doi: 10.1002/hsr2.354.

45. Singh V, Das S, Sharma NK. Iodoform: A boon in disguise. *Open J Stomatol* 2012;2:322–325.

46. Supe NB, Choudhary SH, Yamyar SM, Patil KS, Choudhary AK, Kadam VD. Efficacy of alvogyl (combination of iodoform + butylparaminobenzoate) and zinc oxide eugenol for dry socket. *Ann Maxillofac Surg.* 2018 Jul–Dec;8(2):193–199.

47. Pal US, Singh BP, Verma V. Comparative evaluation of zinc oxide eugenol versus gelatin sponge soaked in plasma rich in growth factor in the treatment of dry socket: An initial study. *Contemp Clin Dent.* 2013 Jan;4(1):37–41. doi: 10.4103/0976-237X.111592.

48. Zakrzewska JM, Linskey ME. Trigeminal neuralgia. *BMJ.* 2014 Feb;348:g474. doi: 10.1136/bmj.g474.

17

Case history: Transalveolar extraction of the mandibular third molars

DARPAN BHARGAVA

PROTOTYPE CASE HISTORY FORMAT

Case Registration Number:
Date:
Patient Name:
Age:
Sex:
Contact Number:
Address:
Referring Doctor:
Chief Complaint:
History of Presenting Illness:
Past Medical/Surgical History:
Personal History:
History of any known allergy:
Drug History:

General Examination

Built/Nourishment:
Gait:
Blood Pressure:
Pulse:
Respiratory Rate:
Any Other Vital Documentation of Relevance:

Systemic Examination

- Cardiovascular system
- Respiratory system
- Abdomen
- Other(s)/miscellaneous (related to history of relevance)

Local Examination

Extra-oral examination
- Face: Symmetrical/asymmetrical
- Inter-incisal opening
- Signs of pathology/deformity

Intra-oral examination
- Oral mucosa
- Tongue
- Dentition: Primary/mixed/permanent
- Occlusion
- Teeth present
- Teeth wear
- Dental caries
- Periodontal status and findings
- Others, any significant

DOI: 10.1201/9781003324034-17

Provisional Diagnosis

Differential diagnosis

Investigations
Haematological parameters
- Haemoglobin
- Complete and differential blood cell counts
- Bleeding time
- Clotting time
- Serological status (HBsAg/HBcAg/HIV)

Radiographic evaluation
- IOPAR
- Orthopantomogram (OPG)
- CBCT

Any other relevant investigation (if required)

Final Diagnosis

Assessment of the Surgical Difficulty:

WAR lines/Winter's lines (Figure 17.1, Table 17.1)

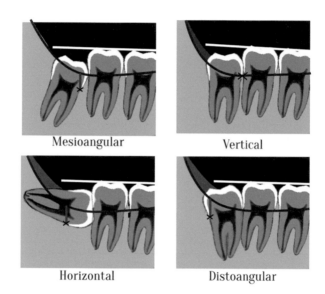

Mesioangular Vertical

Horizontal Distoangular

WAR lines indicating degree of difficulty of removal

Figure 17.1 Winter's WAR lines (Winter, 1926).

Table 17.1 WAR lines

White line	It is drawn along the occlusal surfaces of the mandibular molars and extended posteriorly over the third molar region. This line is used to assess the axial inclination of the impacted tooth.
Amber line	This line is drawn from the surface of the bone lying distally to the third molar to the crest of the interdental septum between the first and second mandibular molars. It indicates the amount of alveolar bone enclosing the impacted tooth.
Red line	The third or "red" line is used to measure the depth at which the impacted tooth lies within the mandible. It is a perpendicular drawn from the "amber" line to an imaginary point of application for an elevator which is usually the cement–enamel (CE) junction on the mesial surface of the impacted tooth. (Distal for distoangular.) If the length of the red line is more than 5 mm, anticipate difficult extraction. For every additional 1 mm beyond 5 mm, the difficulty becomes 3×.

Pell and Gregory's class and position assessment (Figure 17.2, Table 17.2)

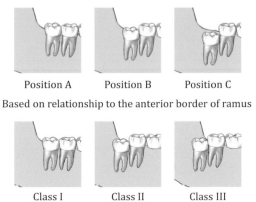

Based on relationship of the occlusal plane of the impacted tooth to that of the second molar

Position A   Position B   Position C

Based on relationship to the anterior border of ramus

Class I   Class II   Class III

Pell and Gregory's classification

Figure 17.2 Pell and Gregory class and position assessment. (Best utilize the panoramic radiograph for this assessment, to visualize the anterior ramus.)

Table 17.2 Pell and Gregory's classification system

Relationship of impacted mandibular third molar to the ramus of the mandible and second molar

Class I	Sufficient amount of space available between the anterior border of ascending ramus and the distal surface of the second molar for the accommodation of the third molar
Class II	The space available between the anterior border of the ramus and the distal side of the second molar is less than the mesio-distal width of the crown of the third molar
Class III	The third molar is totally embedded in the bone from the ascending ramus because of absolute lack of space

According to depth

Position A	The highest portion of the tooth is on a level with or above the occlusal plane
Position B	The highest position is below the occlusal plane, but above the cervical level of the second molar
Position C	The highest position is below the cervical line of the second molar

McGregor's WHARFE assessment (Figure 17.3, Table 17.3)

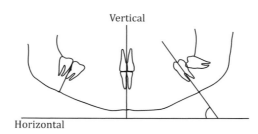

Figure 17.3 Reference lines for radiographic measurements for WHARFE assessment. The height of the mandible is measured from the distal profile of the amelocemental junction of the second molar to the nearest point on the lower border of the mandible. The angle of the second molar is that made by its long axis with a fiducial horizontal line. (Utilize the panoramic radiograph for this assessment.)

Table 17.3 WHARFE surgical difficulty assessment for mandibular third molars

Category	Score
Winters classification (W)	
Horizontal	2
Distoangular	2
Mesioangular	1
Vertical	0
Height of mandible (H)	
1–30	0
30–34	1
35–39	2
Angulation of second molar (degrees) (A)	
1°–59°	0
60°–69°	1
70°–79°	2
80°–89°	3
90° +	4
Root shape and development (R)	
Less than 1/3rd complete	2
1/3rd–2/3rd complete	1
Complex (more than 2/3rd complete)	3
Unfavourable curvature (more than 2/3rd complete)	2
Favourable curvature (more than 2/3rd complete)	1

(Continued)

Table 17.3 (Continued) WHARFE surgical difficulty assessment for mandibular third molars

Category	Score
Follicle size (F)	
Normal	0
Possibly enlarged	−1
Enlarged	−2
Impaction relieved	−3
Exit path (E)	
Space available	0
Distal cusp covered	1
Mesial cusp covered	2
All covered	3
Total	33[a]

[a] More the cumulative score, more would be the difficulty for the surgical extraction. The score indicates the total score that would be captured for an individual case. The maximum score that can be captured is 14

Pederson's difficulty index
(Table 17.4)

Table 17.4 Pederson's surgical difficulty index for mandibular third molars

Classification	Difficulty index
Angulation (A)	
Mesioangular	1
Horizontal/transverse	2
Vertical	3
Distoangular	4
Depth (D)	
Level A	1
Level B	2
Level C	3
Ramus relationship (R)	
Class I	1
Class II	2
Class III	3
Difficulty level (score) (A+D+R)	
Very difficult	7–10
Moderately difficult	5–7
Minimally difficult	3–4

18

Appendix of clinical cases: Transalveolar extraction of the mandibular third molars

VANKUDOTH DAL SINGH AND DARPAN BHARGAVA

A thorough understanding of the step-by-step procedure is vital for appropriate and accurate execution of the transalveolar extraction of the mandibular third molars. The prototype technique is demonstrated for the surgical extraction of the mesioangular, horizontal and distoangular impacted mandibular third molars (Figures 18.1–18.3)

DOI: 10.1201/9781003324034-18

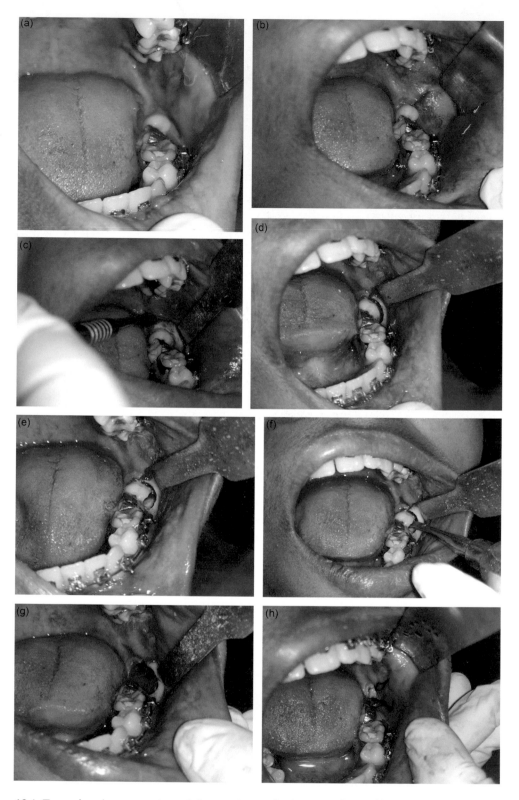

Figure 18.1 Transalveolar extraction of the mesioangular impacted mandibular third molar.
(a) Pre-operative clinical view. (b) Incision. (c) Flap elevation. (d) Bone removal. (e) Tooth sectioning.
(f) Tooth elevation. (g) Socket after toilet of the cavity. (h) Closure using 3–0 sutures.

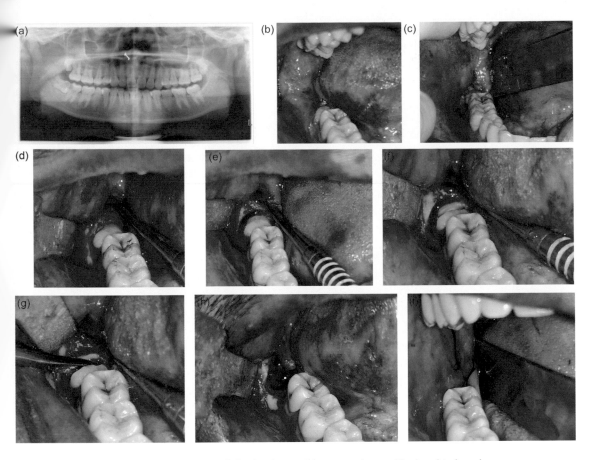

Figure 18.2 Transalveolar extraction of the horizontal impacted mandibular third molar.
(a) Pre-operative orthopantomogram. (b) Pre-operative clinical view. (c) Incision. (d) Flap elevation.
(e) Note the buccal bone guttering. Lingual guard may be used where required to prevent lingual soft
tissue injury. In most situations, it is wise NOT to manipulate lingual tissue but prevent it from injury.
(f) Tooth sectioning. (g) Elevation. (h) Socket after toilet of the cavity. (i) Closure using 3–0 sutures.

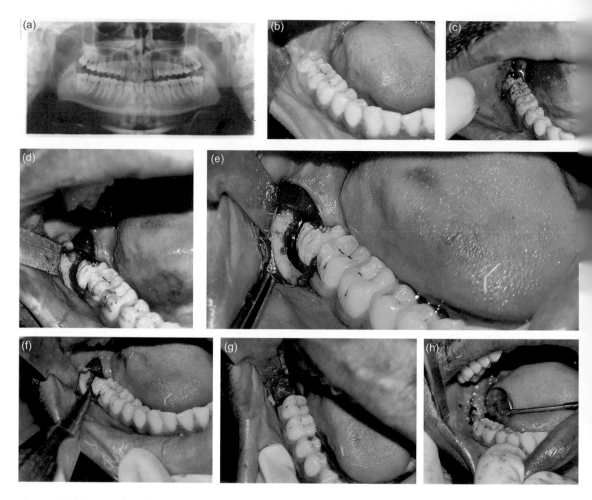

Figure 18.3 Transalveolar extraction of the distoangular impacted mandibular third molar.
(a) Pre-operative orthopantomogram. (b) Pre-operative clinical view. (c) Incision. (d) Flap elevation and buccal bone gutter. (e) Note the buccal and distal bone removal. (f) Tooth elevation. (g) Socket after toilet of the cavity. (h) Closure using 3–0 sutures.

Index

Note: **Bold** page numbers refer to tables and *italic* page numbers refer to figures.

absorbable collagen sponge 129, 162
acetaminophen (paracetamol) 185
adjacent muscles and ligaments
        10–12, *11*
adjacent nerves and innervation
        12–15
adjacent teeth 15
adrenaline in anaphylaxis **138**
airotor handpiece 68
allergies and anaphylaxis 138–139,
        139
Allis tissue holding forceps 75, *77*
alveolar canal, inferior *45*, 45–46,
        46
alveolar nerve, inferior 12–13, *13*
alveolar osteitis 148–149
alvogyl 188–189
American Dental Association
        (ADA) guidelines 103
American Heart Association
        (AHA) guidelines 103
amoxicillin 184
anaerobic gram-negative rods 1836
anaerobic gram-positive cocci 1836
anaesthesia
    inferior alveolar nerve,
        techniques for *100*
    local 99–104
analgesics 185
anaphylaxis management protocol
        139
anti-anxiety 183
antibiotics 183
anti-inflammatory drugs, non-
        steroidal 185
apexo elevator 72, *74*

armamentarium, for transalveolar
        extraction of third molars
        51–85
articaine 182
ascending palatine artery 12
asepsis and patient preparation 99
aspiration of tooth 140
asymptomatic mandibular third
        molar, decision making
        for 173
atraumatic injection techniques 138
atraumatic towel clip 53, *55*
Austin retractor 64, *65*
AXIN2 genes 18

ball burnisher 78, *79*
ball electrode 78
Bard parker blade 60, *61*
benzocaine 181
benzodiazepines 183
bite block 55, *56*
bleeding 141
blood vessels, regional 11
Blumenthal Rongeurs 70, *71*
blunt-ended probe (periodontal
        probe) 52
bone curette 75, *77*
bone file 70, *71*
bone grafts 128
bone removal 105–106,
        106, **107**
    complications during 142–143
    instruments for
        bone file 70, *71*
        Chisel 69, *70*
        Mallet 69, *70*
        physio-dispenser 69, *69*

        Rongeurs 69–70, *71*
        surgical bur 66–68, *67*
        surgical handpiece *68*, 68–69
bone trajectories 8
bone wax 80, *80*
BP handle scalp 60, *61*
bromelain 186–187
BSSO, bad splits during 148
buccal artery 12
buccal corticotomy 110, *110*
buccal fat pad 15
buccal nerve, long 13–14
buccinator 10
bupivacaine 182
bur
    fissure 66, *67*, 68
    round 66, *67*, 68
    surgical 66–68, *67*
    tapered fissure cross-cut 66
    technique 106
    tungsten carbide 66
burnisher 78, *79*

caries 19
cartridge syringe 58, *58*
CBCT *see* cone beam computed
        tomography (CBCT)
CEJ *see* cemento-enamel junction
        (CEJ)
cemento-enamel junction (CEJ) 41
cephalosporins 184
cheek retractor 65–66, *67*
Chisel 69, *70*
chlorhexidine 187
Chompret-L'Hirondel migratory
        abscess 9
chronology of third molars 18

chymotrypsin 187
clavulanic acid 184
clear surgical site, instruments for
    irrigation syringe 59, *59*
    stainless steel bowl 59, *59*
    suction tip 60, *60*
    surgical aspirator 60, *61*
clindamycin 184–185
collagen sponge, absorbable 129,
    162
computed tomography (CT) 135
    cone beam 33, **35**, 36, *36, 37*
computer controlled LA delivery
    system 85
cone beam computed tomography
    (CBCT) 2, 33, **35**, 36, 39,
    127, 135, 136, 140
conventional inferior alveolar nerve
    block (IANB) 100
conventional intraoral periapical
    radiograph 33
coronectomy 110–111, *111, 112*
cortical bone, grain of 8
cortical plates 8
corticosteroids 186
corticotomy, buccal 110, *110*
cotton pliers 53, *54*
Coupland elevator 73, *72*
COVID-19 history,
        immunocompromised
        patients 136
Cowhorn forceps 75, *76*
crown shape 43–44, *44*
Cryer elevator *91*
cryotherapy 5
CT *see* computed tomography (CT)
curette
    bone 75, *77*
        Lucas 75, *77*
        Volkmann 75, *77*
cyclooxygenase (COX) 185
cytochrome-C-oxidase 171
    COX-1 185
cytokine-mediated chemotaxis 153

decision making, for asymptomatic
        mandibular third molar
        173
delayed paraesthesia 147
dental elevators, for exodontia **90**
dental elevators for third molar
        surgery 89

parts of an elevator 90
principles in use of elevators
        90–92
    lever principle 90–91
    wedge principle 91–92
    wheel and axle principle
        92, *92*
rules for use of elevators 89
types of elevators and
        indications 90
dental extraction forceps 88
dental follicle, incomplete removal
        of 145
depressor, tongue 64–65, *65*
dexmedetomidine 183
diazepam 183
difficulty index 30–31
dimitroulis 133
diode laser, soft tissue 85
disposable instruments 51
disposable syringes 58, *58*
distal tilt 44, *45*
Doyen's mouth gag 55, *56*
dry socket (alveolar osteitis)
        148–149

electrocautery 78, *79*
electrosurgery scalpel *62*,
        62–63
elevators 72, *72–74*, 75
    apexo 72, *74*
    Coupland 73, *72*
    straight 72, *72*
endocrinal theory 18
enzyme preparations
    bromelain, trypsin and rutoside
        186–187
    serratiopeptidase 186
    trypsin and chymotrypsin 187
ergonomics 97–98
erythromycin (macrolide
        antibiotic) 184
exodontia **4**
    chair positioning for 97, *97*
    dental elevators used for **90**
    operator positions for *98*
explorer 53, *53*
extraction; *see also specific types*
    dental extraction forceps 88
    mandibular third molar
        flaps for 92–95
        healing after 153–162

medico-legal considerations
        and informed consent for
        177–180
periodontal examination
        records before third
        molar 127
tooth extraction principles
        87–89
    expansion of the bony socket
        87, 87–88
    insertion of wedge or wedges
        88–89, *89*
    use of lever and fulcrum
        88, *88*
transalveolar extraction 92, 99
    of mandibular third molars
        193–197, 199, *200–202*
extra oral technique, nerve block
        103

facial artery *12*
    and vein *12*
facial pain, obscure 19
fasciitis, necrotizing 147
fat pad, buccal 15
Fergusson mouth gag 56, *57,* 58
fibrin, platelet-rich 128, 157
fibrin sealant 83–84
"figure of eight" motion for
        luxation 111
fissure bur 66, *67,* 68
flaps classification of **93**
focal infection theory 20–21
forceps 75, *76*
    Cowhorn 75, *76*
    dental extraction 88
    mandibular third molar 75, *76*
    tissue holding 81, *82*
Forgesy suture cutting scissors 81
formalin 138
fracture of mandible 141–142, *142*
Frazier metal suction tip 60, *60*

GABA analogue 189
gabapentin (for surgical neurogenic
        pain) 189
Gardner Chisel 69, *70*
gelfoam 78, *80*
gel, ozone 5
Gow-Gates technique 100, *101*
guided tissue regeneration (GTR)
        123, 128, *128*

haematoma 139
  organized 145
haemostasis, instruments and
      material for
  bone wax 80, *80*
  burnisher 78, *79*
  electrocautery 78, *79*
  fibrin sealant 83–84
  gelfoam 78, *80*
  hemostatic agents 78, 80
  needle 81, *82*
  needle holder 80–81, *81*
  surgicel 78, *79*
  suture cutting scissors 81, *82*
  suture material 81, *83*
  tissue holding forceps 81, *82*
healing
  after mandibular third molar
      extraction 153–162
  of extraction socket 153
    bone modelling/remodelling
        phase 154
    complications 156
    excessive and prolonged
        trauma 156
    infectious complications 156
    inflammatory phase 153
    pathological states 156–157
    proliferative phase 154
    use of medications 156
  following mandibular third
      molar extraction 154
  tooth socket 153
Heister jaw stretcher 56, *57*
Henry bowdler 65, *66*
high-speed handpieces 68
H$_2$O$_2$ (hydrogen peroxide)138
horizontal angulation 33
Howarth periosteal elevator 63, *64*

IAN *see* inferior alveolar nerve
      (IAN)
IANB *see* inferior alveolar nerve
      block (IANB)
immunocompromised patients
      and missing COVID-19
      history 136
impacted tooth 18
  definition 17
incision
  instruments for placing
    electrosurgery scalpel *62*, 62–63

metzenbaum scissors 62, *62*
  scalpel 60–62, *61*
  and mucoperiosteal flap
      104–105, *105*
inferior alveolar artery and vein 12
inferior alveolar canal *45*, 45–46, *46*
  deroofed *10*
  localization and identification of
      45, 45–46, 46
inferior alveolar nerve (IAN) 12–13,
      13, 110
  anaesthesia techniques for *100*
  canal, mandibular third molar
      roots and 47
  preservation during third molar
      removal surgery 165–169
inferior alveolar nerve block
      (IANB) 99, 137
  conventional 100
informed consent
  for mandibular third molar
      extractions 177–180
  for surgical treatment 177
inhalational sedation 182–183
instruments
  for administration of local
      anaesthesia
    needles 58, *59*
    syringes 58, *58*
  for bone removal and
      odontotomy
    bone file 70, *71*
    Chisel 69, *70*
    Mallet 69, *70*
    physio-dispenser 69, *69*
    Rongeurs 69–70, *71*
    surgical bur 66–68,
        67
    surgical handpiece *68*,
        68–69
  classification 51–52
    area of instrumentation 51
    materials used for
        manufacturing 51
    re-usability of instruments
        51
    types of tissues to be handled
        51
  for clear surgical site
    irrigation syringe 59, *59*
    stainless steel bowl 59, *59*
    suction tip 60, *60*

surgical aspirator 60, *61*
  for diagnosis
    explorer 53, *53*
    mouth mirror 52, *52*
    straight probe 52–53, *53*
    tweezers/cotton pliers 53, *54*
  for placing incision
    electrosurgery scalpel *62*,
        62–63
    metzenbaum scissors 62, *62*
    scalpel 60–62, *61*
  for preparation of surgical site
    swab holder 53, *54*
    towel clip 53, *55*
  for reflection
    Howarth periosteal elevator
        63, *64*
    Molt's no. 9 periosteal
        elevator 63, *63*
    Moon's probe 63, *64*
  for retraction
    Austin retractor 64, *65*
    Henry bowdler 65, *66*
    Laster's maxillary third
        molar and cheek retractor
        65–66, *67*
    tongue depressor 64–65,
        65
  for sterilization and storage
    instrument preparation 84
    instrument storage 84, 85
    monitoring the effectiveness
        of sterilization 84
    sterilization of instruments
        84
  for tooth delivery
    elevators 72, *75*
    forceps 75, *76*
    luxators 75, *75*
    periotome 75, *75*
  used to maintain mouth
      opening
    bite block/mouth prop 55, *56*
    Doyen's mouth gag 55, *56*
    Fergusson mouth gag 56,
        57, 58
    Heister jaw stretcher 56, *57*
instruments and material
  for haemostasis and wound
      closure
    bone wax 80, *80*
    burnisher 78, *79*

instruments and material (*cont.*)
electrocautery 78, *79*
fibrin sealant 83–84
gelfoam 78, *80*
hemostatic agents 78, 80
needle 81, *82*
needle holder 80–81, *81*
surgicel 78, *79*
suture cutting scissors 81, *82*
suture material 81, *83*
tissue holding forceps 81, *82*
for post-operative dressing
ozone gel 84
reso-pac 84
intentional root retention 110–111
intra-oral periapical radiograph
(IOPAR) 39, 40
for assessment of mandibular
third molars
interpretation of IOPAR for
mandibular third molar
surgery 40–46, **41,** *42–46*
patient positioning for the
radiograph 40, *40, 41*
intraoral radiographic technique,
tube shift 33–34
investing bone, texture of *43,* 44
iodoform 188
IOPAR *see* intra-oral periapical
radiograph (IOPAR)
irrigation syringe 59, *59*

Jansen Rongeurs 70, *71*
jaw fracture, prevention of 20

Kelsey Fry technique 106–109, *108*
knotless suture 83
Kurt Thoma technique 102

LA *see* local anaesthesia (LA)
lacerations 140
LA delivery system, computer
controlled 85
laser 85
in mandibular third molar
surgery 169–172, *170*
Laster's maxillary third molar and
cheek retractor 65–66, *67*
lateral trepanation technique
109–110, *109*
lateroalveolar canal 9
lever principle, elevator 90–91

lidocaine 182
ligaments, adjacent muscles and
10–12, *11*
lingual nerve 14–15
injury 148
protection during third molar
removal surgery 165
lingual plat 8
lingual retractor, narrow 1
lingual split technique 1, 106–109,
108
LLLT *see* low level laser therapy
(LLLT)
local anaesthesia (LA) 99–104
intravascular administration
of 138
solution for injection 182
topical local anaesthesia 181–182
local drug delivery 127
long buccal nerve 13–14
low level laser therapy (LLLT) 5,
169, 171
low-speed handpieces 68
Lucas bone curette 75, 77
Luer-lock syringes 58
luxators 75, *75*

magnetic resonance imaging 36
Mallet 69, *70*
mandible, fracture of 141–142,
142
mandibular canal (inferior alveolar
canal/inferior dental
canal) 10, *10, 11*
mandibular impacted tooth
removal
distoangular *116, 117*
horizontal *115*
mesioangular *114, 115*
vertical *112–114*
mandibular nerve block, needle
insertion for extraoral *103*
mandibular, root formation for 21
mandibular third molar
asymptomatic, decision making
for 173
classification systems for
impacted 23–30, *24,*
28–30
mandibular third molar extraction
flaps for 92–95
healing after 153–162

medico-legal considerations
and informed consent for
177–180
mandibular third molar forceps
75, *76*
mandibular third molar impaction
(M3MI) 123
mandibular third molar region 7,
8, *9*
coronal section through *14*
nerves and *13*
mandibular third molar removal
piezosurgery for 172–173
surgical flaps for 163–165,
164
mandibular third molar roots
and inferior alveolar nerve
(IAN) canal 47
mandibular third molars
advances in surgical extraction
of 163–173
benefits and risks of 178–179
CBCT radiological classification
for **35**
contraindications for extraction
for 21
impacted
clinical assessment 39
radiographic assessment 39
indications for extraction for
18–21
orthodontic reasons 20
preparation for orthognathic
surgery 20
presence of pathological
lesion 20
previous attempted
extraction 19
professional, social and
economic factors 20
prosthetic considerations
19–20
periodontal considerations for
impacted 123–129
preoperative and
intraoperative
considerations 125–126,
126
treatment 124
post-surgical instructions after
transalveolar extraction
of **119**

spaces involved with 16
transalveolar extraction of
193–197, 199, *200–202*
transplantation of 119
mandibular third molars, intra-oral
periapical radiographs for
assessment of
difficulty assessment indices 46,
47, **47–49,** *48*
interpretation of IOPAR for
mandibular third molar
surgery 40–46, **41,** *42*
access 40
crown shape 43–44, *44*
inferior alveolar canal *45,*
45–46, *46*
position and depth 40–41
root pattern 43, *43, 44, 45*
texture of the investing bone
43, 44
patient positioning for
radiograph 40, *40, 41*
mandibular third molar surgery
lasers in 169–172, *170*
pharmacology to 181–189
principles and flaps for 87–98
types of incision for *94,* 94–95,
95
mandibular third molar surgery,
complications with
impacted *133,* 133–145,
134
intraoperative complications
137–144
aspiration/swallowing of
tooth 140
bleeding 141
bur breakage/broken
instrument 143
complication during tooth
sectioning 140
complications during bone
removal 142–143
fracture of mandible 141–142
gauze and cotton entrapment
to handpiece bur 144
haematoma 139
importance of surgical area
139
inadequate anaesthesia 137
lack of strict asepsis 137

medical emergencies 144
during nerve block
administration 137–138
pain 138–139
subcutaneous emphysema
143–144
trigemino-cardiac reflex 140
post-operative complications
144–149
bad splits during BSSO 148
complications to surgeon 149
delayed paraesthesia 147
dry socket (alveolar osteitis)
148–149
haematoma/organized
haematoma 145
incomplete removal of dental
follicle 145
infection 147
MRONJ (medicines related
osteonecrosis of the jaw)
145
necrotizing fasciitis 147
nerve injuries 148
oedema 147
osteomyelitis 145–146
periodontal defects 148
pyrexia 146
temporomandibular joint
disorders and dislocations
147–148
trismus 144–145
preoperative complications
133–137
compromising radiographs
and blood investigations
135–136
handling by non-surgical
specialists/lack of
training 136–137
immunocompromised
patients and missing
COVID-19 history 136
improper armamentarium
135
improper patient education
135
inappropriate diagnosis 135
lack of anatomical
knowledge 135
lack of good assistance 136

lack of skill and knowledge
135
patient social, economic &
educational background
137
underestimating the
difficulty of surgery 137
unrealistic expectations 137
maxillary third molar forceps *76*
maxillofacial surgery 136
Mayo-Backhaus works on ratchet
mechanism 53
Mcgregor's WHARFE assessment
31, *31, 48,* **49,** *196*
Mead's mallet 69, *70*
medication related osteonecrosis of
the jaw (MRONJ) 21, 145
Mendelian theory 18
mepivacaine 182
metronidazole (for anaerobic
coverage) 185
metzenbaum scissors 62, *62, 62–63*
micromotor with handpiece *68*
midazolam 183
Miller Colburn bone file *70*
Mitchell's trimmer 75, *78*
M3MI *see* mandibular third molar
impaction (M3MI)
molar extraction, periodontal
examination records
before third 127
molar tooth, role of genetics in
third 3
Molt's no. 9 periosteal elevator 63,
63
monopolar electrode *78*
Moon's probe 63, *64*
Moore/Gillbe Collar Technique 106
mouth mirror 52, *52*
mouth opening
instruments used to maintain
bite block/mouth prop 55, *56*
Doyen's mouth gag 55, *56*
Fergusson mouth gag 56,
57, 58
Heister jaw stretcher 56, *57*
mouth prop 55, *56*
MRONJ *see* medication related
osteonecrosis of the jaw
(MRONJ)
MSX1 genes 18

mucoperiosteal flaps 92
  incision and 104–105, *105*
mucoperiosteum 7–8
  lateral surface 8
  medial surface 8
  posterosuperior mucosal surface
    7–8
    anaesthetic triangle 7
    inferomedial triangle 7
    retromolar triangle 7
    superolateral triangle 7
muco-perisoteal flaps 104
mucosa 7–8, *8*
  lateral surface 8
  medial surface 8
  posterosuperior mucosal surface
    7–8
    anaesthetic triangle 7
    inferomedial triangle 7
    retromolar triangle 7
    superolateral triangle 7
multi-modal approach 5
mylohyoid
  nerve to 15
  ridge 8, 9–10

National Health Service, UK (NHS)
    19
necrotizing fasciitis 147
needle 58, *59,* 81, *82*
  breakage 137–138
  holder 80–81, *81*
  suture 81, *82*
nerve anaesthesia, inferior alveolar,
    techniques for *100*
nerve block, needle insertion for
    extraoral mandibular *103*
nerve injury 148
  partial 116
nerve to mylohyoid 15
neuropraxia 116
neuropraxic nerve injury 186
nitrous oxide (laughing gas) 182
nondisposable cartridge syringe
    58, *58*
non-opioid analgesics 144
non-steroidal anti-inflammatory
    drugs 185
non-surgical therapy 127
non-toothed tissue holding forceps
    81, *82*
NSAIDs 144, 185, **186**

oblique ridges, internal and
    external 8
obscure facial pain 19
obtundents 188
octenidine 187
odondectomy (tooth division)
    111–117
odontogenic cyst development 20
odontotomy, instruments for
  bone file 70, *71*
  Chisel 69, *70*
  Mallet 69, *70*
  physio-dispenser 69, *69*
  Rongeurs 69–70, *71*
  surgical bur 66–68, *67*
  surgical handpiece *68,*
    68–69
oedema 147
OPG *see* orthopantomogram (OPG)
opioids 185
oral agents, topical 187
oral and maxillofacial surgery 136
oral flora 19
organized haematoma 145
orthodontic theory 18
orthodontic treatment 1
orthognathic surgery, preparation
    for 20
orthopantomogram (OPG) 34, 39
osteitis, alveolar 148–149
osteology 9
osteomyelitis 145–146
osteosclerosis 18
ozone gel 5, 84, 187

PABA *see* p-aminobenzoic acid
    (PABA)
pain 138–139
p-aminobenzoic acid (PABA) 181
panoramic radiograph *34,* 34–36,
    35, 39
paraesthesia 19
  delayed 147
paranasal sinus (PNS) X-ray 136
partial nerve injury 116
partial odontectomy 110–111
pathological lesion, presence of 20
pathological theory 18
PDGFs *see* platelet-derived growth
    factors (PDGFs)
Pederson's difficulty index 30, *49,*
    197

Pell and Gregory's class and
    position assessment **48,**
    48, 195
Pell and Gregory's classification
    system **48,** *48,* **195**
pen grasp *93*
penicillin 184
periapical radiograph, conventional
    intraoral 33
pericoronitis, recurrent 19
periodontal defects 148
  formation 123
  post-operative management of
    126–129
  post-operative treatment
    modalities for
    management of 127
  local drug delivery 127
  non-surgical therapy 127
  periodontal surgical
    management 127
periodontal disease 19
periodontal probe 52
periodontal risk predictors 125
periodontal surgical management
    127
periodontal tissues distal to second
    molar
  impaction as a risk factor for
    123–124, *124*
periodontium 15
  effects on, with impaction type
    124
periotome 75, *75*
pharmacology, to mandibular third
    molar surgery 181–189
photobiomodulation therapy 171
phylogenic theory 18
piezoelectric surgical interventions
    5
piezosurgery 85
  for mandibular third molar
    removal 172–173
plasma, platelet-rich 128
plastic instruments 51
platelet-derived growth factors
    (PDGFs) 128
platelet-rich fibrin (PRF) 5, 128,
    157
platelet-rich plasma (PRP) 5,
    128
plumbeum odontogagon 3

polyglactin 910 83
postcoronectomy *112*
post-operative care and follow-up 118–119
povidone iodine 187
PRF *see* platelet-rich fibrin (PRF)
prilocaine 182
propofol 183
PRP *see* platelet-rich plasma (PRP)
pterygomandibular injection, twin mix solution for intra-space **104**
pterygomandibular ligament *11*
pyrexia 146

radiograph
    conventional intraoral periapical 33
    panoramic 34–36
radiographic technique, tube shift intraoral 33–34
randomized control trials (RCT) 168
reactive oxygen species (ROS) 171
recurrent pericoronitis 19
reflection, instruments for
    Howarth periosteal elevator 63, *64*
    Molt's no. 9 periosteal elevator 63, *63*
    Moon's probe 63, *64*
regional blood vessels 11
relief hole 60, *60*
reso-pac 84
    dressings 187
retraction, instruments for
    Austin retractor 64, *65*
    Henry bowdler 65, *66*
    Laster's maxillary third molar and cheek retractor 65–66, *67*
    tongue depressor 64–65, *65*
retromolar fossa 9
retromolar pad 7
retromolar triangle 8–9
Rongeurs 69–70, *71*
root development, impact of 121
root formation, for mandibular 21
root pattern
    of impacted mandibular third molar 43, *43*

and position of second molar 44, *45*
ropivacaine 182
ROS *see* reactive oxygen species (ROS)
round body needle 81, *82*
round bur 66, *67,* 68
rutoside 186–187

Same Lingual Opposite Buccal (SLOB) 33
SARS-COV2 136
scalpel 60–62, *61*
scissors
    Forgesy suture cutting 81
    metzenbaum 62, *62*
    suture cutting 81, *82*
sealant, fibrin 83–84
sedation, inhalational 182–183
sedatives 183
serratiopeptidase 186
silk, suture material 81, *83*
skeletal anatomy 8–10
SLOB *see* Same Lingual Opposite Buccal (SLOB)
socket management, instruments for
    Allis tissue holding forceps 75, *77*
    curette 75, *77*
    Mitchell's trimmer 75, *78*
socket toilet 117
soft tissue diode laser 85
soft tissue injuries 140
split bone technique 106–109, *108*
sponge holder 53
stabilized chlorine dioxide 187
stainless steel bowl 59, *59*
stainless steel instruments 51
sterilization of instruments 84
    burs 84
    handpiece 84
steroids 144
straight elevator 72, *72*
straight handpieces 68
straight probe 52–53, *53*
streptococci 183
stylet 60, *60*
styptics 188, **188**
suction tip 60, *60*
superior pharyngeal constrictor 10

surgery, underestimating the difficulty of 137
surgical bur 66–68, *67*
surgical flaps, for mandibular third molar removal 163–165, *164*
surgical handpiece 68, *68*–69
surgical irrigant 189
surgical loupes 85
surgical site
    instruments for preparation of
        swab holder 53, *54*
        towel clip 53, *55*
surgicel 78, *79*
suture cutting scissors 81, *82*
suture material 81, *83*
suture needle 81–83
    silk 81, *83*
    vicryl *83*
suturing 117–118, *118*
suturing priciples 95–96, *96, 97*
suturing technique 126, *126*
swallowing of tooth 140
syringes 58, *58*

TAE *see* transalveolar extraction (TAE)
tapered fissure cross-cut burs 66
TCR *see* trigemino-cardiac reflex (TCR)
Teflon-coated mallet 69
temporalis 10
temporomandibular disorders (TMD) 148
temporomandibular joint (TMJ) disorders 147–148
tetracaine 181
third molar impaction, causes for 17–18
third molar removal surgery
    inferior alveolar nerve (IAN) preservation during 165–169, *166,* **167–168**
    lingual nerve protection during 165
third molars
    armamentarium for transalveolar extraction of 51–85
    chronology of 18
third molar surgery, dental elevators for 89

third molar surgery, dental (*cont.*)
    parts of an elevator 90
    principles in use of elevators
        90–92
        lever principle 90–91
        wedge principle 91–92
        wheel and axle principle
            92, *92*
    rules for use of elevators 89
    types of elevators and
        indications 90
tissue holding forceps 81, *82*
tongue depressor 64–65, *65*
tooth delivery
    instruments for
        elevators 72, 75
        forceps 75, *76*
        luxators 75, *75*
        periotome 75, *75*
toothed tissue holding forceps 81,
    82
tooth extraction principles 87–89
    expansion of the bony socket *87*,
        87–88
    insertion of wedge or wedges
        88–89, *89*
    use of lever and fulcrum 88, *88*
tooth impaction 112, 123
    causes for 33
    theories of 18
tooth removal 111–117, *112–117*
tooth socket, healing of 153
topical local anaesthesia 181–182
topical oral agents 187
topical wound dressings 187
TORS *see* transoral robotic surgery
    (TORS)
towel clip 53, *55*
tramadol hydrochloride 185
transalveolar extraction (TAE) 92, 99

of mandibular third molars
    193–197, 199, *200–202*
transoral robotic surgery (TORS) 5
transplantation, of mandibular
    third molars 119
trauma 20
trigemino-cardiac reflex (TCR) 140
triiodomethane 188
trismus 144–145
trypsin 186–187
tube shift intraoral radiographic
    technique 33–34
tungsten carbide
    burs 66
    instruments 51
tweezers 53, *54*
Twin Mix mandibular anesthesia
    (TM) 99

vague pain 19
vasoconstrictor 181
    standard local anaesthetic
        solution with **104**
Vazirani Akinosi closed mouth
    technique insertion *102*
vein, facial artery and 12
vicryl, suture needle *83*
Volkmann's curette 75, *77*

Walter's retractor 1–2
Ward's incision 94–95, *95*, 105, *105*
WAR lines 46, 194, *194*
    amber line 41, **47**
    red line **7**, 41
    white line 41, **47**
    Winter 40, *42*
wedge elevators 91
wedge principle, elevator 91–92
WHARFE assessment **31**, *31*, *48*, **49**
WHARFE surgical difficulty
    assessment **196**

wheel and axle principle, elevator 92, *9.*
Winter Cryer
    crossbar pattern 72, *73*
    straight pattern 72, *74*
Winter's WAR lines 40, *42*
wound closure, instruments and
    material for
    bone wax 80, *80*
    burnisher 78, *79*
    electrocautery 78, *79*
    fibrin sealant 83–84
    gelfoam 78, *80*
    hemostatic agents 78, 80
    needle 81, *82*
    needle holder 80–81, *81*
    surgicel 78, *79*
    suture cutting scissors 81, *82*
    suture material 81, *83*
    tissue holding forceps 81, *82*
wound dressings, topical 187
wound healing
    after mandibular third molar
        extraction 157
        absorbable collagen sponge
            162
        clinical assessment 154–155
        dentin autologous graft and
            other graft materials 157,
            158–161, 162
        histological assessment 156
        platelet-rich fibrin 157
        radiographic assessment
            155–156
        suturing 157
        suturing with buccal
            drainage 157

Yankauer suction tip 60, *60*

zinc oxide eugenol (ZOE) dressing
    188